A Late Mamluk Medical Regimen for Travellers

Sir Henry Wellcome Asian Series

VOLUME 22

The titles published in this series are listed at *brill.com/was*

A Late Mamluk Medical Regimen for Travellers

Ibn al-Amshāṭī's al-Isfār ʿan ḥikam al-asfār
Critical Edition, Translation, and Commentary

By

Zsuzsanna Csorba

BRILL

LEIDEN | BOSTON

The Sir Henry Wellcome name is used under licence from the Wellcome Trust. The volumes in this series are published with financial support from the Wellcome Trust Centre for the History of Medicine at UCL.

The peacock logo of the series was drawn by the artist Phyllida Legg.

Cover illustration: Caravan of pilgrims on the way to Mecca from the Schefer Maqāmāt (*Maqāmāt al-Ḥarīrī*, dated 634/1237, illustrated by Yaḥyā ibn Maḥmūd ibn al-Wāsiṭī). MS Paris, Bibliothèque nationale de France, Arabe 5847, f. 94v.

The Library of Congress Cataloging-in-Publication Data is available online at https://catalog.loc.gov
LC record available at https://lccn.loc.gov/2024044144

Typeface for the Latin, Greek, and Cyrillic scripts: "Brill". See and download: brill.com/brill-typeface.

ISSN 1570-1484
ISBN 978-90-04-70819-8 (hardback)
ISBN 978-90-04-70820-4 (e-book)
DOI 10.1163/9789004708204

This book is printed on acid-free paper and produced in a sustainable manner.

Contents

Acknowledgements

Since this book is a revised version of my PhD dissertation, I am indebted to my supervisor, Zoltán Szombathy, for his invaluable guidance throughout my doctoral studies. My deep appreciation goes out to the reviewers of my dissertation, Anne Regourd and Elaine van Dalen, as the process of revision greatly benefited from their suggestions.

I also owe a great debt of gratitude to the Avicenna Institute of Middle Eastern Studies for providing numerous research and travel grants. Without the constant guidance and support of the director of the Institute, Professor Miklós Maróth, and the help of the director of finance of the Institute, Éva Molnárné Mayer, this work would have been impossible.

I am also pleased to thank the staff of the Dār al-Kutub and the Maʿhad al-Makhṭūṭāt al-ʿArabiyya, where I was able to consult the manuscripts and microfilms that serve as the basis of this book. I am also thankful for all the help and support I received at the Dominican Institute of Oriental Studies during the months I spent in their Scholar's House.

I would also like to thank my teachers at the Eötvös Loránd University (Budapest) for sharing their scholarly knowledge and providing help and suggestions with various aspects of my research. I also owe thanks to all my colleagues at the Avicenna Institute for all our stimulating discussions.

I would like to express my sincere appreciation to the editorial board of the Sir Henry Wellcome Asian Series for including my book as well as Brill's Patricia Radder and TAT Zetwerk's Manon Vrolijk.

Also, I would like to express my sincere gratitude for the anonymous reviewers who helped me improve the manuscript tremendously. I am especially grateful for all their suggestions on how to better render certain phrases and technical terms into English, as well as their meticulous reading of the whole text.

Last but by no means least, I wish to thank my husband for always being by my side throughout the writing of this book and encouraging me every step of the way. This book is dedicated to you.

Zsuzsanna Csorba
March 2024, Budapest

List of Tables

Tables

Introduction

The text edited in the present book, Ibn al-Amshāṭī's travel regimen entitled *al-Isfār ʿan ḥikam al-asfār* is quite interesting for numerous reasons. For one, the author, Ibn al-Amshāṭī born in 810/1407–1408 and died in 902/1496 in Cairo, is not only a jurist-physician of the late Mamluk period but he also travelled and participated in military campaigns. While his name is not known to us, he was a close friend of the well-known *ḥadīth* scholar and prosopographer al-Sakhāwī (d. 902/1497) and a member of the learned Cairene elite of their time. According to one of his biographers, he held the position of chief physicianship as well. All in all, his life and studies also contribute to our understanding of the physicians and their education in the postclassical period. As for his travel regimen, while not explicitly tailored to the needs of those embarking on the pilgrimage to Mecca, like Qusṭā ibn Lūqā's (d. 300/912) regime,[1] it was most likely written for the occasion of the pilgrimage of Ibn al-Amshāṭī's patron, Kamāl al-Dīn al-Bārizī (d. 856/1452) who was the head of the Chancery. Thus, compared to Qusṭā's work, it is a general travel regimen written by a physician for another layman. Its closer examination reveals many aspects of the text that contribute to our refutation of the decline narrative[2] and understanding of the postclassical medical literature. Moreover, it also sheds light on the tradition of medieval Arabic travel regimens which were not studied comprehensively on their own right since Bos's edition of Qusṭā's work.

To emphasise the importance of this literature, it might be worth to examine what travel medicine is and situate this study of medieval Arabic travel regimens in the field of history of travel medicine. For a brief definition, "Travel medicine is a new interdisciplinary field [...]. The primary goal of travel medicine is to protect travelers from disease and death; the secondary one is to minimize the impact of illness and accidents through principles of self-treatment."[3] Although the birth of the modern scientific field is usually linked to 1988 and 1991,[4] the few histories of this discipline already recognise that "travel medicine as an interdisciplinary concept is not new."[5] One such historical summary mentions some examples for this from ancient and medieval Europe and focuses on

1 Available in an edition and English translation with a commentary by Bos. See Qusṭā ibn Lūqā, *Qusṭā ibn Lūqā's medical regime*.

2 See for example Brentjes, *The prison of categories*.

3 Steffen—DuPont, *Manual of travel medicine*, 1.

4 Kozarsky—Keystone, *Introduction*, 1.

5 Buck—Steffen, *History of the development of travel medicine*, 7.

 DOI:10.1163/9789004708204_002

the developments of the period between the 1740s and 1905 as well as from the 1960s to 1991.[6] Considering the aim and focus of this and similar brief overviews, they warrant commendation for many reasons. Still, examined from the point of view of the history of medicine, there are many shortcomings that are to be addressed by historians of medicine. The temporal and geographical focus of these summaries is quite narrow, however, this is most likely due to the fact that comprehensive discussions on the history of travel medicine are not readily and widely available. Moreover, it would likely be a better choice to talk about histories of travel medicines in the plural first,[7] which would provide grounds for more comparative approaches. In this sense, in the present book I aim to offer a preliminary history of a limited tradition of travel regimens: those written in Arabic between the 3rd/9th and the 9th/15th centuries.

The importance of this literature can also be viewed from the point of the phenomenon of travel. While for most, travel in the medieval Islamic world most likely conjures up the travelogues of Ibn Baṭṭūṭa, Ibn Faḍlān, and Ibn Jubayr,[8] there are additional forms of travel to be mentioned, such as trade, military campaigns, or travel in search of knowledge or to obtain education. While one could argue that these types of travel are relevant only to specific strata of the population, we must also not forget about the pilgrimage, an obligatory religious duty of every Muslim if they have the means to perform it, in addition to other religious travels of both Muslims and non-Muslims. Still, this is only a fraction of the possible aims and types of travel; this is best illustrated by a taxonomy of travel proposed by Toorawa.[9] Besides the travelogues mentioned in this paragraph, the most well-studied types of travel seem to be the pilgrimage (*ḥajj*), travelling in search of knowledge (*riḥla fī ṭalab al-ʿilm*), and trade, based on the number of scholarly volumes and articles dedicated to them.[10] In modern scholarly studies of various kinds of travel, it is not travelling itself or the circumstances of journeying that are important but rather the aim or goal of the travel which defines the focus of such studies. A day-to-day aspect of travel which is less-studied is health and sickness, ever-present in any kind of travel, regardless its type or purpose. This neglect of how travellers stayed healthy

6 Buck—Steffen, *History of the development of travel medicine*.

7 For some different examples, see Brentjes, *Research foci*, esp. section 4.

8 As pointed out in Toorawa, *Travel in the medieval Islamic world*, 53.

9 Toorawa, *Travel in the medieval Islamic world*, 66–67.

10 For some examples, see the entry for *riḥla* in the Encyclopaedia of Islam's second edition (Netton, *Riḥla*), which deals with travelogues for the most part, or Touati's *Islam and travel in the Middle Ages* which is (purposely) dedicated to travelling in search of knowledge, despite the more generic title.

or overcame illness on the road is, however, not to be condemned without acknowledging that there is not much information on it in the sources on which studies on various types of travel rely. Lambourn finds, in another context, that "[t]he everydayness of travel and luggage-making may partly explain why travel knowledges remain largely invisible […]";[11] I would argue that this point is very much valid for travel in the medieval Islamic world in general as well. Still, in there is a body of sources where we should expect to find some information that should acknowledge the everyday health-concerns, namely medical literature, and more precisely travel regimens.

However, some limitations mark the scope of my research. Whenever using the term medieval, I refer to the period from the *hijra* to the fall of the Mamluk Sultanate (1–923/622–1517). By Arabic, I mean 'written in Arabic language'. When talking about the 'medical tradition', I have in mind the scholarly medical tradition based in its technical texts. Moreover, my sources come from the medieval Arabic scholarly medical literature only. While I realise the numerous shortcomings of these limitations, I hope that this study can facilitate further research that is more befitting to the current approaches to the study of the history of medicine and also show that undertaking even such a research and editing a single text can yield some interesting results, maybe even inspiring inquiries into other travel medicines.

In order to present a preliminary history of medieval Arabic travel regimens and contextualise Ibn al-Amshāṭī's *Isfār* in this tradition, in Chapter *1 Travel Regimens in the Medieval Arabic Medical Tradition* I gather a corpus of texts belonging to this genre and then survey their characteristics, the topics they discuss, and their relationships. In Chapter *2 The Author, Ibn al-Amshāṭī*, I point out the problems present in our sources on Ibn al-Amshāṭī's life, then, solving as much of these as possible, present his biography in depth, together with his oeuvre and its manuscript tradition. In Chapter *3 Al-Isfār ʿan ḥikam al-asfār*, I first describe the manuscripts in which Ibn al-Amshāṭī's travel regimen is preserved alongside the textual tradition of the text, then offer an approximate dating of the treatise. Before the Arabic edition and the English translation, I also include a brief summary of the contents of the work.

The second part of this book is a commentary of Ibn al-Amshāṭī's travel regimen. To better accommodate the various parts of the work, the commentary is separated into three parts. In Chapter *1 Preface: A Literary Analysis*, I examine the preface of the work as a piece of literary text, following the tripartite struc-

11 Lambourn, *Abraham's luggage*, 33.

ture of the preface with a focus on its functions and topoi and with special attention dedicated to the *sajʿ* or 'rhymed prose' in which the preface is written. In Chapter 2 *Introduction and Chapters 1–8: The Isfār as a Travel Regimen*, I take under scrutiny the introduction and eight chapters of the work, comparing it to the tradition of travel regimens as studied in the first part of the book. In Chapter 3 *Epilogue: Simple and Compound Medicaments for Travellers*, I take a look at a unique feature of Ibn al-Amshāṭī's text, namely a list of simples and a 'mini-pharmacopoeia' at the end of the treatise, examining the simples and the recipes before attempting to identify the sources of the epilogue. Then I move on to my *Concluding Remarks*.

1 Travel Regimens in the Medieval Arabic Medical Tradition

To discuss the travel regimens of the medieval Arabic medical tradition, it is necessary to first identify as many of its specimens as possible. Some are already referenced in previous scholarship but even more can be found in other encyclopaedias, manuscripts (such as Ibn al-Amshāṭī's *al-Isfār ʿan ḥikam al-asfār*), or as references in bio-bibliographical works.

Then it is possible to try and uncover what makes these texts belong together in their own genre, what topics they deliberate and how, how they relate to each other, and how the texts change over time.

As a main purpose of this study is to better know the tradition to which Ibn al-Amshāṭī's *Isfār* belongs, this specific treatise is listed as the last text of the corpus, chronologically speaking, but left out from the subsequent analyses. Nevertheless, in the Commentary, it is compared and connected to the whole tradition.

1.1 *The Corpus of Travel Regimens*

To better understand the genre of medieval Arabic travel regimens, it is necessary to locate its specimens present in the medical literature first. Looking for this corpus of texts, we find mentions of some of them in previous scholarly literature.

Already in 1910, Karl Sudhoff mentions in his article entitled *Ärztliche Regimina für Land- und Seereisen aus dem 15. Jahrhundert* four Arabic travel regimens, namely the ones in al-Rāzī's *Ḥāwī* and *Manṣūrī*, al-Majūsī's *Malakī*, and Ibn Sīnā's *Qānūn*.[12] His aim with these texts is to look at how the frameworks found

12 Sudhoff, *Ärztliche Regimina*, 263–265.

in them and in some Hippocratic observations and Paul of Aegina's advice expanded in medieval Europe and to search in them for the antecedents of some points in a medieval European travel regimen in manuscript form that he reproduces in his article. Hans Schadewaldt's *Ärztliche Regimina für Pilgerreisen* from 2006 can be mentioned here, as he reflects on Sudhoff's article;[13] however, from the point of view of Arabic travel regimens, we do not learn much more from it.

The third volume of Fuat Sezgin's *Geschichte des arabischen Schrifttums*, dedicated to medicine, pharmacy, zoology, and veterinary medicine, was published in 1970. In the title index of the volume, Sezgin lists under "*tadbīr al-musāfir*", 'regimen of travellers' five works: a treatise by Ibn Mandawayh, three treatises by Qusṭā ibn Lūqā, and Ibn al-Jazzār's encyclopaedia.[14] Due to the temporal scope of Sezgin's volume and the fact that he does not list chapters of encyclopaedias, we do not find here the texts listed by Sudhoff.

While Manfred Ullmann's *Die Medizin im Islam*, also published in 1970, remains silent on travel regimens, his *Islamic medicine* published in 1978 contains a passing mention of such writings. There is a paragraph of particular interest for our purposes in chapter seven, "Dietetics and Pharmaceutics"[15] in which Ullmann discusses books on hygiene and mentions that shorter treatises on "the way of life of the traveller" also belong here.[16] Despite the fact that there is no further discussion of these topics in Ullmann's work, nor examples given of such works, they are positioned in the medical tradition as they are mentioned in the sub-chapter on dietetics or, more closely, in the paragraph on books on hygiene.

Gerrit Bos prepared a critical edition, translation, and commentary of Qusṭā ibn Lūqā's *Risāla fī tadbīr safar al-ḥajj*, published in 1992. This treatise, to the best of our knowledge, remains the only travel regimen written in Arabic specifically for those undertaking the pilgrimage. This is of special importance as it sets this treatise apart from 'general' travel regimens. Besides this fact and the edition and the translation, the extensive and detailed commentary, as well as the indices, a quite short section of the introduction of the volume is also of great importance when surveying the literature, namely the section where Bos reviews the "literary genre to which the Risāla belongs".[17] Here, Bos

13 Schadewaldt, *Ärztliche Regimina*.

14 GAS III/483. For the individual titles, see GAS III/271 (Qusṭā ibn Lūqā), 305 (Ibn al-Jazzār), 329 (Ibn Mandawayh).

15 Ullmann, *Islamic medicine*, 97–106.

16 Ullmann, *Islamic medicine*, 99.

17 Qusṭā ibn Lūqā, *Qusṭā ibn Lūqā's medical regime*, 5–6.

mentions ancient Greek and Byzantine authors besides several authors writing in Arabic who wrote about "the preservation of one's health during a journey".[18] While this is a brief survey, it nevertheless supplements the information present in the works of Sezgin and Ullmann besides showing that the discussion of this topic in the medieval Arabic medical tradition has antecedents, which is especially clearly articulated in the commentary of Qusṭā's *Risāla* where, amongst other things, Bos clearly identifies Paul of Aegina's influence on Qusṭā's text.

Peregrine Horden's article *Regimen and travel in the Mediterranean*[19] was published in 2004 and largely repeated in 2005 as *Travel sickness, Medicine and mobility in the Mediterranean from Antiquity to the Renaissance*. The questions posed by Horden and the aim and framework of his articles are quite far from our present purposes, still he mentions Ibn al-Jazzār's *Zād al-musāfir*,[20] Ibn Sīnā's *Qānūn*, al-Rāzī's *Ḥāwī* and *Manṣūrī*,[21] and Qusṭā ibn Lūqā's *Risāla*, and refers his reader to its edition by Bos "for other writings in Arabic in the genre".[22]

Peter Pormann's and Emilie Savage-Smith's *Medieval Islamic medicine*, published in 2007, also mentions travel regimens. In the second chapter of their book dedicated to "medical theory", we find a sub-section dedicated to "regimen and diet", where they list the common regimens and topics contained in medical encyclopaedias: "Medical compendia routinely had sections devoted to regimens for infants and for the elderly, both groups requiring special adjustments in diet and other routines. Occasionally regimen for travellers would be treated in a separate section. Another subtopic that attracted particular attention was that of sexual hygiene, with a considerable number of monographs devoted to the topic. […]"[23] In the fourth chapter of the book dedicated to "practice", there is a sub-section discussing "regimen, circumcision, and personal hygiene"[24] but here there is no reference to travelling or travel regimens. Altogether, Pormann's and Savage-Smith's *Medieval Islamic medicine* places travel regimens into the whole of the Arabic medical tradition, even slightly

18 Qusṭā ibn Lūqā, *Qusṭā ibn Lūqā's medical regime*, 5. For example, while the Greek original of the travel regimen of Rufus of Ephesus is lost, a fragment in Arabic is preserved by the 5th/11th-century Ibn al-Mubārak.

19 Horden, *Regimen and travel*.

20 Horden, *Travel sickness*, 184.

21 Horden, *Travel sickness*, 193–194.

22 Horden, *Travel sickness*, 195–196, 196 n. 66.

23 Pormann—Savage-Smith, *Medieval Islamic medicine*, 50.

24 Pormann—Savage-Smith, *Medieval Islamic medicine*, 135–138.

more precisely than Ullmann's *Islamic medicine*, but does not discuss them in any detail, similarly to Ullmann's volume, undoubtedly due to the scope of their volume as well as the fact that travel regimens are a hitherto less studied aspect of the history of medieval Islamic medicine.

Mention must also be made of Elizabeth Lambourn's volume *Abraham's luggage, A social life of things in the medieval Indian Ocean world*, published in 2018. In it, Lambourn embarks on a quest to reconstruct various aspects of life in Malibarat, India and the details of a voyage from there to Ifrīqiyya based on the luggage list of a 12th-century Jewish trader, Abraham Ben Yiju, which is "the only surviving list of luggage and travel provisions known from the medieval Indian Ocean".[25] Besides the appeal of the whole volume for a quite broad audience, of special interest here is the volume's eighth chapter, "The balanced body, On vinegar and other sour foods",[26] where Lambourn is "asking whether any of the foods in Abraham's luggage list might be understood as "medicinal foods" and so as evidence for the self-prescription of ordinary travelers."[27] Throughout this inquiry focusing on how to deal with nausea and vomiting and the various uses of vinegar and sour foodstuffs, Lambourn references and makes excellent use of some Arabic medical works and practices which are discussed in detail later in this book.

To sum up, we find that in the volumes serving as standard reference works of medieval Islamic medicine (the works of Sezgin, Ullmann, and Pormann–Savage-Smith), the topic of travel regimens is mentioned but not discussed in any detail. For works dedicated to travel regimens (the articles of Sudhoff and Horden), the focus is either on medieval European examples or answering questions pertaining to a broader issue, where the regimens written in Arabic appear more as antecedents to mention but are not studied in their own right. The only example for this is the work of Bos; while he offers only a brief survey of the genre of travel regimens, his commentary of Qusṭā's *Risāla* is the most complete analysis of travel regimens to date. Lambourn's work shows how a knowledge of the theoretical framework present in medical travel regimens can be used to 'reverse-engineer' the practicalities of travel medicine and better understand and contextualise an altogether different type of source.

Turning our attention from the scholarly literature to our primary sources, it becomes obvious that the corpus of medieval Arabic travel regimens contains even more texts than mentioned so far. Broadly, speaking, they fall into

---

25 Lambourn, *Abraham's luggage*, 10.

26 Lambourn, *Abraham's luggage*, 219–239.

27 Lambourn, *Abraham's luggage*, 220.

two categories: they are either parts of encyclopaedias or separate treatises. We also have evidence of travel regimen(s) lost to us to date, which are included in the list that follows. Despite my best efforts, this list is not a definitive one, as there are surely even more sections in encyclopaedias as well as treatises in manuscript form that are not known or edited, still in manuscript form. The list is arranged chronologically according to the dates of death of the authors. The focus is on the sources themselves in accordance with their characteristics, while, for the sake of brevity, the account of their authors is in all cases only a short summary with references to more exhaustive works on them. Notably, Ibn al-Jazzār's *Zād al-musāfir wa-qūṭ al-ḥāḍir* is absent from this list, being a medical handbook of diseases *a capite ad calcem* and therefore not intrinsically related to the genre of travel regimens, although it does contain some chapters relevant to certain topics of travel regimens.[28]

1.1.1 Al-Ṭabarī (d. ca. 250/864): *Firdaws al-ḥikma*

Abū al-Ḥasan ʿAlī ibn Sahl Rabban al-Ṭabarī was born most probably around the year 174/790 and died in 250/864 or shortly after. He served the governor of Ṭabaristān, Māzyār ibn Qārin, after whose execution in 225/840 he gained admission to the Abbasid court in Samarra and served the caliphs al-Muʿtaṣim, al-Wāthiq, and al-Mutawakkil. He was Christian but converted to Islam in or after 235/850. Most of his works discuss various medical topics.[29]

Al-Ṭabarī completed his most famous work, the *Firdaws al-ḥikma* ('Paradise of Wisdom') in 235/850. It is available in only one printed edition.[30]

Browne was the first to acquaint the scholars with the "general plan of the book" by outlining the contents with a summarized translation of the parts' and chapters' titles.[31] It is divided into seven thematic parts (*nawʿ*), thirty treatises (*maqāla*), and 360 chapters (*bāb*). The 1st part is on the theoretical background

---

28 On Ibn al-Jazzār's *Zād al-musāfir*, see also sub-chapter *1.2 The Genre of Travel Regimens*' part *1.2.17 A Remark on Misleading Titles*.

29 On his life and works, see al-Ṭabarī, *Health regimen*, 4–13; Wakelnig, *Al-Ṭabarī and al-Ṭabarī*, 219–222; al-Ṭabarī, *The polemical works*, 2–24; Olsson, *Design, determinism and salvation*, 11–28; Thomas, *al-Ṭabarī*; Ullmann, *Die Medizin*, 119–122; GAS III/236–240; GAL S I/414–415.

30 Bibliographical details: *Firdaws al-ḥikma* = *Firdausu'l-Ḥikmat or Paradise of Wisdom of ʿAlī b. Rabban-al-Ṭabarī*, ed. Muḥammad Zubayr Ṣiddiqī, Berlin-Charlottenburg: Buch- u. Kunstdruckerei "Sonne" G.m.b.H., 1928. For the descriptions of the manuscripts used in the edition, see pages *kāf-jīm–kāf-zā'*. For the list of additional manuscripts, see GAS III/239 (No. 1.—*Firdaus al-ḥikma*). On the edition, its translations, and the manuscripts of the *Firdaws*, see Olsson, *Design, determinism and salvation*, 20–26.

31 Browne, *Arabian medicine*, 42–44.

of medicine. The 2nd part has five treatises. The 1st is on embryology, pregnancy, the organs, the ages and seasons; the 2nd is on the issues of the souls, the senses, and the faculties; the 3rd is on the temperaments, emotions, some movements, dreams, visions, and the evil eye; the 4th is on nursing, general hygiene and diet; the 5th is on the ideal diet according to the seasons, travel, and some aspects of the diet itself. The 3rd part of the work is on nutrition and dietetics. The 4th part has twelve treatises, dealing with the diseases *a capite ad calcem*, the muscles, nerves, veins, as well as phlebotomy, pulse, and uroscopy. The 5th part is on the properties of ailments and remedies, flavours, scents, colours, and causes of various changes. The 6th part, in brief, deals with simple and compound medicaments in six chapters. The 7th part discusses assorted, quite interesting topics in four treatises, a summary of Indian medicine being the subject matter of the last one.[32]

The arrangement of the book partially follows the Greek compendiums, and it served as an example for later physicians. Many early and some later medical authors quoted parts of the book.[33] According to Ṣiddiqī, the *Firdaws al-ḥikma* is the first medical compendium written in Arabic.[34] Meyerhof refuted this just a few years later; however, he recognised that this was "so far the earliest Arabic medical compendium published in print".[35]

For our purposes, the 2nd part, specifically the 5th treatise[36] is especially significant, which comprises seven chapters. Chapters 1–4 deal with the regimen for spring, summer, autumn, and winter, respectively. Chapter 5 is on the regimen for travellers and armies. Chapter 6 is on fattening, thinning, and appetizing things. Chapter 7 is on atrophy and useful and harmful things for the organs.[37]

32 A detailed translation of the chapters' titles is given in Meyerhof, *'Alî aṭ-Ṭabarî's "Paradise of Wisdom"*, 100–132. The last treatise on Indian medicine is available in a recent critical edition with an annotated Enlgish translation, introduction, and glossaries: Kahl, Oliver, *'Alī ibn Sahl Rabban aṭ-Ṭabarī: The Indian Books*, Leiden–Boston: Brill, 2022.

33 For a list of these, see Meyerhof, *'Alî aṭ-Ṭabarî's "Paradise of Wisdom"*, 96–97.

34 Al-Ṭabarī, *Firdaws al-ḥikma, alif–bāʾ*, as well as in the English preface.

35 Meyerhof, *'Alî aṭ-Ṭabarî's "Paradise of Wisdom"*, 91.

36 Al-Ṭabarī, *Firdaws al-ḥikma*, 105–114.

37 Al-Ṭabarī's *Health regimen* or *Book of the pearl*, "is deliberately designed for the profit of the educated (and affluent) layman" and "on the level of informational content, is a redesigned abstract of his much larger *Paradise of Wisdom*", al-Ṭabarī, *Health regimen*, 1–4. Unfortunately, al-Ṭabarī does not offer a version of his travel regimen in this work; the regimens for the seasons are followed by the regimen in bathhouses and travel is mentioned only once throughout the work. See al-Ṭabarī, *Health regimen*, 19–21 for a comparison of the contents of the *Health regimen* and the *Paradise of wisdom* and al-Ṭabarī, *Health regimen*, 124, 125 (§ 132) for the mention of travel.

1.1.2 Ibn Māhān Yaʿqūb al-Sīrāfī: *Kitāb al-safar wa-al-ḥaḍar fī al-ṭibb*

There is not much we know about Ibn Māhān. Ibn Abī Uṣaybiʿa's account of him in the chapter of early Abbasid physicians is rather short. As translated in the new edition of Ibn Abī Uṣaybiʿa's *ʿUyūn al-anbāʾ*: 'Ibn Māhān was known as Yaʿqūb al-Sīrāfī. He is the author of a work entitled *The Book of Medicine for Travelling and Residing* (*K. al-safar wa-l-ḥaḍar fī l-ṭibb*).'[38] The translators note that Ibn Abī Uṣaybiʿa's source for this biography is Ibn al-Nadīm's *Fihrist*. The only additional information there is that the book, according to Ibn al-Nadīm, is 'fine' (*laṭīf*);[39] the same adjective found its way into Ibn al-Qifṭī's account of Ibn Māhān as well.[40]

Unfortunately, there is not much we can gather from these brief accounts regarding the content of his work. Therefore, it might be that the book is more of a general, theoretical work, and it might or might not contain sections on practical aspects of medicine (possibly regarding travel regimens as well).[41]

1.1.3 Qusṭā ibn Lūqā (d. 300/912): *Risāla fī tadbīr safar al-ḥajj*

Qusṭā ibn Lūqā al-Baʿlabakkī was born around 205/820. He was a Melkite Christian with a knowledge of Greek, Syriac, and Arabic. He likely travelled to the Byzantine Empire when he was young. He was preparing new translations of Greek scientific works and revising old ones in Baghdad under the caliph al-Mustaʿīn. Later he moved to Armenia, composing works for several patrons. Besides translating, he wrote numerous medical works.[42]

Being unable to accompany al-Ḥasan ibn Makhlad, a secretary of Christian origin serving al-Mutawakkil and a vizier under al-Muʿtamid,[43] on his pilgrimage, Qusṭā decided to write a treatise for him, the *Risāla fī tadbīr safar al-ḥajj* ('Epistle on the regimen of the journey of pilgrimage'). The treatise is available in a critical edition with an English translation and commentary.[44]

The treatise consists of 10 chapters (*bāb*). The 1st chapter is on eating, drinking, sleeping, and sexual intercourse; the 2nd chapter is on fatigue; the 3rd

---

38 LHOM, 8.38.

39 Ibn al-Nadīm, *Fihrist*, II/303.

40 Ibn al-Qifṭī, *Taʾrīkh al-ḥukamāʾ*, 378.

41 On the possibility of this being a misleading title, see also sub-chapter *1.2 The Genre of Travel Regimens*' part *1.2.17 A Remark on Misleading Titles.*

42 On his life and works, see Qusṭā ibn Lūqā, *Qusṭā ibn Lūqā's medical regime*, 1–2; Ullmann, *Die Medizin*, 126–128; GAS III/270–274.

43 On his life, see Sourdel, *Ibn Makhlad.*

44 Bibliographical details: *Qusṭā ibn Lūqā's medical regime for the pilgrims to Mecca, The Risāla fī tadbīr safar al-ḥajj*, ed., transl. Gerrit Bos, Leiden–New York–Köln: E.J. Brill, 1992. The manuscripts used for the edition are described in Qusṭā ibn Lūqā, *Qusṭā ibn Lūqā's medical regime*, 3–5. For other manuscripts of the work, see GAS III/271.

chapter is on massages and rubbing of the foot; the 4th chapter is on the diseases caused by winds; the 5th is on earache; the 6th is on rheum, defluctions, and cough; the 7th is on eye diseases; the 8th is on waters; the 9th is on how to improve contaminated water; the 10th is on thirst; the 11th is on the prevention of vermin; the 12th is on the treatment of stings and bites; the 13th is on the prophylaxis against *Dracunculus medinensis*; the 14th is on the treatment of *Dracunculus medinensis*.[45] So far, the work is "the only known health guide for the pilgrim to Mecca".[46]

So far this treatise is the only published regimen for travellers (and especially for those going on the pilgrimage), it was written by a physician well-acquainted with the ancient and Byzantine sources, and to our current knowledge, this is the first standalone travel regimen written in Arabic. Therefore, not just the text itself, but also the selection of the discussed topics and their arrangements are important regarding the history and evaluation of these regimens.

1.1.4 Al-Rāzī (d. 313/925 or 323/935): *al-Kitāb al-Manṣūrī fī al-ṭibb*

The biographical accounts of Abū Bakr Muḥammad ibn Zakariyyāʾ al-Rāzī's life are short and do not mention exact dates.[47] He was born around 250/865 in Rayy and practised medicine there and in Baghdad. Biographical accounts on him elaborate on his merits as a physician, hospital director, and teacher as well. Some of them give well-known anecdotes illustrating his knowledge besides the list of his works.[48]

One of his most important works is the *al-Kitāb al-Manṣūrī fī al-ṭibb* ('The book dedicated to al-Manṣūr on medicine'), a systematic and complete work on medicine. It is available in an edition based on four manuscripts.[49] Its first part is available with a French translation as well.[50] It was translated into Latin

---

45 For a survey and evaluation of the chapters' contents, see Qusṭā ibn Lūqā, *Qusṭā ibn Lūqā's medical regime*, 7–12.

46 Qusṭā ibn Lūqā, *Qusṭā ibn Lūqā's medical regime*, 1.

47 For a summary of these, see Meyerhof, *Thirty-three clinical observations*, 2–4.

48 For his life and works, see Ullmann, *Die Medizin*, 128–136; Ranking, *The life and works of Rhazes*, 82–104; GAS III/274–294; GAL I/267–271; GAL S I/417–421; Adamson, *Al-Rāzī*, esp. ch. 7. Medicine.

49 Bibliographical details: *al-Manṣūrī fī al-ṭibb*, ed. Ḥāzim al-Bakrī Ṣiddīqī, al-Kuwayt: Maʿhad al-Makhṭūṭāt al-ʿArabiyya, 1987. For the list of the manuscripts of the *Manṣūrī*, see GAS III/281–282 (2.—*al-Kitāb al-Manṣūrī fī ṭ-ṭibb*); GAL I/269; GAL S I/419.

50 Bibliographical details: ed., transl. Pieter de Konig, *Trois traités d'anatomie arabes*, Leiden: E.J. Brill, 1903 (repr. Frankfurt am Main: Institute for the History of Arabic-Islamic Sciences at the Johann Wolfgang Goethe University, 1996).

in 1175 by Gerardus Cremonensis, as well as into Hebrew. The 9th book was frequently acknowledged and commented upon.[51]

The book has ten treatises (*maqāla*). The 1st is an introduction to medicine, discussing the various organs; the 2nd is on the humours, the organs, and physiognomy; the 3rd is on the properties of food and medicaments; the 4th is on the preservation of health; the 5th is on cosmetics (*zīna*); the 6th is on the regimen of the travellers; the 7th is on bonesetting, wounds, and ulcers; the 8th is on poisons and pests; the 9th is on various diseases *a capite ad calcem*; the 10th is on fevers.

As the list shows, there is a complete treatise written on the regimen of the travellers.[52] This treatise deals with the issues of hot weather, poisons, thirst, cold weather, freezing, fainting due to hunger, preservation of the limbs, eye afflictions due to the snow, cold, or wind, exhaustion, the proper way of eating, prevention of the harms caused by different waters, the regimen of military camps, the regimen of those who travel on sea, lice, paleness of the face, fissures of the lower parts of the leg, the scraping off of the skin due to riding, shoes, and sandals, and falling and hitting the head or other parts of the body.

1.1.5 Al-Rāzī: *al-Ḥāwī fī al-ṭibb*

Another significant work of al-Rāzī is the *al-Ḥāwī fī al-ṭibb* ('The comprehensive [book] on medicine'), an enormous collection of medical notes and extracts for his use as an aide-mémoire, believed to be arranged in part by his students after his death.[53] It is available in three editions.[54] Like the *al-Kitāb al-Manṣūrī*, this work was also translated into Latin by the Jewish author Faraj ibn Sālim in 1279.[55]

As for the contents of the *Ḥāwī*, its 23 parts (*juzʾ*) follow an *a capita ad calcem* arrangement of diseases, namely those of the head, the eyes, the ears, nose, and teeth, the lungs, and the gullet and stomach. After a part on purgatives, the arrangement continues with the diseases of the breasts, heart, liver, and

---

51 Ullmann, *Die Medizin*, 132; GAS III/282.

52 Al-Rāzī, *al-Manṣūrī*, 281–300.

53 The work is often referred to as a collection of case notes, which is not true. However, al-Rāzī did write a work containing case histories under the title *Kitāb al-tajārib*. The *Ḥāwī* contains notes based on al-Rāzī's readings and practice which is, for the most part, not structured in a way that would suggest that it was intended for other readers.

54 One printed in Hyderabad, two in Beirut; bibliographical details of the edition used here: *al-Ḥāwī fī al-ṭibb*, ṭabʿa jadīda muṣaḥḥaḥa, 23 vols. in 7, ed. Haytham Khalīfa Ṭuʿaymī, Beirut: Dār Iḥyāʾ al-Turāth al-ʿArabī, 2002.

55 Ullmann, *Die Medizin*, 131. On the relationship of the Arabic text and the Latin translation, as well as on lost chapters of the work, see Witt, *Al-Rāzīs Kitāb al-Ḥāwī*.

spleen, the intestines, and the womb. From part 12, the focus shifts to conditions affecting more organs or the whole body. The following chapters are on cancer and cancerous ulcers, then bruises, dislocation of joints, and ulcers of the reproductive and other organs. Various kinds of fevers are discussed in three parts, followed by parts on smallpox, measles, and plagues, the crisis, and urine. Parts 20–22 are on simple medicaments and pharmacology. The last part is a varied collection of notes on practical matters.

It is here, in part 23 of the *Ḥāwī*, that al-Rāzī dedicates a chapter to discussing issues of travel with the title 'On the regimen of travellers and armies on the land and the sea, the protection against hot and cold, the phenomena of the air, hunger, thirst, and what protects the face from the burning of the sun and splitting open from the cold'.[56] Due to the nature of the *Ḥāwī*, the topics discussed in this chapter are a collection of quotations and notes from previous works (sometimes attributed, sometimes left anonymous), with additional observations by al-Rāzī introduced by the phrase *lī*, 'by me'. It is important to note that this is the only regimen on which al-Rāzī collected notes; we do not find any parallels for pregnant women or any age group from newborns to the elderly.

1.1.6 Al-Majūsī (4th/10th Century): *Kāmil al-ṣināʿa al-ṭibbiyya / al-Kitāb al-malakī*

Very little is known of ʿAlī ibn al-ʿAbbās al-Majūsī's life. Based on his *nisba*s, he was born into an old Persian Zoroastrian family which originated in the town of Arrajān and practised medicine in Shīrāz. The exact dates of his birth and death are not known.[57]

He wrote his famous *Kāmil al-ṣināʿa al-ṭibbiyya* ('The complete [book] of the medical art') before 366/977 and dedicated it to the Būyid emir and king, ʿAḍud al-Dawla, this being the reason for the other well-known title of this work, *al-Kitāb al-malakī* ('The royal book'). It was printed in Būlāq,[58] and there is a facsimile as well.[59] Parts of it are available in French and German translations.[60]

---

56 Al-Rāzī, *al-Ḥāwī*, VII/396–401.

57 On his life and works, see Micheau, *ʿAlī b. al-ʿAbbās al-Majūsī*; Ullmann, *Die Medizin*, 140–146; GAS III/320–322; GAL I/272; GAL S I/423.

58 Bibliographical details: *Kāmil al-ṣināʿa al-ṭibbiyya*, 2 vols, Būlāq, 1294/1877 (repr. Frankfurt am Main: Institute for the History of Arabic-Islamic Sciences at the Johann Wolfgang Goethe University, 1996).

59 Bibliographical details: *Kāmil al-ṣināʿa al-ṭibbiyya*, 3 vols, Frankfurt am Main: Institute for the History of Arabic-Islamic Sciences at the Johann Wolfgang Goethe University, 1985 (facsimile of Istanbul University Library, MS A.Y. 6375, MS A.Y. 4713a).

60 Bibliographical details: ed., trans. Pieter de Konig, *Trois traités d'anatomie arabes*, Leiden:

The work consists of two parts. The first is on theory and the second is on practice, both in ten treatises (*maqāla*). The first part's 1st treatise is on the theoretical background of medicine; the 2nd treatise is on the anatomy of homogeneous organs; the 3rd on the heterogeneous organs; the 4th on the faculties; the 5th on the non-naturals; the 6th on the classification and causes of diseases; the 7th on the symptoms of diseases and various ways of diagnostics; the 8th on the external diseases; the 9th on the internal diseases; and the 10th on various symptoms. The second part's 1st treatise is on the preservation of health; the 2nd is on simple medicaments; the 3rd on fevers; the 4th on the curing of skin diseases, ulcers, bites, and poisons; the 5th on the diseases of the head; the 6th on the respiratory organs; the 7th on the digestive organs; the 8th on the genitalia; the 9th on surgery, bloodletting, cauterization etc.; and the 10th on complex remedies. Until Ibn Sīnā's *Qānūn* 'overshadowed' it, the work was quite popular, with more than a hundred manuscript copies of it being still available. However, the extant manuscripts generally contain only parts of the work.[61] It was translated into Latin, partially by Constantinus Africanus before 1086, and the whole work by Stephen of Antioch in 1127. It was used by Jewish physicians as well.[62]

The second part's 1st treatise begins with general chapters on preserving the health according to the seasons of the year, with various activities, in certain conditions, and the different ages of life. The following chapters deal with specific issues connected to preserving one's health (exercise, fatigue, bathing, nourishment, water, wine, sleeping, intercourse, mental symptoms, cleansing the body, customs, temperaments, appearance). Chapters 19–24 discuss various regimens, from that of pregnant women to that of the elderly. Chapters 25–29 are on the regimen for the convalescent, safeguarding against infectious diseases, and how to stop various causes of illnesses, while chapter 30 discusses

E.J. Brill, 1903 (repr. Frankfurt am Main: Institute for the History of Arabic-Islamic Sciences at the Johann Wolfgang Goethe University, 1996); Sezgin, Fuat (ed.), *ʿAlī b. al-ʿAbbās al-Majūsī (4th/10th cent.), Texts and studies*, Frankfurt am Main: Institute for the History of Arabic-Islamic Sciences at the Johann Wolfgang Goethe University, 1996.

61 According to Troupeau's lists to which Micheau also refers, there are [at least] 128 manuscripts of the *Kāmil al-ṣināʿa*. Out of these, 50 are dated. While the majority of these are from the 12th and 13th centuries (8 and 13, respectively), there are also 4 dated copies from the 14th century and 3 from the 15th century. See Troupeau, *Manuscripts*, esp. 313–315. Despite Micheau's remark that the *Kāmil al-ṣināʿa* 'was overshadowed by Ibn Sīnā's *Qānūn*' for which he refers to Ibn al-Qifṭī's *Taʾrīkh al-ḥukamāʾ*, the two works (that is the *Kāmil al-ṣināʿa* and the *Qānūn*) were obviously used side by side to complement each other still in the 15th century, at least by one author for one of his compilations, as I will show throughout the analysis of Ibn al-Amshāṭī's *Isfār*.

62 Micheau, *ʿAlī b. al-ʿAbbās al-Majūsī*; Ullmann, *Die Medizin*, 146.

cosmetics (*zīna*). The last, 31st chapter contains the regimen of the travellers on land and sea (pp. 81–84).[63]

1.1.7 Ibn Mandawayh (d. 410/1019): *Risāla ilā Abī al-Qāsim Aḥmad ibn ʿAlī ibn Baḥr fī tadbīr al-musāfir*

Abū ʿAlī Aḥmad ibn ʿAbd al-Raḥmān ibn Mandawayh was a renowned physician born in Iṣfahān, who served several rulers and dignitaries. Besides poetry, he composed numerous works on medicine.[64] Most of these are a collection of 40 epistles he addressed to fellow physicians. One of them is the *Risāla ilā Abī al-Qāsim Aḥmad ibn ʿAlī ibn Baḥr fī tadbīr al-musāfir* ('Epistle to Abū al-Qāsim Aḥmad ibn ʿAlī ibn Bahr on the regimen of the traveller'). Here, the title implies a travel regimen without a doubt.

Unfortunately, while at least 18 of Ibn Mandawayh's medical works have extant manuscript copies, this epistle is not one of them.[65] Nevertheless, it is a fascinating piece of information, since this is the only work in this list dedicated solely to travel regimens which was written for another physician instead of being dedicated to a patron who is a layman.

1.1.8 Ibn Sīnā (d. 428/1037): *al-Qānūn fī al-ṭibb*

The first 30 years of Abū ʿAlī al-Ḥusayn ibn ʿAbd Allāh Ibn Sīnā's life are known from his autobiography, and an account of his later years was written by one of his students.[66] He was born in 370/980, in Afshana, close to Bukhārā. His father paid great attention to his studies, and according to some sources, Ibn Sīnā was well-versed in all the sciences of his age by the time he was 18. After the death of his father, he started working and was consulted not only as a physician but also for his political opinions, the latter sometimes leading to stints in exile. He died in 428/1037 in Hamadān, while accompanying the Kākūyid ruler ʿAlāʾ al-Dawla. Most of his writings are philosophical and medical works, but he wrote on all other sciences as well. More than 200 works are attributed to him; approximately half of these considered genuine.[67]

The enormous *al-Qānūn fī al-ṭibb* ('The canon of medicine') served as a basis of Muslim and European medical theory and practice for seven centuries. It is

---

63 Al-Majūsī, *Kāmil al-ṣināʿa*, II/81–84.

64 For his biography and list of his works, see LHOM, 11.16.

65 See GAS III/328–329.

66 For its edition and English translation, see Gohlman, William E., *The life of Ibn Sina, A critical edition and annotated translation*, Albany, NY: State University of New York Press, 1974.

67 On his life and writings, see Gutas, *Avicenna*, 387–540, esp. 512–522 for the medical works; Goichon, *Ibn Sīnā*; Ullmann, *Die Medizin*, 152–156; GAL I/590–600; GAL S I/812–828.

available in many printed editions.[68] The encyclopaedia consists of five books (*kitāb*), which are further subdivided into several layers (*funūn, taʿālīm, jumal,* and *fuṣūl*). The 1st book is on the fundaments of medicine; the 2nd details medical substances and pharmacology; the 3rd is on pathology arranged according to the organs *a capite ad calcem*; the 4th contains various topics, for example fevers, diagnostics, minor surgery, poisons etc.; the 5th is a pharmacopoeia. Numerous manuscripts of the work are known,[69] with even more versifications, commentaries, and abridgements.[70]

The first book of the *Qānūn* contains four parts (*fann*), the third of these has only one chapter (*al-faṣl al-mufrad fī sabab al-ṣiḥḥa wa-al-maraḍ wa-ḍarūrat al-mawt*) and five more discourses (*taʿlīm*). The 1st is on the upbringing of children in four chapters; the 2nd is on the regimen of adults in seventeen chapters; the 3rd is on the regimen of the elderly in six chapters; the 4th is on the regimen of those with bad temperaments; and the 5th is on the changes.[71] This last discourse has one chapter dealing with the effects of the seasons, and a clause (*jumla*) on the regimen of travellers. This clause has eight chapters. The 1st is on various symptoms indicating diseases; the 2nd is on the regimen for travellers in general; the 3rd is on the protection against the harmful effects of heat and the regimen of those travelling in hot weather; the 4th is on the regimen of those travelling in cold weather; the 5th is on the preservation of the limbs against the cold; the 6th is on the preservation of the complexion; the 7th is on the harmful effects of different waters and how to prevent them; the 8th is on the regimen for the traveller on the sea. As can be seen, scrutinizing this clause with all its chapters is necessary for an outline of a history of these regimens.

1.1.9 Ibn Sīnā: *Tadbīr manzil al-ʿaskar*

This treatise, 'Regimen of military camps', survives in three known manuscripts.[72] It is available in a printed edition as well.[73] Although the treatise is not written for travellers in general but rather with the preservation of the health of the military in mind, it is nevertheless included in this list, considering that elements of military regimens found their way into the regimens for ordinary travellers.

---

68 Biographical details of the edition used here: *al-Qānūn fī al-ṭibb*, 4 vols., ed. Saʿīd Laḥḥām, Beirut: Dār al-Fikr, 1994.

69 For the list of its manuscripts, see Gutas, *Avicenna*, 512–513.

70 See the references given in Gutas, *Avicenna*, 512.

71 Ibn Sīnā, *al-Qānūn*, 1/318–326.

72 Gutas, *Avicenna*, 518 (GMed 12).

73 Bibliographical details: Shams al-Dīn, ʿAbd al-Amīr, *al-Madhhab al-tarbawī ʿinda Ibn Sīnā, Min khilāl falsafatihi al-ʿamaliyya*, Beirut: al-Sharika al-ʿĀlamiyya li-l-Kitāb, 1988, p. 280.

1.1.10 Ibn Sīnā: *Risāla fī tadbīr al-musāfirīn*

The treatise 'Regimen for travellers' is extant in six known manuscripts. It is available in edited form as well.[74] Even though Gutas listed the treatise amongst the authentic works of Ibn Sīnā, he notes that the attribution is doubtful.[75]

1.1.11 Ibn al-Quff (d. 684/1286): *Jāmiʿ al-gharaḍ fī ḥifẓ al-ṣiḥḥa wa-dafʿ al-maraḍ*

Amīn al-Dawla Abū al-Faraj ibn Muwaffaq al-Dīn Yaʿqūb ibn Isḥāq Ibn al-Quff al-Malakī al-Masīḥī al-Karakī was born in 630/1233 in Karak. Ibn Abī Uṣaybiʿa taught him medicine in Ṣarkhad. Ibn al-Quff became acquainted with the other sciences in Damascus besides gaining medical experience in hospitals. He was the first appointed surgeon-physician in ʿAjlūn, and later, the Mamluk sultan al-Ẓāhir Baybars called him back to Damascus to serve as a physician and surgeon in the citadel. He died there in 684/1286. Respected amongst his fellow physicians and his students, he wrote treatises upon their requests as well.[76]

His *Jāmiʿ al-gharaḍ fī ḥifẓ al-ṣiḥḥa wa-dafʿ al-maraḍ* ('The comprehensive [book] of the effects on preserving health and preventing illness') was written around 674/1275. He dedicated it to his patron Fakhr al-Dīn Muḥammad and offered a copy of it to the Cairene library of al-Ṣāḥib Bahāʾ al-Dīn ʿAlī ibn Muḥammad ibn Ḥinnā, a long-serving vizier of al-Ẓāhir Baybars. The work is available in a printed edition.[77]

It consists of 60 chapters. The 1st of these is on embryology; the 2nd is on the ages and their temperaments; the 3rd is on the preservation of health in general; chapters 4–11 deal with the preservation of the health according to age groups, from pregnant women to the elderly; chapters 12–13 are on the preservation of the health of travellers on land and sea; the following chapters up to chapter 30 deal with various circumstances and activities with regard to preserving one's health; and the second 30 chapters deal with the use of foodstuffs, medicaments, oils, clothing, stones, buying slaves, and physiognomy.[78] This book was also translated into Latin and circulated in the West.[79]

As obvious from this overview, chapters 12–13[80] contain Ibn al-Quff's travel regimen.

---

74 Shams al-Dīn, *al-Madhhab al-tarbawī*, 285–294.

75 Gutas, *Avicenna*, 518 (GMed 13).

76 For his life and works, see Hamarneh, *Ibn Al-Quff's writings*; Hamarneh, *Ibn al-Ḳuff*.

77 Bibliographical details: *Jāmiʿ al-gharaḍ fī ḥifẓ al-ṣiḥḥa wa-dafʿ al-maraḍ*, ed. Sāmī Khalaf al-Ḥamārnah, ʿAmmān: Manshūrāt al-Jāmiʿa al-Urduniyya, 1989. For the description of the manuscripts used in the edition, see Ibn al-Quff, *Jāmiʿ al-gharaḍ*, 92–95.

78 For a more detailed summary of the chapters, see Ibn al-Quff, *Jāmiʿ al-gharaḍ*, 76–92.

79 Hamarneh, *Ibn Al-Quff's writings*, 377–378.

80 Ibn al-Quff, *Jāmiʿ al-gharaḍ*, 168–172.

1.1.12 Ibn al-Khaṭīb (d. 776/1374–1375): *Kitāb al-wuṣūl li-ḥifẓ al-ṣiḥḥa fī al-fuṣūl*

Abū ʿAbd Allāh Lisān al-Dīn Ibn al-Khaṭīb was born in 713/1313 near Granada, where he later completed his education. He made a successful career under the Naṣrid sultans Muḥammad IV, Yūsuf I, and Muḥammad V. His fortune was tied to Muḥammad V, as he was forced into exile with the dethroned sultan to Fez. Then Ibn al-Khaṭīb settled in Salé, where he wrote many of his works. Later, after Muḥammad V returned to power, he called Ibn al-Khaṭīb back to Granada. Some years later, due to court intrigues and politics, the physician fled to Ceuta, Tlemcen, then Fez. Eventually, his enemies managed to have him sentenced to death for apostasy, and he was strangled in prison before his execution. He is well-known mostly as a biographer, historian, and poet, even though he was a prolific writer in many other fields, amongst them medicine.[81]

According to Ibn Khaldūn, whom he met and befriended in exile, "he excelled in medicine", writing ten works on the subject.[82] His *Kitāb al-wuṣūl li-ḥifẓ al-ṣiḥḥa fī al-fuṣūl* ('The book of obtaining the preservation of health during the seasons') is available in a critical edition with Spanish translation.[83]

The book comprises two parts (*juzʾ*), which are divided into principles (*qāʿida*) and subdivided into chapters (*bāb*), which are sometimes further split into sections (*faṣl*). The first part is on theory. Its first principle is on the seasons in five chapters (on the seasons, their characteristics, their effects on the body, the changes characteristic of them, and their extents). Its second principle is on the general things determining further division in seven chapters (on the elements of which the body is comprised, the temperaments, the humours, the organs, the essences, the potencies, and the actions). The third and last principle of the first part is on the things necessary for people in six chapters, covering the six non-naturals (air, food and drinks, retention and excretion, sleeping and wakefulness, movement and rest, and mental movements). The second part of the book is on practice. Its first principle is on the characteristics of the temperaments in four chapters (in general and in detail, on the signs of fullness and the signs of diseases which can be avoided). Its second principle is on the regimens according to the seasons and the four temperaments. The third and last principle contains specified regimens in three chapters: the first

---

81 On his life and works, see Bosch-Vilá, *Ibn al-Khaṭīb*; Vidal-Castro, *Ibn al-Khaṭīb*.

82 Vidal-Castro, *Ibn al-Khaṭīb*, 120.

83 Bibliographical details: *Libro del cuidado de la salud durante las estaciones del año o "Libro de la higiene" = Kitāb al-wuṣūl li-ḥifẓ al-ṣiḥḥa fī al-fuṣūl*, ed. transl. María de la Concepción Vázquez de Benito, Salamanca: Ediciones Universidad de Salamanca, 1984. The manuscripts used for this edition are discussed in Ibn al-Khaṭīb, *al-Wuṣūl*, 22–24.

for children (from birth to growing up), the second for the elderly, and the third for travellers.[84] This chapter is divided into seven sections. The 1st of these is on the preparations before travelling; the 2nd is on nutrition in general; the 3rd on the different kinds of water; the 4th on safeguarding against the harms of hot and cold weather, thirst, and fatigue; the 5th on the issues of the eye; the 6th on choosing the campsite; and the 7th on travelling on the sea. After this chapter, there is an epilogue on medical terminology. While the regimen of travellers comes at the very end of the work, it is nevertheless included and detailed, unlike the regimen of the elderly, a chapter without further sub-division, or the regimen for pregnant women and those in childbed, omitted in this work but regularly appearing in other encyclopaedias.

1.1.13 Ḥājjī Bāshā (d. 810s or early 820s/1410s or early 1420s): *Shifāʾ al-aqsām wa-dawāʾ al-ālām*

Ḥājjī Bāshā Jalāl al-Dīn al-Khiḍr ibn ʿAlī ibn al-Khaṭṭāb al-Aydīnī was born in Konya but travelled to Cairo to study religious sciences. Due to an illness he suffered there, he became interested in learning medicine. In time it became his primary occupation, and he even worked in the Manṣūrī hospital. Later, in the last quarter of the 14th century, he returned to Anatolia and served his patron, ʿĪsā Bey, as *qāḍī*, teacher, and physician, after whose death he moved to Konya and Birgi, where he died. He wrote on Quranic exegesis, mysticism, and philosophy, chiefly in Arabic, but he owes his renown to his medical works.[85]

He wrote short medical essays, but his main work is the *Shifāʾ al-aqsām wa-dawāʾ al-ālām* ('Recovery from illnesses and remedy for pains'), a compendium dedicated to his patron. He composed abridgements and summaries of this compendium both in Arabic and Turkish, and his works enjoyed popularity due to the clarity and simplicity of his style. As for the *Shifāʾ* itself, it is divided into four sections (*maqāla*). The 1st is an introduction to medical theory and practice. The 2nd is on foodstuffs, beverages, and simple and compound medicaments. The 3rd discusses diseases *a capita ad calcem*. The 4th section deals with conditions affecting more than one organ or the whole body.[86] The 1st *maqāla* of the compendium is available in edited form.[87] In its second half, dedicated to the practical side of medicine, we find regimens associated with the

84 Ibn al-Khaṭīb, *al-Wuṣūl*, 130–134 and 261–267 in the Spanish translation.
85 On his life and works, see Walsh, *Ḥādjdjī Pasha*; Shefer-Mossensohn, *Ḥājjī Pasha*.
86 Shefer-Mossensohn, *Ḥājjī Pasha*, 23.
87 Bibliographical details: *Shifāʾ al-aqsām wa-dawāʾ al-ālām, al-Maqāla al-ūlā, Fī ʿilm al-ṭibb*, ed. Sayyida Ḥāmid ʿAbd al-ʿĀl—Mahā Maẓlūm Khiḍr, Cairo: Maṭbaʿat Dār al-Kutub wa-al-Wathāʾiq al-Qawmiyya, 2016.

ages from childbirth to childhood, followed by the regimens relating to foodstuffs, beverages and drinks, movement and rest, sleeping and wakefulness, emptying and retaining, bathing, intercourse, diuresis, sweating, nasal discharge, saliva, the health-preserving *siwāk*, kohl, and snuff, and clothing. These topics are followed by the regimen for the seasons, the elderly, those recuperating from diseases, pregnant mothers and those in childbed, and those who menstruate during pregnancy, with some medicaments against miscarriage and advice on easing childbirth. The regimen for travellers comes after all these topics.[88] However, it is still followed by numerous additional parts on healing diseases and health in general, about the regimen for various ailments and procedures (vomiting, venesection, cupping, leeching, cauterisation, retention, fatigue), and signs of diseases. A summary of the most common weights and measurements completes the work.

1.1.14 Ibn al-Amshāṭī (d. 902/1496): *al-Isfār ʿan ḥikam al-asfār*

The Cairene jurisprudent and physician Muẓaffar al-Dīn Maḥmūd Ibn al-Amshāṭī's treatise, *al-Isfār ʿan ḥikam al-asfār* ('Unveiling of the wisdoms of the books') belongs in the category of treatises dedicated solely to the regimen of travellers. Though lesser-known to us, Ibn al-Amshāṭī was very much in the midst of the network of the learned Cairene elite of his time. His travel regimen proves to be an excellent example of how a jurist-physician of the post-classical period engages with his sources from the classical period while adding much new and original, in some cases quite ingenious features to them both in terms of arrangement and content, as will be shown.

1.2 *The Genre of Travel Regimens*

Looking at the corpus of texts listed in the previous section, it is important to note what they share in common that makes them part of the same genre. This is for the most part the main theme of the works and the topics they discuss, or to put it more plainly, their content.

Although these topics, being the most important factors in this regard are the backbone of the analysis that follows, the style or language of the regimens can also be mentioned as a common point. It does not matter if a travel regimen is part of an encyclopaedia or a separate treatise, nor is it important whether it was written for physicians or dedicated to laymen, the texts seem to use the same style and expressions if one looks behind the unique voices of the different authors. Still, this style does not really differ from that of other regimens,

88 Ḥājjī Bāshā, *Shifāʾ al-aqsām*, 324–329.

say those written for pregnant women or young children, and so it is most likely governed by the practical nature of regimens in general.

In the following analysis, I start with the topics discussed by travel regimens in general, then move on to an in-depth study of each and every topic. Since some overall observations get lost between the topics, I also summarise these and point out the relationships between the text in this corpus besides giving some examples of misleading titles which suggest a travel regimen but are in fact not travel regimens and discussing the place of travel regimens in encyclopaedias at the end of this sub-chapter.

1.2.1 The Topics of Travel Regimens

In the introduction to his *Risāla fī tadbīr safar al-ḥajj*, Qusṭā ibn Lūqā presents a survey of the topics which general travel regimens and travel regimens written for pilgrims should include. This list is the only one of its kind in all the extant travel regimens listed in the previous sub-chapter. Therefore, I quote this part in its English translation by Bos below:

> I will now give you a description of the regimen which must be applied during journeys in general and of the needs of the body during this journey in particular. What one must know about the regimen of the body during journeys in general can be classified according to four points:
> 1. Knowledge of the regimen in regard to resting, eating, drinking, sleeping and sexual intercourse.
> 2. Knowledge of the different kinds of fatigue and their cure.
> 3. Knowledge of the diseases which are caused by the blowing of the different winds and their treatment.
> 4. Knowledge of the prophylaxis against vermin and of the treatment of the injuries caused by them.
>
> These are the things of which practical knowledge is necessary during journeys in general. The pilgrimage to Mecca, however, is, apart from the four points mentioned, distinguished, by four other points:
> 1. Knowledge of the different waters and of the improvement (of the quality) of contaminated water.
> 2. (Knowledge of) the expedients with which one can quench one's thirst in the case of lack or paucity of water.
> 3. Knowledge of the prophylaxis against the matter from which the *dracunculus medinensis* and hemorrhoids arise.
> 4. (Knowledge of) the prophylaxis against snakes and of the treatment of the injuries caused by them.[89]

89 Qusṭā ibn Lūqā, *Qusṭā ibn Lūqā's medical regime*, 19 (Arabic text: 18, 21).

Comparing this division to the topics discussed by all the other travel regimens shows that the rest of the physicians do not agree with Qusṭā ibn Lūqā's list. As the rest of the travel regimens are general and not specific, they fall in the first category. They generally do not mention the *dracunculus medinensis*, while fatigue, winds (more precisely solely the *samūm*), and vermin are discussed only occasionally. However, water and thirst are always included in the guides, with the single exception of al-Majūsī who does not write about waters. Therefore, even if later physicians used Qusṭā ibn Lūqā's material when compiling their own guides, they disregarded Qusṭā's division.

Some of the topics that are discussed in the travel regimens are general in the sense that they are almost always included in the regimens, while some are more particular, included in only half of the regimens or less. Additionally, there are some more miscellaneous and unique topics discussed by certain authors only. When referring to the encyclopaedias in enumerating these topics, I mean the texts of the corpus that are not standalone treatises but parts of encyclopaedias.

The more general topics are the following. Preparation (what to do before embarking on a journey) and some additional general advice for the traveller are discussed in all the encyclopaedic travel regimens, except for al-Ṭabarī. Regimens for travelling in cold weather or wintertime and in hot weather or summertime are staple elements of travel guides. These are chiefly based on instructions and recommendations regarding some of the six non-naturals (air, food and drinks, retention and excretion, sleeping and wakefulness, movement and rest, and mental movements). Protection of the limbs against the effects of the cold is also more of a general topic (al-Ṭabarī and Ibn al-Khaṭīb are the ones excluding this), similarly to thirst, discussed either in its own chapter or section, included in the regimen for summertime travel, or more broadly in the form of general advice. Waters and improving their quality are another general topic included in all encyclopaedic regimens, except for al-Majūsī's guide. The regimen of seafarers is the same, as it is excluded only by al-Ṭabarī. Similarly, fatigue is discussed in more or less detail by all except for al-Ṭabarī and Ibn Sīnā who refers his readers to a separate chapter on fatigue. The last of the general topics is hunger, treated in more detail by two encyclopaedias but also included in three other encyclopaedic guides, meaning that it is omitted only by two authors (al-Ṭabarī and al-Majūsī).

The more particular topics are the following. Protecting the eyes chiefly against the whiteness of the snow is discussed by al-Rāzī and Ibn al-Khaṭīb and mentioned to a lesser degree by al-Majūsī and Ḥājjī Bāshā. Preserving the complexion and safeguarding the skin against the cold has a similar rate of inclusion, as this issue is examined by al-Rāzī and Ibn Sīnā and to some extent by al-Majūsī. Prophylaxis against the *samūm* and treating its effects are included in the regimens of al-Rāzī, Ibn Sīnā, and Ḥājjī Bāshā. The last of the particular topics is the regimen for armies. It is included in al-Ṭabarī's and al-Rāzī's guide, and some elements of it found their way into Ibn al-Khaṭīb's regimen as well. In addition to these, there is Ibn Sīnā's shorter essay on the regimen of armies.

The more miscellaneous and unique topics are taking care not to swallow leeches or vermin when drinking mentioned by al-Ṭabarī and al-Rāzī, bruising of the skin and injuries due to falling off the mount discussed by al-Rāzī, or the chapter on various signs indicating specific diseases included in Ibn Sīnā's regimen in his *Qānūn*.

In the following sections, I group the topics regardless of their generality or particularity. I start with preparation, then move on to travelling in warm weather and connecting topics (thirst and *samūm*), cold weather and related topics (preserving and treating the limbs, the eyes, and the complexion), the waters and their improvement, hunger, fatigue, and the regimen for sea travel. The instructions for armies and unique topics come at the end.

1.2.2 Preparation and General Advice

Preparing oneself for the journey is one of the general topics, included in all the encyclopaedic travel regimens except for al-Ṭabarī's guide and also omitted by Qusṭā ibn Lūqā.[90] While it would make sense to begin travel regimens with instructions on how to prepare for a journey, this is not always the case. Only half of the authors start their regimens with the necessary preparations, namely al-Majūsi, Ibn al-Khaṭīb, and Ḥājjī Bāshā. In al-Rāzī's guide, travelling in hot weather and cold weather with all the connected topics come before preparation. In Ibn Sīnā's *Qānūn*, preparation is included in his travel guide's second chapter containing general advice regarding health-related issues of travelling, and even in this section preparation does not come first. Lastly, Ibn al-Quff discusses preparation after writing about the different waters and their improvement.

There are three essential components of preparation. The first of these is purification of the body. The physicians recommend two methods for this, purgation (*ishāl*) and bloodletting (*faṣd*). Al-Rāzī, al-Majūsī, and Ibn al-Khaṭīb deem this especially important if the traveller's last purification was a long time ago; the wording of this remark is quite similar in all three cases (*lā siyyamā*

90 Al-Rāzī, *al-Manṣūrī*, 292–293; al-Majūsī, *Kāmil al-ṣināʿa*, II/81; Ibn Sīnā, *al-Qānūn*, I/321; Ibn al-Quff, *Jāmiʿ al-gharaḍ*, 168–169; Ibn al-Khaṭīb, *al-Wuṣūl*, 130; Ḥājjī Bāshā, *Shifāʾ al-aqsām*, 324.

in kāna baʿīd al-ʿahd bi-himā,[91] *wa-kāna ʿahduhu bi-hi baʿīdan*,[92] *lā siyyamā in kāna ʿahduhu bi-dhālika baʿīdan*,[93] respectively; 'especially if a long time has passed since these'). Al-Rāzī and al-Majūsī provide additional overall explanation to underline the importance of purging, which is getting rid of excess and bad humours that can cause fevers, ulcers, swellings, pustules, abscesses, and the like. Ibn al-Khaṭīb mentions fevers only. Al-Majūsī recommends purgative medicaments that one is accustomed to taking, while Ḥājjī Bāshā advises bloodletting first, then taking purging medicaments if the traveller's body is full of excess humours. Interestingly, Ibn Sīnā remains completely silent about the issue of purification.

The second main component of preparation is gradually getting accustomed to the anticipated circumstances of the journey. The physicians give general examples, such as eating, sleeping, sleeplessness, moving, thirst, hunger, abstinence, and so on. While the guides of Ibn al-Quff, Ibn al-Khaṭīb, and Ḥājjī Bāshā present the above general statement and a list of examples, the earlier encyclopaedic guides provide slightly more details. For example, al-Majūsī explains the importance of getting accustomed to sleeplessness: one might need to travel during the night-time, in which case the traveller is better equipped to endure this. Al-Rāzī and al-Majūsī advise changing the mealtimes in accordance with that expected during the journey, while al-Rāzī and Ibn Sīnā suggest eating the kinds of foodstuffs that will be available on the road even before the journey.

The third major part of preparation is exercise. All physicians writing about preparation recommend either a gradually increased amount of exercise prior to the journey, or to more specifically walk or ride more and more each day depending on the mode of travel. While this point falls into the previous category, it nevertheless draws more attention and is discussed somewhat separately in the regimens.

A unique detail can be found in al-Rāzī's section on preparation: he recommends the traveller to stockpile the medicaments he is accustomed to for his journey.[94] This advice is not present in any other travel regimen; although, as mentioned before, there is precedent for a somewhat similar approach, namely al-Majūsī recommending purging medicaments one is accustomed to.

Besides preparation, the physicians also give more general advice. It is generally recommended to not travel, move, or hurry on a full stomach as it would

---

91 Al-Rāzi, *al-Manṣūrī*, 292.
92 Al-Majūsī, *Kāmil al-ṣināʿa*, II/81.
93 Ibn al-Khaṭīb, *al-Wuṣūl*, 130.
94 Al-Rāzi, *al-Manṣūrī*, 292.

lead to diseases and swellings,[95] only eat once resting,[96] eat foodstuffs with high nutritional values but of smaller quantities,[97] and some additional nutritional advice more connected to the topic of hunger and therefore discussed in their section. Al-Majūsī offers some general advice for those who will travel on foot: he instructs to wrap the muscles of the traveller's thighs with wraps and bandages, tighten the traveller's trunk with stays (*mishadd*) to strengthen the back for movement, and to bring a staff or stick (*ʿukkāza*) to lean on it occasionally as it eases fatigue.[98] This advice is also present in Ibn al-Quff's guide,[99] the difference between them being that Ibn al-Quff simply writes to tighten the thighs and wrap the trunk, omitting the tools al-Majūsī mentions (wraps, bandages, stays).

1.2.3 Travelling in Hot Weather

The regimen for travelling in hot weather is one of the staple topics of travel guides.[100] While there is a definable core content in the parts of travel regimens discussing this topic, there are noticeable differences between the authors.

The more general advice for travelling in hot weather is focused on balancing eating and moving, avoiding thirst, and protecting the body from the sun and the heat. Regarding the first, the general consensus is to avoid travelling on a full or an empty stomach. It is al-Rāzī who explains the underlying reasons to his reader: when the stomach is full of food or drinks, moving shakes up the stomach's contents and this leads to indigestion. Instead of moving with an empty stomach, it is better to eat a small amount of cold and thirst-quenching food or soup and digest for a while before moving out. According to al-Rāzī, travelling on an empty stomach is more harmful for exhausted bodies or those with diseases but less harmful for chubby ones; in some cases of the latter, it can even be beneficial. To avoid thirst, consuming cold or cooling foodstuffs and avoiding thirst-inducing foodstuffs (such as salty, spicy, or sweet food) is recommended; however, this will be discussed in more detail in the section on thirst. The last of the general advice is protecting the body from the sun and the heat. The main way to do so is dressing up properly, taking special care when

---

95 Al-Rāzi, *al-Manṣūrī*, 293; Ḥājjī Bāshā, *Shifāʾ al-aqsām*, 324.

96 Ibn Sīnā, *al-Qānūn*, I/321; Ḥājjī Bāshā, *Shifāʾ al-aqsām*, 324.

97 Al-Rāzī, *al-Manṣūrī*, 293; Ibn Sīnā, *al-Qānūn*, I/321; Ibn al-Khaṭīb, *al-Wuṣūl*, 130; Ḥājjī Bāshā, *Shifāʾ al-aqsām*, 324.

98 Al-Majūsī, *Kāmil al-ṣināʿa*, II/81.

99 Ibn al-Quff, *Jāmiʿ al-gharaḍ*, 169.

100 Al-Ṭabarī, *Firdaws al-ḥikma*, 109–110; al-Rāzī, *al-Manṣūrī*, 281–282; al-Majūsī, *Kāmil al-ṣināʿa*, II/81–82; Ibn Sīnā, *al-Qānūn*, I/322–323; Ibn al-Quff, *Jāmiʿ al-gharaḍ*, 169–170; Ibn al-Khaṭīb, *al-Wuṣūl*, 131; Ḥājjī Bāshā, *Shifāʾ al-aqsām*, 325.

covering the head and the chest. Al-Majūsī also adds that properly covering the head and the face prevent the traveller to inhale much hot air; this statement is copied by Ḥājjī Bāshā. Ibn Sīnā, Ibn al-Quff, and Ḥājjī Bāshā recommend coating the chest or other parts of the body with certain oils or mucous materials besides covering the body with garments.

There is some additional advice usually included in most of the guides. These are to travel during the night and rest during the daytime (al-Majūsī, Ibn al-Quff, Ḥājjī Bāshā) and to consume certain cooling, moistening, and thirst-quenching foodstuffs and drinks before journeying in hot weather (al-Majūsī, Ibn Sīnā, Ibn al-Quff). The most detailed instructions for resting are provided by al-Ṭabarī and al-Rāzī who recommend washing oneself with cold or lukewarm water, anointing the body with specific oils, eating cooling and moistening food, sleeping in an airy, ventilated space, and avoiding intercourse.[101] In contrast, Ibn al-Quff advises to wash the limbs with diluted water and then drink some diluted white wine.[102]

Al-Majūsī gives a list of typical illnesses caused by travelling in hot weather: headache, hectic fever (*ḥummā al-diqq*), dryness and withering of the body, and other hot and dry illnesses. He states that these are more likely to occur in travellers of hot and dry temperaments and thin bodies.[103] Al-Majūsī's list of diseases is faithfully reproduced by Ḥājjī Bāshā,[104] making it apparent that the latter relied on al-Majūsī's text greatly when compiling this part.

Some additional issues to point out are the following. It is only al-Rāzī who gives advice on treating headache and fever, not just on how to prevent these. Ibn Sīnā is the only one mentioning that swimming in cold water suddenly causes many problems so the traveller should wait patiently and enter the cold water gradually. Ibn al-Khaṭīb provides general advice for travelling in hot weather, however, his text is worded and arranged in a greatly different manner than all the other texts.

1.2.4 Preventing and Quenching Thirst

Thirst is chiefly discussed as a section of the regimen for travelling in hot weather. The exceptions are al-Rāzī with a separate sub-section on thirst and to a smaller extent al-Majūsī and Ḥājjī Bāshā who write about thirst in more length. Al-Ṭabarī, Ibn Sīnā, Ibn al-Quff and Ibn al-Khaṭīb are more succinct

101 Al-Ṭabarī, *Firdaws al-ḥikma*, 110; al-Rāzī, *al-Manṣūrī*, 282.
102 Ibn al-Quff, *Jāmiʿ al-gharaḍ*, 170.
103 Al-Majūsī, *Kāmil al-ṣināʿa*, 11/81.
104 Ḥājjī Bāshā, *Shifāʾ al-aqsām*, 325.

regarding thirst.[105] In the case of Ibn Sīnā, this is due to the fact that he refers his reader to a separate chapter on thirst and provides only the most important information in his travel regimen.

The general advice is to not eat much and avoid eating things that cause thirst, such as salty, spicy, or sweet foodstuffs and rather consume meals that have moistening and cooling properties, such as dishes prepared with vinegar, sour grapes, and *dūgh*, buttermilk. These instructions are included in all of the guides and sometimes with examples of specific dishes, except for al-Ṭabarī who only writes that in case of thirst, the traveller should wash his face and legs and then drink sip by sip. Another general advice is to not speak much and avoid opening the mouth, noted by al-Rāzī, Ibn Sīnā, and Ibn al-Quff.[106] Al-Rāzī advises not to hurry as hurrying leads to frequent and heavy breathing, resulting in thirst.[107] Moreover, Ibn al-Quff and Ḥājjī Bāshā mention *dūgh* cooled with ice as a drink useful for preventing thirst.[108]

Some authors recommend drinking specific drinks before travelling to prevent getting thirsty. Al-Majūsī recommends mucilage of psyllium seeds and juice of purslane seeds with some sour pomegranate juice, almond oil, or pumpkin oil.[109] Ibn al-Quff recommends barley *sawīq*.[110] Ḥājjī Bāshā relies here on al-Majūsī again, listing the same materials as al-Majūsī, except that instead of juice of purslane he writes milk of purslane seeds.[111] Al-Rāzī gives the longest list of drinks and foodstuffs to consume before travelling to ward off thirst.[112] While this is never explicitly explained, the idea is to consume these moistening and cooling drinks before the journey as well and not only during it to push the body of the traveller more towards moistness and coolness pre-emptively so that it cannot become so warm and dry as to feel strong thirst.

A widely recommended method of quenching thirst is to put things into one's mouth; either a specific pill for which al-Majūsī, Ibn al-Quff, and Ḥājjī Bāshā all provide a recipe or alternative things if the pill is not available or cannot be prepared.[113] The recipe is the same in all three cases. Ḥājjī Bāshā again

---

105 Al-Ṭabarī, *Firdaws al-ḥikma*, 110; al-Rāzī, *al-Manṣūrī*, 284–286; al-Majūsī, *Kāmil al-ṣināʿa*, II/82; Ibn Sīnā, *al-Qānūn*, I/321–322, 323; Ibn al-Quff, *Jāmiʿ al-gharaḍ*, 170; Ibn al-Khaṭīb, *al-Wuṣūl*, 131; Ḥājjī Bāshā, *Shifāʾ al-aqsām*, 325–326.

106 Al-Rāzī, *al-Manṣūrī*, 284; Ibn Sīnā, *al-Qānūn*, I/322; Ibn al-Quff, *Jāmiʿ al-gharaḍ*, 170.

107 Al-Rāzī, *al-Manṣūrī*, 284.

108 Ibn al-Quff, *Jāmiʿ al-gharaḍ*, 170; Ḥājjī Bāshā, *Shifāʾ al-aqsām*, 326.

109 Al-Majūsī, *Kāmil al-ṣināʿa*, II/82.

110 Ibn al-Quff, *Jāmiʿ al-gharaḍ*, 170.

111 Ḥājjī Bāshā, *Shifāʾ al-aqsām*, 325.

112 Al-Rāzī, *al-Manṣūrī*, 284–286.

113 Al-Majūsī, *Kāmil al-ṣināʿa*, II/82; Ibn al-Quff, *Jāmiʿ al-gharaḍ*, 170; Ḥājjī Bāshā, *Shifāʾ al-aqsām*, 325.

likely copied it directly from al-Majūsī, as their recipe is five dirhams of pumpkin seed kernel, serpent melon kernel, cucumber kernel, and purslane seed, two dirhams of corn-starch, tragacanth, and chalk, all pulverised together neatly, then kneaded with mucilage of psyllium seeds[114] and formed into pills.[115] Ibn al-Quff mentions serpent melon seed kernels, cucumber seeds, and purslane seeds from the first group of materials but adds white poppy, and for the second group of materials he lists corn-starch and chalk and adds sugar. He does not provide measurements or preparation methods.[116] Alternatives for the pill are quince (al-Majūsī, Ḥājjī Bāshā), a coin made of lead or a dirham coin (al-Majūsī), a similarly shaped thing prepared from tragacanth and gum Arabic (Ḥājjī Bāshā), or generally a piece of silver, crystal, pearl (Ibn al-Khaṭīb, Ḥājjī Bāshā), or any smooth pebble (Ibn al-Khaṭīb). In addition, Ḥājjī Bāshā recommends 3 dirhams of purslane put into vinegar if nothing else is available. It is al-Rāzī once more who provides the longest list of such alternatives, even if in his case, we do not find the recipe for the above-mentioned thirst-quenching pill. Instead, he provides the recipe for a pill which, in addition to its usefulness against thirst also alleviates fever. It is one part cucumber seeds and pumpkin seeds each, half part lettuce seeds and purslane seeds each, and quarter part pure liquorice rob pulverised finely, then kneaded with juice of purslane or mucilage of psyllium seeds, shaped into small pills like lupin beans.[117] In addition to the recipe, al-Rāzī also provides instructions regarding dosage for thirst-quenching and for fevers both, noting that the pill is also useful against burning urine in his experience.[118]

The last interesting advice is to drink water with vinegar if water is scarce, as this is especially good for quenching thirst. While this practice is mentioned only by Ibn Sīnā and Ḥājjī Bāshā, they either used the same source or Ḥājjī Bāshā copied from Ibn Sīnā as the two sections are almost exactly the same: *wa-idhā shariba al-māʾ bi-al-khall kāna al-qalīl minhu kāfiyan fī taskīn al-ʿaṭash ḥaythu lā yūjadu māʾ kathīr*[119] is how Ibn Sīnā phrases his advice, compared to which Ḥājjī Bāshā only changes *minhu* to *min al-māʾ*[120] ('and if he drinks water with vinegar, a small amount of it suffices in quenching thirst if there is not a lot of water').

114 The edition of Ḥājjī Bāshā has *qaṭūn* instead of *qaṭūnā* which is likely a typo or mistake: Ḥājjī Bāshā, *Shifāʾ al-aqsām*, 325.

115 Al-Majūsī, *Kāmil al-ṣināʿa*, 11/82; Ḥājjī Bāshā, *Shifāʾ al-aqsām*, 325.

116 Ibn al-Quff, *Jāmiʿ al-gharaḍ*, 170.

117 Al-Rāzī, *al-Manṣūrī*, 285.

118 Al-Rāzī, *al-Manṣūrī*, 285.

119 Ibn Sīnā, *al-Qānūn*, 1/322.

120 Ḥājjī Bāshā, *Shifāʾ al-aqsām*, 325.

1.2.5 The *samūm*

Qusṭā ibn Lūqā deems discussion of the various winds, their effects and curing of their harms, a necessary element of all health guides. Accordingly, he dedicates chapter 4 of his travel regimen written for the pilgrims to this topic,[121] advising to cover the head, ears, nose, and mouth with a turban and if the ears are weak to plug them with some cotton soaked in oils. Qusṭā ibn Lūqā recommends this against hot and cold winds alike and against much sand. Without any specification of various types of winds, he recommends warm remedies against the cold winds and cold remedies against the warm winds and discusses some of the illnesses caused by the winds separately. The discussion of the effects of winds is heavily influenced by Hippocrates and Galen, as shown by Bos.[122] Despite this, only three of the travel regimens (those of al-Rāzī, Ibn Sīnā, and Ḥājjī Bāshā)[123] include anything regarding winds, more specifically on the *samūm* only without any reference to other kinds of winds.

The *samūm* is "a hot wind of the desert accompanied by whirlwinds of dust and sand [...] especially characteristic of the Sahara, in Egypt, in Arabia and in Mesopotamia". In the *ḥadīth* literature we find that Hell's taking breath in summer is the *samūm* and in the Quran (15:27) that the *jinn* were created from the fire of the *samūm*.[124] Even Ibn Baṭṭūṭa (d. 770/1368–1369 or 779/1377), the famous traveller mentions this wind as it blows two months a year in a desert he crosses during his travels, killing all who travel in it. He even recounts that whoever perishes in the *samūm*, his limbs fall apart when his friends attempt to wash him for burial.[125] In a medical sense, the dangers of the *samūm* lie in the fact that it is, as an extremely hot and dry wind, considered to have strong warming and drying qualities besides the addition of dust and sand it carries. This means that when travelling in the *samūm* is unavoidable, the recommended precautions (and treatment for the afflictions it causes as well) are aimed at countering the *samūm*'s warming and drying properties with cooling and moistening drinks and foodstuffs besides some physical protection to prevent the heat and sand from getting to and into the body.

Al-Rāzī dedicates a subsection of his travel regimen to the *samūm* that is approximately half the length of his subsections on travelling in hot weather or that on thirst. Most of al-Rāzī's subsection on the *samūm* focuses on prevention. He recommends eating balanced foodstuffs prepared with fats and not

---

121 Qusṭā ibn Lūqā, *Qusṭā ibn Lūqā's medical regime*, 39, 41 (Arabic text: 38, 40).

122 Qusṭā ibn Lūqā, *Qusṭā ibn Lūqā's medical regime*, 8, 96–97 n. 65.

123 Al-Rāzī, *al-Manṣūrī*, 283; Ibn Sīnā, *al-Qānūn*, I/322–323; Ḥājjī Bāshā, *Shifāʾ al-aqsām*, 326.

124 Wensinck, *Samūm*, 1056.

125 Gibb, *The travels of Ibn Baṭṭūṭa*, II/404.

drinking a lot after eating, covering one's face with a turban, secluding oneself from the direction of the wind's blowing if possible, and rinsing the mouth with water hourly and drinking it only when it is cold. A lot of al-Rāzī's advice pertains to preparing before journeying in the *samūm*, such as coating the chest and stomach with mucilage of psyllium seeds and juice of purslane with pumpkin seed oil and egg whites, sucking on purslane as well as eating lots of dishes prepared with it and cooked with *rā'ib* (a kind of yoghurt) or whey and butter, drinking pumpkin oil, and eating chopped up onions soaked in *rā'ib* for a night and then drinking the *rā'ib* as this allows the traveller to only rinse with water, and when he drinks water he is able to drink only a little and eat only a minimal amount of food with cooling properties as to avoid dangerous thirst. While it is possible to heed this advice once on the journey, as all the materials recommended have cooling and moistening properties, al-Rāzī phrases these more as things to do prior to starting travel in the *samūm*. If the damage caused by the *samūm* grows stronger then al-Rāzī advises hiding one's head in his garments and seeking shelter from the wind hourly, sniffing sweet pumpkin oil and almond oil.

In Ibn Sīnā's travel guide, the discussion of the *samūm* is the second half of chapter 3 which is on travelling in hot weather. This section also contains preventative advice and instructions for treatment but, unlike in the case of al-Rāzī, the treatments are discussed in greater length. Ibn Sīnā's preventive advice is wrapping the nostrils and mouth with a turban and veil and abstaining from demanding physical activity in the meantime, eating onions in *dūgh* before the journey and also drinking the said *dūgh*, sniffing rose oil and pumpkin seed oil as well as drinking pumpkin oil. Ibn Sīnā gives some detailed information regarding the onions in *dūgh*: the onions are to be finely chopped before they are put into the *dūgh*, then it should soak there for a night or they are to be left in there to be preserved like a jam. Interestingly, coating the chest and belly is not mentioned here. For treating the afflictions of the *samūm*, Ibn Sīnā recommends pouring cold water on the limbs and also washing the face with cold water, preparing one's meal from cooling herbs, putting cooling oils and saps on one's head such as rose oil and sap of houseleek tree, then washing oneself and avoiding intercourse. Curiously, Ibn Sīnā recommends salty fish once the traveller's body calms down, despite the fact that salty foods, especially fish, are commonly advised against in general due to its thirst-inducing drying qualities. Additionally, Ibn Sīnā recommends mixed wine, milk if the traveller does not have fever, and sour *dūgh* if the traveller has fever but not a putrid one. Ibn Sīnā's last advice is regarding drinking: if the traveller gets thirsty while sleeping in recovery, he is to rinse his mouth only as drinking a lot leads to immediate death. If drinking is unavoidable, it should be sip by sip until the traveller's body calms down so his thirst can be quenched. The best method is to drink water mixed with rose oil first and only then pure water.

Ḥājjī Bāshā's discussion of the *samūm* also consists of preventive measures and advice on treatment. He recommends covering the nose and mouth and enduring this, eating chopped onion which was soaked in buttermilk (he uses the word *mukhīḍ* instead of *dūgh*) for a day and a night as well as drinking the buttermilk used for this, sniffing cooling and moistening oils (without providing any examples), and drinking pumpkin oil prior to the journey. For treatment, Ḥājjī Bāshā advises pouring cold water on the body and legs, putting rose oil and rose water on the head, then sitting in cold water, and eating dishes prepared with lettuce, cucumbers, purslane and the like (all are moistening and cooling) thereafter, rinsing with cold water and drinking only after that, as well as sleeping after consuming buttermilk if the traveller is not feverish. For the issues regarding travelling in hot weather, Ḥājjī Bāshā was shown to consistently work from al-Majūsī's travel regimen. As al-Majūsī does not write about the *samūm*, here, Ḥājjī Bāshā had to look for another source which was in this case Ibn Sīnā's section on the *samūm*, which is especially apparent when inspecting the methods of treatments more closely.

1.2.6 Travelling in Cold Weather

The regimen for travelling in cold weather is the other staple topic of travel guides, as all the encyclopaedic guides include a subchapter or section dedicated to this matter.[126] The issues discussed regarding travelling in the cold are what to eat and drink before and during the journey, how to protect one's body from the cold, and what to do once resting, besides some general advice.

The more general points mentioned by al-Majūsī, Ibn al-Quff, and Ḥājjī Bāshā are to travel during the daytime and rest during the nighttime.[127] It is worth pointing out that these are the same authors that recommended the opposite for travelling in hot weather. Ibn al-Quff even notes that walking is a more beneficial way of travelling in the cold than riding.[128] While he does not explain the otherwise obvious reason for this, al-Majūsī does write that walking warms the legs; this is his reason for suggesting wrapping the legs even more if

126 Al-Ṭabarī, *Firdaws al-ḥikma*, 109; al-Rāzī, *al-Manṣūrī*, 286–287; al-Majūsī, *Kāmil al-ṣināʿa*, II/82–83; Ibn Sīnā, *al-Qānūn*, I/323–324; Ibn al-Quff, *Jāmiʿ al-gharaḍ*, 170–171; Ibn al-Khaṭīb, *al-Wuṣūl*, 131–132; Ḥājjī Bāshā, *Shifāʾ al-aqsām*, 326–327.

127 Al-Majūsī, *Kāmil al-ṣināʿa*, II/82; Ibn al-Quff, *Jāmiʿ al-gharaḍ*, 170; Ḥājjī Bāshā, *Shifāʾ al-aqsām*, 327.

128 Ibn al-Quff, *Jāmiʿ al-gharaḍ*, 170.

one is riding.[129] Another general point of the physicians is to not travel on an empty stomach. Al-Rāzī is the most specific regarding this when he writes that one should eat until full and drink a sufficient amount of wine as well and then move only to a degree that keeps the consumed foodstuffs in one's stomach warm while any outbursts or flare-ups that might be caused by too excessive movement on a full stomach are avoided.[130] This can be found in two more regimens. Ibn Sīnā also presents this same advice in a different way but in the case of Ḥājjī Bāshā, it is an obvious copying of al-Rāzī's material.[131]

The recommended foodstuffs are concurrent for the most part. Most of the advice regarding dishes focuses on listing the ingredients to include that have strong warming properties. These are garlic, onion (especially raw onion), almonds, butter (made from milk of cattle according to Ḥājjī Bāshā), assafetida, pepper, ginger, mustard (listed only by Ibn al-Khaṭīb), leek (*kurrāth*, listed by al-Rāzī only), and *isfīdabāj*.[132] Al-Rāzī praises garlic especially, for it has such strong warming properties that it ignites the innate heat until it spreads into the whole body and forms a surplus even in the limbs.[133] Ibn Sīnā says that garlic is especially useful when the brain and mental faculties are affected by the cold.[134] Assafetida is recommended by al-Rāzī and Ibn Sīnā: they advise mixing a *dirham* of it into wine. Ḥājjī Bāshā also gives this advice but it seems to be a copy of Ibn Sīnā's words.[135] Ibn al-Quff is the only one who lists specific types of meats to use, namely game meat, such as meat of gazelle, rabbit, and duck, or if the traveller finds that these do not agree with him, then meat of sheep or young goats are preferable with the above-mentioned warming herbs.[136]

Moving on to drinks, the consensus is to consume strong, mostly unmixed, and not sour wine. Al-Rāzī writes that it is possible to mix the wine with some lukewarm water to warm it up a little before consuming it.[137] It is also generally recommended to mix pepper and ginger into the wine as to add additional warming properties to it via the herbs.

129 Al-Majūsī, *Kāmil al-ṣināʿa*, 11/83.

130 Al-Rāzī, *al-Manṣūrī*, 286.

131 Ibn Sīnā, *al-Qānūn*, 1/323–324; Ḥājjī Bāshā, *Shifāʾ al-aqsām*, 327.

132 A dish prepared from meat, onions, butter, oil, parsley, and coriander or a white stew. A great collection of sources and studies regarding *isfīdabāj* is presented by Bos in Maimonides, *On the elucidation of some symptoms*, 60–31 n. 117.

133 Al-Rāzī, *al-Manṣūrī*, 286–287.

134 Ibn Sīnā, *al-Qānūn*, 1/324.

135 Al-Rāzī, *al-Manṣūrī*, 287; Ibn Sīnā, *al-Qānūn*, 1/324; Ḥājjī Bāshā, *Shifāʾ al-aqsām*, 327.

136 Ibn al-Quff, *Jāmiʿ al-gharaḍ*, 171.

137 Al-Rāzī, *al-Manṣūrī*, 286.

The advice on how to protect the body from the cold from the outside is also similar in nature in all the encyclopaedic regimens; nonetheless, some differences between the texts are easy to discern and enable grouping of the sources. Ibn Sīnā is the most succinct on this issue, writing that the pores should be closed, and the cold is to be prevented from entering the nose and mouth.[138] Ibn al-Khaṭīb shortened a section from Ibn Sīnā's guide which contained this advice.[139] Al-Rāzī is also briefer in this case as he writes that the traveller should wrap himself excessively especially if he travels in the wind's eye; however, doing so should be avoided if there is pain, coarseness, or coughing in the chest or if the traveller has weaker chest or lungs, as doing so leads to excessive breathing which results in strong coughing and maybe even coughing up blood.[140] Ibn al-Quff gives some more details on clothing: he recommends fluffy, fuzzy garments made from cotton, wool, or goat hair, cotton turbans, and excessively covering the limbs by making gloves and leg-covers from wool with fur lining.[141] The most detailed instructions for properly dressing up is provided by al-Majūsī. He recommends napped and fur garments for the whole body, caps and turbans for the head and face, and wool or silk wraps for the limbs. For travelling in even colder areas with snow or wind, al-Majūsī advises putting goat hair between the fingers, wrapping them in paper (*kāghad*), putting on socks, then shoes, then fur boots or fur gloves in case of the hand. He also recommends to not wear too tight boots as to allow for some movement of the limbs.[142] Here, Ḥājjī Bāshā obviously copies al-Majūsī's material once again. Ḥājjī Bāshā adds covering the pores, nose, mouth, and ears to prevent the cold reaching them.[143] Al-Majūsī is more specific about covering the pores: he recommends using Egyptian willow oil, lily oil, and bay laurel oil as these all close the pores and therefore keep the warmth of the body inside and the cold outside.[144] Ibn al-Quff lists violet oil, lily oil, and chamomile oil,[145] while Ibn al-Khaṭīb names iris oil as an example of warming oils to use.[146] Al-Ṭabarī and Ibn Sīnā advise using warming oils in general without examples.

Another more significant topic of regimens for travelling in cold is resting. Al-Rāzī and Ibn Sīnā give the most detailed instructions on how to rest prop-

138 Ibn Sīnā, *al-Qānūn*, 1/323.
139 Ibn al-Khaṭīb, *al-Wuṣūl*, 131.
140 Al-Rāzī, *al-Manṣūrī*, 286.
141 Ibn al-Quff, *Jāmiʿ al-gharaḍ*, 170.
142 Al-Majūsī, *Kāmil al-ṣināʿa*, 11/83.
143 Ḥājjī Bāshā, *Shifāʾ al-aqsām*, 327.
144 Al-Majūsī, *Kāmil al-ṣināʿa*, 11/82.
145 Ibn al-Quff, *Jāmiʿ al-gharaḍ*, 171.
146 Ibn al-Khaṭīb, *al-Wuṣūl*, 132.

erly after travelling in cold weather,[147] although Ibn Sīnā focuses mostly on what to eat. Gradually warming up by a fire is advised instead of rushing to the fire straightaway. Al-Rāzī then recommends taking a long bath and getting massaged or if a bathhouse is not available, then simply massage in a heated dwelling until the skin of the face becomes red is appropriate. After this, a long sleep under many blankets helps prevent fever. In Ibn Sīnā's opinion, warming oils should be used after gradually warming up and it is actually [physically] hot foods that cause a sensation similar to being feverish, therefore he recommends eating dishes with warming properties instead. It is quite curious that Ibn Sīnā recommends adding whey and butter to the dishes to make the garlic and almonds agreeable; while butter is amongst the warming ingredients listed in general, whey is cooling and moistening so while it might make dishes with a lot of garlic taste more acceptable it should also decrease the warming properties of any dish which seems counterintuitive at first glance. Ḥājjī Bāshā mentions warming oneself with garments before approaching a fire as well as using euphorbium oil,[148] one of the warming oils on the body and the legs.[149] Ibn al-Khaṭīb recommends bathing in hot water when the traveller is tired and using oils in which chamomile or dill was boiled with a gentle massage. While this advice is located in his section on travelling in cold, it is more focused on tiredness as he also writes that violet and rose oil are to be used if this occurs in the summer.[150]

Al-Rāzī dedicates a separate subchapter to what to do if the traveller becomes frozen in general and al-Majūsī, Ibn al-Khaṭīb, and Ḥājjī Bāshā also write about this in greater length. As treatment of frozen limbs is a separate issue, these discussions focus on freeze or chill manifesting as hypothermia or a state close to it with rigid or firm skin. Al-Rāzī recommends resting in a warm, leeward place, getting a good massage with warm hands on the whole body except for the head, and drinking strong wine with assafetida, myrrh, and pepper. Once the life comes back to the frozen traveller, he is to eat some *isfīdabāj* and drink a moderate amount of wine, then sleep for a long time under warm blankets until he is ready to take a long, hot bath followed by massage and using iris oil or narcissus (*narjis*) oil in which costus (*qusṭ*), castoreum, musk, and euphorbium was put.[151] The advice of al-Majūsī is similar

147 Al-Rāzī, *al-Manṣūrī*, 287; Ibn Sīnā, *al-Qānūn*, 1/323.

148 *Furbiyūn*, inspissated sap of plants of the *Euphorbia* genus. The edition has *duhn al-furfiyūn* and identifies it as purslane: Ḥājjī Bāshā, *Shifāʾ al-aqsām*, 326.

149 Ḥājjī Bāshā, *Shifāʾ al-aqsām*, 326.

150 Ibn al-Khaṭīb, *al-Wuṣūl*, 132.

151 Al-Rāzī, *al-Manṣūrī*, 287–288.

in nature, albeit shorter. He recommends warming up by a fire before bathing, then using dill oil or lily oil, dressing up still in the bathhouse and staying in a warm place afterwards, eating meat broth and *isfīdabāj*, and lastly taking a long nap under blankets. He does not mention massaging.[152] Ibn al-Khaṭīb does recommend massage and the use of oils with pepper, euphorbium, and pellitory added to them, also coating the limbs with garlic and galbanum in addition to using the oils. A unique advice from him is to put the limbs in water of rapeseed in which fig, chamomile, cabbage, and basil was boiled if the innate heat starts to dissipate from the limbs, as this treatment prevents putrefaction and therefore the need of surgery.[153] Ḥājjī Bāshā copies al-Majūsī but he also adds the use of warm compresses, the putting of dill oil, Egyptian willow oil, lily oil, and bay laurel oil on the traveller's body and his garments. He also adds that tar is the best to coat the limbs with, as it prevents putrefaction.[154]

Unique features in these regimens can also be observed. While al-Ṭabarī provides his reader with only a few words on travelling in the cold which he bases on Galen, he shares a personal account: he saw people from the mountains of Tabaristan overcoming the cold by eating garlic and kebabs and drinking so much pure wine that some of them became drunk and as a result fell asleep on the snow that continued to fall on them, but they did not notice a thing.[155]

Al-Rāzī gives a list of typical diseases befalling those travelling in the cold, namely freezing (*jumūd*), hunger, fainting (*al-jūʿ wa-al-ghashy*, likely hungry fainting, *al-ghashy al-jūʿī*), apoplexy (*sakta*), limpness (*istirkhāʾ*), spasms (*kuzāz*), decay or putridity of the limbs (*ʿafan al-aṭrāf*), numbness (*khadhar*), and constipation (*ʿaql al-baṭn*). He also states that occurrence of these diseases or afflictions is less likely in those accustomed to the cold and those with a temperament more resistant against such diseases.[156] Additionally, al-Rāzī dedicates a short subchapter to hungry fainting, a strong hunger resulting in fainting and slumber which can lead to death. It can be treated with providing specific foods and strong wine with warming spices, massage of the cardia and limbs but al-Rāzī provides some additional methods of treatment for when the affliction does not subside.[157]

---

152 Al-Majūsī, *Kāmil al-ṣināʿa*, II/83.
153 Ibn al-Khaṭīb, *al-Wuṣūl*, 132.
154 Ḥājjī Bāshā, *Shifāʾ al-aqsām*, 328.
155 Al-Ṭabarī, *Firdaws al-ḥikma*, 110.
156 Al-Rāzī, *al-Manṣūrī*, 286.
157 Al-Rāzī, *al-Manṣūrī*, 288.

Ibn Sīnā also emphasises at the beginning of his regimen for wintertime travel that travelling in the cold is dangerous and even if prepared, many travellers die because of the cold. He also lists typical related diseases and afflictions. Some of these are familiar from al-Rāzī's list, such as convulsion (*tashannuj*), spasms (*kuzāz*), freezing (*jumūd*), and apoplexy (*sakta*); however, Ibn Sīnā also adds dying from drinking opium and mandragora and also being affected by the hunger called bulimia (*būlīmūs*).[158] In this part of his travel regimen, he offers more overall advice as he writes about the above afflictions in more detail separately.

The last of the more unique features can be found in Ibn al-Quff's writing, as he dedicates a few sentences on what to do if one must travel during the night or in much snow. It is in this latter part where we find some additional methods and materials, namely the use of warm compresses on the limbs when resting made with water in which turnip (*lift*), a kind of mint (*nammām*), and wormwood (*shīkh*) was boiled, in addition to using warming oils with castoreum, assafetida, and euphorbium, as well as drinking pure wine in which some great theriac is added.[159]

1.2.7 Preserving and Treating the Limbs

Apart from al-Ṭabarī and Ibn al-Khaṭīb, all the authors who wrote on wintertime travel dedicate either a separate section to the protection and treatment of the limbs (al-Rāzī, Ibn Sīnā) or include a section on it in their regimen for travelling in the cold (al-Majūsī, Ḥājjī Bāshā).[160] Ibn al-Quff focuses on how to properly protect the limbs as it was shown in the previous subchapter, but he does not include instructions for treatment. While the instructions of these authors regarding covering and wrapping the limbs discussed in the previous subchapter also pertain to this issue, here the focus is the discussion of the various treatments and only partially on additional preventive methods.

For prevention, generally the use of warming oils is recommended before wrapping, padding, and covering the limbs. Al-Rāzī recommends oils of lily, Sambac jasmine (*rāziqī*), Egyptian willow, iris, and bay laurel.[161] All four authors agree that it is not recommended to endure the painful cold instead of applying additional warming oils, layers of clothes, or warming oneself up. Al-Majūsī notes that it is better to walk than ride and Ibn Sīnā advises against

158 Ibn Sīnā, *al-Qānūn*, 1/323.

159 Ibn al-Quff, *Jāmiʿ al-gharaḍ*, 171.

160 Al-Rāzī, *al-Manṣūrī*, 288–290; al-Majūsī, *Kāmil al-ṣināʿa*, 11/83; Ibn Sīnā, *al-Qānūn*, 1/324–325; Ḥājjī Bāshā, *Shifāʾ al-aqsām*, 328–329.

161 Al-Rāzī, *al-Manṣūrī*, 289.

too tight shoes, as not moving the feet or restricting their movement results in a more severe affliction by the cold.[162] They also advise taking additional care if the traveller stops feeling the pains due to the cold without him changing his covers or the cold subsiding, as this signals a loss of sense in the limbs. Al-Rāzī recommends immediately changing the covers on the limb followed by a gentle massage and covering the limb once more, followed by some walking.[163] Al-Majūsī advises the use of Egyptian willow oil, lily oil, or bay laurel oil, in addition to padding the space around and between the fingers with pieces of squirrel, sable, or goat hair, and then putting on goat fur socks or stockings as to prevent new or further harm due to the cold.[164] Ibn Sīnā recommends using paper (*kāghad*), hair, or fur as padding. His choice for preventive treatment at this stage is the use of warming and fragrant oils, such as oil of iris or Egyptian willow, or if these are not available then oil with pepper and pellitory, euphorbium, assafetida, or castoreum, in addition to dressings prepared with galbanum and garlic.[165] Ḥājjī Bāshā faithfully copies al-Majūsī's advice yet again on this issue.[166]

More serious afflictions of the limbs are separated into two cases. The first is if the affected limb started to decay without discolouration and the second is if the limb turned green or black.

In case of limbs that are not discoloured, only al-Majūsī provides an additional symptom, namely swelling of the limb.[167] Nevertheless, the treatment to follow is fairly similar in all four regimens. Putting the affected limb into warm water in which various things with dissolving qualities were boiled is one of the treatments. Al-Rāzī lists chaff or wheat, rapeseed, cabbage, dill, chamomile, raw wormwood (*shīkh khām*), melilot, flax seed, and fenugreek (*ḥulba*) to be used on their own or combined.[168] Al-Majūsī names chamomile, melilot, and dill as examples of warming and dissolving materials to boil in the water.[169] Ibn Sīnā mentions snow water or water in which fig, cabbage, basil, dill, chamomile, wormwood, pennyroyal (*fūdanaj*), or a kind of mint (*nammām*) was boiled.[170] Here, Ḥājjī Bāshā seems to combine al-Rāzī's and Ibn Sīnā's advice, leaving out

162 Al-Majūsī, *Kāmil al-ṣināʿa*, II/83; Ibn Sīnā, *al-Qānūn*, I/324.
163 Al-Rāzī, *al-Manṣūrī*, 289.
164 Al-Majūsī, *Kāmil al-ṣināʿa*, II/83.
165 Ibn Sīnā, *al-Qānūn*, I/324.
166 Ḥājjī Bāshā, *Shifāʾ al-aqsām*, 328.
167 Al-Majūsī, *Kāmil al-ṣināʿa*, II/83.
168 Al-Rāzī, *al-Manṣūrī*, 289.
169 Al-Majūsī, *Kāmil al-ṣināʿa*, II/83.
170 Ibn Sīnā, *al-Qānūn*, I/324.

the word *khām* and pennyroyal but adding marjoram (*marzanjūsh*) to the list.[171] In addition to putting the affected limb into such warm water, all authors agree that the traveller should also use warming oils and to go near a fire a few times to warm up somewhat, although al-Majūsī does not mention the latter instruction explicitly. Ibn Sīnā has some further recommendations, namely, to walk a bit to move and exercise the legs and limbs a bit, then massage them, anoint them, coat them, and also use warm compresses. He also notes that some people put the affected limb into cold water and find this useful as it drives the pain away and compares this treatment to the act of putting a frozen fruit into cold water, resulting in the extremities of the fruit turning level and smooth, while putting the frozen fruit near the fire would ruin it.[172]

In case the affected limb turns green or black, the authors also agree on the general treatment for the most part. It is to make a deep incision on the limb without delay and allow the blood to flow out of the incision freely. To do so, the physicians recommend putting the limb into warm water to prevent the blood from clotting and disrupting its own flow. Once the flow of the blood subsides, the limb is to be coated with Armenian bole on its own (Ḥājjī Bāshā), mixed with vinegar (Ibn Sīnā), water and vinegar (al-Rāzī), or rose water and vinegar (al-Majūsī). This coating is to be left on for a day and a night, then washed off and coated again until the treated part becomes firm, solid, and wrinkly and the tissue starts to regrow.[173] Ibn Sīnā recommends this treatment for when the limbs turn a dull colour.[174]

If putrefaction sets in, a more severe treatment is necessary. Instead of incisions, the putrid parts should be removed before the putrefaction spreads to the healthy tissue (al-Rāzī, Ibn Sīnā) or dressings are to be used that help these putrefied parts fall off (al-Rāzī, al-Majūsī, Ḥājjī Bāshā). The recommended dressings are a warm dressing made with boiled beet and cabbage mixed with hot butter (al-Rāzī)[175] and a warm dressing made with marshmallow, mallow, or gooseberry leaves pulverised and mixed with violet oil (al-Majūsī).[176] These dressings or bandages are to be changed multiple times a day for as long as all the discoloured tissue falls off, then medicaments that promote tissue growth can be used. If the putrefaction reached the bones, while some authors

171 Ḥājjī Bāshā, *Shifāʾ al-aqsām*, 328.
172 Ibn Sīnā, *al-Qānūn*, I/324.
173 Al-Rāzī, *al-Manṣūrī*, 289; al-Majūsī, *Kāmil al-ṣināʿa*, II/83; Ḥājjī Bāshā, *Shifāʾ al-aqsām*, 328–329.
174 Ibn Sīnā, *al-Qānūn*, I/325.
175 Al-Rāzī, *al-Manṣūrī*, 290.
176 Al-Majūsī, *Kāmil al-ṣināʿa*, II/83.

briefly write that the affected part needs to be removed, they agree that this treatment pertains to surgery.

1.2.8 Protecting the Eyes

Protection of the eyes from the harsh whiteness of the cold is mentioned briefly by al-Majūsī and Ḥājjī Bāshā.[177] Both recommend putting a black veil in front of the eyes and wearing black, dark blue, or green outer garments. It is only al-Majūsī who writes that the reason for this is that the above-mentioned colours collect the seeing light (*al-nūr al-bāṣir*) and prevent it from scattering.[178]

Ibn al-Khaṭīb dedicates a short but separate chapter to the protection and treatment of the eye. For protection, he also recommends black, blue, and green garments in general, and turbans and headcloths in particular. Additionally, he instructs the traveller to look at a [dark coloured] cloth carried in his hand. For ophthalmia (*ramad*) and swelling from the wind and dust Ibn al-Khaṭīb advises bending over steam of wheat chaff and venesection of the cephalic vein (*qīfāl*).[179]

Not surprisingly, the longest discussion of the topic is provided by al-Rāzī in two parts, the first on protecting the eye against the harsh whiteness of the snow, the second on relieving the pain of the eyes caused by the wind or cold.[180] Against the snow, al-Rāzī recommends wearing a black turban, headband, some eye covers, and carrying a black cloth in one's hands to look at them.[181] This latter advice might be Ibn al-Khaṭīb's source for the same recommendation in his own text; however, it is worded in a different manner, therefore Ibn al-Khaṭīb either rephrased the instruction, or added it from another source or based on his own experience. For the burning sensation and strong pains of the eye, the movement and roughness of the eyelids, and the possibly resulting ophthalmia, al-Rāzī advises to cover and protect the eyes, first and foremost. It is also beneficent to lean over the vapours of boiling wheat chaff, marjoram (*marzanjūsh*), camomile, or dill on their own or together, or leaning over the vapours of aged wine heated by throwing hot stones into it. In case of redness of the eye, al-Rāzī recommends venesection of the cephalic vein (*qīfāl*), followed by bathing the next day, eating, drinking strong wine, and sleeping for a long time. This recommendation strengthens the theory that Ibn al-Khaṭīb used al-Rāzī's passages regarding the eye but instead of simply copying, Ibn

177 Al-Majūsī, *Kāmil al-ṣināʿa*, II/83; Ḥājjī Bāshā, *Shifāʾ al-aqsām*, 328.
178 Al-Majūsī, *Kāmil al-ṣināʿa*, II/83.
179 Ibn al-Khaṭīb, *al-Wuṣūl*, 132.
180 Al-Rāzī, *al-Manṣūrī*, 290, 291.
181 Al-Rāzī, *al-Manṣūrī*, 290.

al-Khaṭīb paraphrased and significantly simplified his source material. Finally, al-Rāzī writes that applying a hot compress on the eyes afflicted by the cold is a grave mistake, but one might resort to this if the redness of the eyes does not subside after the treatment he recommended.[182]

1.2.9 Preserving the Complexion

One of the least frequently discussed topics is preserving the complexion and taking care of the facial skin of the traveller. Al-Rāzī and Ibn Sīnā have short and succinct recommendations for some frequent skincare-related issues of travellers,[183] obviously building on the tradition of cosmetics (*zīna*) contained in their encyclopaedias. The basic idea behind prevention is the same in case of both authors.

Al-Rāzī is concerned with paleness (*shuḥūb*) of the face due to the sun or wind, and quite simply states that seeking shade and covering oneself prevents this. If doing so is not possible, he recommends covering the face with a mixture of tragacanth, cornstarch, gum Arabic, dried mucilage of psyllium seeds, and mucilage of quince seeds admixed with egg white or purslane water and washing this mixture off once resting. Al-Rāzī notes that only one of these materials is useful, just like dry biscuits (*kaʿk*) dissolved in water or egg white with tragacanth alone. For treatment, he advises coating the face with cerate, that is a cream made of wax (*qīrūṭī*), chicken fat, and milk, then washing it off the next day with warm water and flour of chickpea (*ḥimmiṣ*). In case of more serious affliction, al-Rāzī directs the reader to his chapter on cosmetics.[184]

Ibn Sīnā focuses solely on prevention, advising the traveller to coat his face with sticky things, such as mucilage of psyllium seeds, mucilage of the arfaj plant (*ʿarfaj, Rhanterium epapposum*), tragacanth or gum Arabic dissolved in water, egg white, semolina biscuits (*al-kaʿk al-samīdh*) soaked in water, flat bread or pastry (*qurṣ*), and "the recipe of Crito". Ibn Sīnā refrains from mentioning even the simplest treatment and rather refers his reader to his chapter on cosmetics.[185]

1.2.10 The Different Waters

The issue of the different waters and their improvement is a fundamental topic of all travel regimens, as al-Majūsī is the only one who does not write about it.[186]

182 Al-Rāzī, *al-Manṣūrī*, 291.
183 Al-Rāzī, *al-Manṣūrī*, 296–297; Ibn Sīnā, *al-Qānūn*, 1/325.
184 Al-Rāzī, *al-Manṣūrī*, 296–297.
185 Ibn Sīnā, *al-Qānūn*, 1/325.
186 Al-Ṭabarī, *Firdaws al-ḥikma*, 110–111; al-Rāzī, *al-Manṣūrī*, 293–295; Ibn Sīnā, *al-Qānūn*,

The discussion of this topic in the Arabic-Islamic medical tradition relies on the Hippocratic treatise *Airs, waters, and places* heavily. This text entered the Arabic medical literature through the translation of Galen's commentary of it made by Ḥunayn ibn Isḥāq's (d. 260/873) circle.[187] One aspect of how the ideas in it pertaining to waters developed in the Arabic medical tradition is present in the section of travel regimens concerned with the different waters.

The importance of the issue of different waters is underlined by the statement of Ibn Sīnā and Ibn al-Khaṭīb that the difference of waters causes more diseases than the difference of foodstuffs.[188] The rest of the authors start with their advice straightaway.

The chapters or subsections of travel regimens on the issue of waters generally consist of two types of advice: general and specific according to exact types of waters. One of the more general points which al-Rāzī, Ibn Sīnā, Ibn al-Quff, and Ibn al-Khaṭīb all make is that bringing water and clay from one's home and mixing either of them into the water found at the first resting place of the journey is good practice. Then, some from this water can be mixed again into water from the following resting place and so on until the traveller reaches his destination. While waters are simply to be mixed, if clay is thrown into the water, the authors do not fail mentioning that it should be left to settle and meanwhile it purifies the water.[189] Ibn al-Quff and Ibn al-Khaṭīb also mention taking food from one's home. Al-Rāzī and Ḥājjī Bāshā generally recommend mixing wine or vinegar into the waters one comes across but Ibn Sīnā is more specific, stating that wine is useful if the corruption of the water is not strong, and vinegar is useful in the summer when water is scarce.[190] Ibn al-Khaṭīb also advises mixing pure vinegar into the water during the summer but using oxymel during the winter, without offering any explanation like that of Ibn Sīnā.[191] Another generally useful regimen according to Ibn Sīnā is to mix sour robs into any kind of water.[192] The other general advice on how to repel the harms of the different waters is connected to foodstuffs. All authors praise the qualities of onion in this regard, especially with vinegar. Ibn Sīnā goes even further and writes

---

1/325–326; Ibn al-Quff, *Jāmiʿ al-gharaḍ*, 168; Ibn al-Khaṭīb, *al-Wuṣūl*, 131; Ḥājjī Bāshā, *Shifāʾ al-aqsām*, 329.

187 See for example Strohmaier, *Galen the pagan*, Strohmaier, *Galen's not uncritical commentary*, Jouanna, *Water, health and disease*.

188 Ibn Sīnā, *al-Qānūn*, 1/325; Ibn al-Khaṭīb, *al-Wuṣūl*, 131.

189 Al-Rāzī, *al-Manṣūrī*, 293; Ibn Sīnā, *al-Qānūn*, 1/326; Ibn al-Quff, *Jāmiʿ al-gharaḍ*, 168; Ibn al-Khaṭīb, *al-Wuṣūl*, 131.

190 Al-Rāzī, *al-Manṣūrī*, 293; Ibn Sīnā, *al-Qānūn*, 1/325; Ḥājjī Bāshā, *Shifāʾ al-aqsām*, 329.

191 Ibn al-Khaṭīb, *al-Wuṣūl*, 131.

192 Ibn Sīnā, *al-Qānūn*, 1/326.

that onion is like theriac against the harms of the different waters.[193] Besides onion and vinegar, al-Rāzī and Ibn Sīnā recommend garlic and lettuce,[194] Ibn al-Quff mentions garlic and aged wine,[195] Ibn al-Khaṭīb mentions only onion and vinegar,[196] and Ḥājjī Bāshā recommends onion, garlic, and vinegar.[197]

Before moving on to how to make specific waters potable, Ibn Sīnā discusses in some length what he means by carefully dealing with the different waters: abundant purification (*tarwīq*), abundant filtering (*istirshāḥ*) from earthenware vessels, and boiling, as these methods purify the water and separate the pure water from the contaminants. Ibn Sīnā deems distillation (*taqṭīr*) by vaporisation (*taṣʿīd*) to be the best of these methods. The next method is putting one end of a twisted wool cord into a vessel which is full to the brim and putting the other end of the cord into an empty vessel, waiting for it to dribble the pure water into the empty vessel. Ibn Sīnā praises this method as well, especially if done repeatedly. For boiling, he recommends putting warm clay and wool balls into the boiling water and then taking those out and squeezing them, as they collect pure water. Lastly, Ibn Sīnā mentions using warm, preferably sundried clay to be put in the water generally as it breaks the water's corruption.[198] Although other authors advise to purify, filter, and boil various waters, they do not compare these methods or describe them in more detail, like Ibn Sīnā does.

There are 12 different types of waters mentioned by the authors with some further variation in case of certain types. The following part of this subchapter presents these types and the recommendations of the physicians on how to make these safe for consumption. Ḥājjī Bāshā does not write about any kind of water, but generally recommends using things with opposing qualities than those of the waters, following the principle *contraria contrariis curentur*.

Salty (*māliḥ*) water is discussed by al-Ṭabarī, al-Rāzī, Ibn Sīnā, Ibn al-Quff, and Ibn al-Khaṭīb.[199] All of these authors recommend putting carob, myrtle seeds, or azerole (*zuʿrūr*) into salty water, although Ibn al-Quff advises to eat azerole after drinking salty water instead of throwing it into the water like carob or myrtle seeds. Al-Ṭabarī recommends azerole to be thrown into the water and also eaten after drinking salty water, in addition to drinking wine before and

193 Ibn Sīnā, *al-Qānūn*, 1/326.
194 Al-Rāzī, *al-Manṣūrī*, 293; Ibn Sīnā, *al-Qānūn*, 1/326.
195 Ibn al-Quff, *Jāmiʿ al-gharaḍ*, 168.
196 Ibn al-Khaṭīb, *al-Wuṣūl*, 131.
197 Ḥājjī Bāshā, *Shifāʾ al-aqsām*, 329.
198 Ibn Sīnā, *al-Qānūn*, 1/325.
199 Al-Ṭabarī, *Firdaws al-ḥikma*, 110; al-Rāzī, *al-Manṣūrī*, 293; Ibn Sīnā, *al-Qānūn*, 1/325; Ibn al-Quff, *Jāmiʿ al-gharaḍ*, 168; Ibn al-Khaṭīb, *al-Wuṣūl*, 131.

after and eating quince after drinking salty water. He also advises to put clay (*ṭīn khūzī*, clay from the Khuzestan region) or stalk (without specifying which plant's stalk) into salty water. Al-Rāzī, however, recommends eating quince before drinking salty water. He also recommends putting clay into the water, but he mentions warm clay in general. Ibn al-Khaṭīb, too, mentions eating quince in general. Mixing vinegar or oxymel into salty water appears first in al-Rāzī's guide, and later it is also found amongst the advice of Ibn Sīnā, Ibn al-Quff and Ibn al-Khaṭīb. Another interesting method is that offered by Ibn al-Quff, namely putting a pericarp into the water, since it will fill with sweet water only.

Muddy and thick (*kadir*, *ghalīẓ*) water is mentioned by the same authors, namely al-Ṭabarī, al-Rāzī, Ibn Sīnā, Ibn al-Quff (only muddy), and Ibn al-Khaṭīb.[200] The methods they recommend show more variety than in the case of salty water. Al-Tabarī simply and solely recommends eating garlic. However, he shares two of his personal experiences: he asked people from Egypt how they make the muddy water of the Nile safe to consume and they throw pulverised kernel of peach (*khawkh*) and apricot (*mishmish*) into the water. He also saw bleachers (*qaṣṣārīn*) purify muddy water by adding alum into a bowl and pouring water onto it, and once it dissolved, they poured that into a water pit or container, and they moved the dissolved mixture around in it to purify the place and make it appropriate for washing. Similarly to al-Ṭabarī, Ibn Sīnā also recommends eating garlic after drinking muddy water but also mentions that Yemeni alum purifies it. The latter advice appears in al-Rāzī's guide (Yemeni alum filters and purifies muddy water fast), making it a possible source for this addition. However, this is only a last measure for al-Rāzī, as he recommends pouring muddy water from vessel to vessel and he advises other methods only if this is too difficult. One of these is using Yemeni alum, and the other is filtering the water through a cloth stained with moist biscuits (*kaʿk*). Ibn al-Quff recommend various methods of purification, namely shaking the water, boiling it, or filtering it. Ibn al-Khaṭīb adds to these methods evaporation and filtering it from a vessel into another via a wool cord.

Bitter (*murr*) water is discussed briefly by al-Ṭabarī, al-Rāzī, Ibn Sīnā, Ibn al-Quff, and Ibn al-Khaṭīb.[201] The general recommendation is to mix something sweet into bitter water or eat sweet things; al-Ṭabarī and Ibn al-Quff say nothing more. Al-Rāzī's advice is the same, although he names rose water (*julāb*) and sugar as examples. Ibn Sīnā recommends drinking water of chickpea and sim-

200 Al-Ṭabarī, *Firdaws al-ḥikma*, 110–111; al-Rāzī, *al-Manṣūrī*, 293; Ibn Sīnā, *al-Qānūn*, 1/326; Ibn al-Quff, *Jāmiʿ al-gharaḍ*, 168; Ibn al-Khaṭīb, *al-Wuṣūl*, 131.

201 Al-Ṭabarī, *Firdaws al-ḥikma*, 111; al-Rāzī, *al-Manṣūrī*, 294; Ibn Sīnā, *al-Qānūn*, 1/326; Ibn al-Quff, *Jāmiʿ al-gharaḍ*, 168; Ibn al-Khaṭīb, *al-Wuṣūl*, 131.

ilar things before drinking bitter water as well as eating chickpeas, in addition to the previous advice. Ibn al-Khaṭīb does not mention any of these, however, he recommends consuming quince and similar things.

Stagnant (*qāʾim*) water is mentioned by al-Rāzī, Ibn Sīnā (also swampy, *ājamī*), Ibn al-Quff (also sour, *ḥāmiḍ*), and Ibn al-Khatib (also putrid, *ʿufūna*).[202] The general advice of all these physicians is to mix into such waters robs of sour and costive fruits or to simply eat such fruits. The examples they provide are sour grapes, pomegranate, apple, quince, ribes, and azerole. Al-Rāzī and Ibn Sīnā also advise against warm foodstuffs.

Al-Ṭabarī, al-Rāzī, Ibn Sīnā, and Ibn al-Khaṭīb include waters in which there are leech, or in the case of al-Rāzī, leech, vermin, weeds, and grass.[203] With the exception of al-Ṭabarī, they all recommend drinking such water through some kind of a filter as to not swallow leeches or other vermin by accident. In the opinion of Ibn Sīnā, this also helps prevent nausea due to the bad humours of such waters. Al-Rāzī adds eating fatty foods and purifying the water as additional advice for travellers who must consume such waters. Ibn al-Khaṭīb mentions eating fatty foods and fat if one drank leech or vermin by accident. Al-Ṭabarī also has advice on what to do if one swallowed leech by accident: drink sour vinegar, salt, wormwood (*shīkh*), or garlic. It is also al-Ṭabarī who presents a more elaborate method to make poisoned water or water full of deadly vermin safe to consume. It is to throw little fir spurge (*shubrum*) into it, burn the surrounding trees and the vermin dwelling in them, and smoke the place with galbanum or antler of red deer, since those make vermin flee. His other advice is to put speedwell (*ḥabaq al-māʾ*), wild thyme (*ṣaʿtar*), or wormwood (*shīkh*) into the wine one consumes.

Alumic and acrid (*shabbī*) water is included in the list of various waters by Ibn Sīnā (also acrid, *ʿafiṣ*) and Ibn al-Quff.[204] Ibn Sīnā advises one to drink after it something that soothes the disposition, such as wine, while Ibn al-Quff recommends eating anything one desires after drinking alumic water. The latter also writes to put *sukk*, a kind of perfume,[205] into alumic water.

Al-Rāzī and Ibn al-Khaṭīb mention waters that urge one to pee shortly after consumption or in an otherwise uncomfortable manner.[206] In this case, al-Rāzī

---

202 Al-Rāzī, *al-Manṣūrī*, 294; Ibn Sīnā, *al-Qānūn*, 1/326; Ibn al-Quff, *Jāmiʿ al-gharaḍ*, 168; Ibn al-Khaṭīb, *al-Wuṣūl*, 131.

203 Al-Ṭabarī, *Firdaws al-ḥikma*, 111; al-Rāzī, *al-Manṣūrī*, 294; Ibn Sīnā, *al-Qānūn*, 1/326; Ibn al-Khaṭīb, *al-Wuṣūl*, 131.

204 Ibn Sīnā, *al-Qānūn*, 1/326; Ibn al-Quff, *Jāmiʿ al-gharaḍ*, 168.

205 See al-Ṭabarī, *Health regimen*, 160–161 n. 138.

206 Al-Rāzī, *al-Manṣūrī*, 294–295; Ibn al-Khaṭīb, *al-Wuṣūl*, 131.

recommends drinking wine with the water or consuming it with boiled celery seeds and fennel. Ibn al-Khaṭīb recommends eating butter and sugar besides boiled celery and fennel.

The same authors, al-Rāzī and Ibn al-Khaṭīb include unpotable (*zuʿāq*) water.[207] Al-Rāzī advises the traveller who is forced to drink such water to purify it with the following method: put the water into a clean earthenware pot, cover it with twigs, throw a piece of clean, fluffy wool on top of it, then put the pot onto kindled embers, and once the wool is moist, squeeze the water out of it and drink only that. Ibn al-Khaṭīb, perhaps reflecting on this somewhat complicated procedure, writes that simple evaporation and oxymel is enough to make unpotable waters potable.

Al-Ṭabarī mentions two kinds of waters only found in his guide, namely dirty (*qadhir*) and stinking (*muntin*) waters.[208] For the first one, he advises throwing azerole and thyme (*ṣaʿtar*) into the water, and for the second one, he recommends boiling it, then throwing into it lupine (*būmūs*, n. 1 *turmus*), celery root, mountain fennel, or rue.

Al-Rāzī also has unique mentions, namely waters that either loosen the stomach or cause nausea.[209] For the first one, he recommends eating foodstuffs that agree with the stomach, and for the second one, he recommends drinking it with rob of pomegranate.

1.2.11 Hunger and Nutrition

Al-Rāzī, Ibn Sīnā, Ibn al-Quff, Ibn al-Khaṭīb, and Ḥājjī Bāshā all discuss hunger in varying detail and provide instructions regarding nutrition and eating during a journey in general.[210] The discussions are heavily focused on the proper diet to follow on a journey in general besides additional related, nevertheless general advice. Al-Rāzī dedicates a separate short subchapter to hungry fainting.[211] In addition, Ḥājjī Bāshā's section on this matter clearly seems to be a copy of Ibn Sīnā's text, consequently the name of the former is not mentioned every time the latter's is.

All four authors recommend eating foodstuffs with high nutritional value paired with small quantities. Ibn Sīnā explains briefly that this serves to make the digestion of the traveller good and prevents excess materials building up in

---

207 Al-Rāzī, *al-Manṣūrī*, 294; Ibn al-Khaṭīb, *al-Wuṣūl*, 131.

208 Al-Ṭabarī, *Firdaws al-ḥikma*, 110–111.

209 Al-Rāzī, *al-Manṣūrī*, 294, 295.

210 Al-Rāzī, *al-Manṣūrī*, 292–293; Ibn Sīnā, *al-Qānūn*, 1/321; Ibn al-Khaṭīb, *al-Wuṣūl*, 130; Ḥājjī Bāshā, *Shifāʾ al-aqsām*, 324.

211 Al-Rāzī, *al-Manṣūrī*, 288.

the veins. Ibn al-Quff offers examples for the best of such foodstuffs: roasted livers and good birds, from which he deems liver of sheep, liver of two-year-old goats, chicken, and francolin the best besides ground meat.

Apart from al-Rāzī, the physicians advise to not travel on a full or empty stomach. Ibn Sīnā and Ibn al-Quff give some explanations. Riding on a full stomach spoils the food and the digestion and leads to drinking more water while there is still much undigested food in the stomach, which can possibly cause vomiting. Ibn al-Quff notes that for a certain body figure, travelling on a full stomach is permittable. He also writes that if one travels on an empty stomach it can lead to excess heat dissolving in the body. All five physicians who write about nutrition agree that therefore the traveller should eat only when he is resting. If it is not possible for him to wait for this occasion, al-Rāzī and Ibn Sīnā recommend eating only a little instead of a full meal.

Except for Ibn al-Quff, the physicians advise to avoid herbs and fruits that generate moist humours in general and only consume them if they are needed to counter the effects of hot weather or treat an affliction. Ibn al-Khaṭīb lists some additional foodstuffs to avoid, namely anything that makes one thirsty, that is all the salty or sweet foodstuffs. Al-Rāzī generally advises not eating food that is not from one's own country.

Ibn Sīnā has a general list of foodstuffs useful against hunger: anything prepared from roasted livers, kebab made with grease, fat, almonds, or almond oil. In his opinion, eating one piece from such a kebab wards off hunger for a long time. He records a more radical method as well: 'it is said' (*qīla*) that if a person drinks a *raṭl* (approximately 450 grams) of violet oil mixed with wax so it becomes like a cerate (*qīrūṭī*), that person will not feel hunger for ten days.[212] While Ḥājjī Bāshā compiled his own text most likely from Ibn Sīnā's chapter, he omitted repeating this part.

1.2.12 Fatigue

While the longest discussion of fatigue is provided by al-Rāzī, al-Majūsī, Ibn al-Quff, Ibn al-Khaṭīb, and Ḥājjī Bāshā all offer advice on how to treat fatigue,[213] and Ibn Sīnā refers his reader to a separate chapter on fatigue.[214]

Al-Rāzī advises those afflicted by severe fatigue (*iʿyāʾ*, *taʿab*) in the following way. They are to rest for a while when they stop the journey and then go to the bath if possible. If the traveller cannot find a bath, then he is to bathe in warm

212 Ibn Sīnā, *al-Qānūn*, I/321.

213 Al-Rāzī, *al-Manṣūrī*, 292; al-Majūsī, *Kāmil al-ṣināʿa*, II/81; Ibn al-Quff, *Jāmiʿ al-gharaḍ*, 169; Ibn al-Khaṭīb, *al-Wuṣūl*, 132; Ḥājjī Bāshā, *Shifāʾ al-aqsām*, 325.

214 Ibn Sīnā, *al-Qānūn*, I/321.

water so that it relaxes and reddens his skin. This is to be followed by a gentle massage, especially around the joints. Then the traveller is to anoint his body, again with special care regarding the joints, with oils in which dill and chamomile were boiled if it is wintertime and with violet oil in summertime. Then the traveller is to rest and sleep for a long time in warmth and under blankets. Once he wakes up, he is to repeat massaging, bathing, and anointing himself and only then return to his usual regimen.[215]

In comparison to these instructions, al-Majūsī uses only the word *iʿyāʾ* for fatigue and *ghamz* for massage instead of *dalak*. He recommends massage and anointing only, the latter with fine and warm violet oil with a focus on the legs and back as to moisten these organs that were overtaken by dryness. He then instructs the traveller to follow the regimen of those affected by fatigue (here using both *iʿyāʾ* and *taʿab*).[216]

Ibn al-Khaṭīb offers a quite faithful version of al-Rāzī's advice, and while he omits the details about the joints, he uses both *dalak* and *ghamz* when mentioning massaging the body.[217] Meanwhile, Ḥājjī Bāshā relied on al-Majūsī, although he amended the list of oils with oil of chamomile and lily and omitted the importance of anointing the legs and back.[218] Ibn al-Quff uses the word *taʿab* for fatigue and he is the one who deviates most from the general advice outlined above: he recommends resting, relaxing the thighs, and anointing the thighs with oil of violet, pumpkin, or snake (*ḥayya*) to moisten them, besides putting the traveller on guard regarding anything that might befall the thighs due to fatigue.[219]

1.2.13 Regimen for Sea Travel

All encyclopaedic travel regimens include a regimen for seafarers, except for al-Ṭabarī's text.[220] Besides some words on preparation, these regimens mostly focus on preventing nausea (*ghathayān*) and vomiting (*qayʾ*) and the regimen to follow if these preventive methods fail. In addition to these, al-Majūsī includes a small section on lice, often troubling those travelling on ships. The most unique feature of these regimens is found in Ibn al-Khaṭīb's guide who discusses in length his explanation of dizziness (*mayd*).

215 Al-Rāzī, *al-Manṣūrī*, 292.
216 Al-Majūsī, *Kāmil al-ṣināʿa*, II/81.
217 Ibn al-Khaṭīb, *al-Wuṣūl*, 132.
218 Ḥājjī Bāshā, *Shifāʾ al-aqsām*, 325.
219 Ibn al-Quff, *Jāmiʿ al-gharaḍ*, 169.
220 Al-Rāzī, *al-Manṣūrī*, 295–296; al-Majūsī, *Kāmil al-ṣināʿa*, II/83–84; Ibn Sīnā, *al-Qānūn*, I/326; Ibn al-Quff, *Jāmiʿ al-gharaḍ*, 172; Ibn al-Khaṭīb, *al-Wuṣūl*, 132–133; Ḥājjī Bāshā, *Shifāʾ al-aqsām*, 329.

Al-Rāzī's instructions on how to prepare for travelling on sea are to eat less in the days prior to embarking, eat foodstuffs that strengthen the cardia, and once embarking, avoid looking at the water. Additionally, he recommends bringing some provisions of robs and medicine the traveller is accustomed to.[221] Ibn al-Quff advises purging the body before embarking with the purgatives one is used to, as this helps preventing nausea, repeated vomiting, and mixing of the healthy humours with the putrid ones.[222]

The physicians recommend some further ways to prevent nausea and vomiting once on board. These are to sniff pleasant-smelling things and 'take thing after thing from those [things] that soothe nausea', according to al-Rāzī.[223] Al-Majūsī is more specific, recommending drinks made of sour grapes, minted pomegranate, apple, tamarind, sucking on sour pomegranate and sour quince or sniffing these.[224] Ibn Sīnā mentions various additional methods. For eating, he recommends quince, apple, pomegranate, foodstuffs prepared with costive things strengthening the cardia, foodstuffs that prevent vapours from rising to the head, such as lentils (*ʿadas*) with vinegar, sour grapes, pennyroyal (*fūdanaj*), and thyme (*ḥāshā*), or bread cooled or sopped in odorous wine or thymed cold water. As for drinks, Ibn Sīnā mentions drinks with seeds of celery or wormwood (*afsatīn*, probably a typo of *afsantīn*), as both prevent and calm nausea. Additionally, he advises to cover the inside of the nose (*anfus*, likely a typo for *unf*) with white lead. Ḥājjī Bāshā faithfully copies Ibn Sīnā's recommendations of eating the lentil-based meal and sopped bread, all the drinks, and covering the inside of the nostrils.[225] The rest of Ḥājjī Bāshā's regimen relies on the texts of al-Rāzī and al-Majūsī. Ibn al-Quff advises consuming robs that strengthen the cardia and prevent nausea once the traveller embarks the ship, such as rob of sour grapes and pomegranate or rob of ribes and barberry (*barbārīs*), besides a drink prepared from tamarind. He recommends sucking on quince and sour pomegranate, sniffing myrtle and rose, and eating costive foodstuffs but a smaller amount in general than usual.[226]

If these methods fail and the traveller becomes nauseous or vomits, Ibn Sīnā notes that this subsides after the first few days, recommending fighting

221 Al-Rāzī, *al-Manṣūrī*, 295–296.

222 Ibn al-Quff, *Jāmiʿ al-gharaḍ*, 172.

223 Al-Rāzī, *al-Manṣūrī*, 296.

224 Al-Majūsī, *Kāmil al-ṣināʿa*, II/83.

225 Ibn Sīnā, *al-Qānūn*, I/326; Ḥājjī Bāshā, *Shifāʾ al-aqsām*, 329. The edition of the *Qānūn* has cooled bread while the *Shifāʾ* has sopped bread. The *Shifāʾ* has nostrils (*minkhar*) instead of the *Qānūn*'s nose (*anfus*, likely for *unf*).

226 Ibn al-Quff, *Jāmiʿ al-gharaḍ*, 172.

nausea and vomiting as long as possible but vomit without restraint if it happens.[227] Al-Rāzī states that vomiting multiple times is not harmful. If it occurs frequently, his advice is to consume robs, sumac (*summāq*), and pomegranate seeds. If vomiting is excessive, he instructs to follow the treatment of summer cholera.[228] Al-Majūsī recommends sniffing sandalwood, rose water, or warm clay moistened with vinegar and vine, and eating costive meals such as cooked meat steeped in vinegar (*maṣūṣ*), jelly (*hulām*), foodstuffs prepared with sorrel (*ḥummāḍ*), sumac, and chickpeas, besides applying the preventive methods and avoiding looking at the water.[229] Ibn al-Quff even recommends drinking warm water if necessary in order to truly empty one's stomach once vomiting. Curiously, his advice is to strengthen the thighs and upper arms, anointing the feed and head excessively, bandaging these with vinegar, sandalwood, and rose water, consuming the generally recommended drinks with celery seeds, and bandaging the cardia with water of myrtle, vinegar, and sandalwood. Moreover, he advises following this regimen as long as the traveller is on the sea, not just for the time he is afflicted by severe vomiting.[230] These instructions are not found in the other regimens.

It is only Ibn al-Quff who writes on what to do after arriving at one's destination. He recommends resting, going to the bath, restoring one's original diet, and strengthening the brain [likely with an appropriate diet] until the mind returns to his pre-travel ways.[231]

Al-Majūsī states that lice often afflict the seafaring traveller due to perspiration, dirt, and scarceness of bathing. He advises to coat the body with a mixture of lily, long aristolochia, smearwort, lice-bane (*maywīzaj*), and oleander (*diflā*). Then the afflicted person is to go to the bath the following day, cleaning his body well, washing his head with marshmallow, beet, and borax, and then dressing in clean and fine cotton garments.[232] The rest of the authors do not write about this issue at all.

As for Ibn al-Khaṭīb, he admittedly summarises the opinion of the rest of the physicians (*qāla al-aṭibbā'*, 'the physicians said'), which is to withhold vomiting but let it occur once it happens, except if it is excessive, eating costive foodstuffs that strengthen the cardia (quince, apple, and pomegranate), drink seeds of celery and wormwood, consume foods that prevent vapours rising to the

227 Ibn Sīnā, *al-Qānūn*, 1/326.
228 Al-Rāzī, *al-Manṣūrī*, 296.
229 Al-Majūsī, *Kāmil al-ṣināʿa*, 11/83.
230 Ibn al-Quff, *Jāmiʿ al-gharaḍ*, 172.
231 Ibn al-Quff, *Jāmiʿ al-gharaḍ*, 172.
232 Al-Majūsī, *Kāmil al-ṣināʿa*, 11/83–84.

brain (lentils with vinegar, sour grapes, pennyroyal, and thyme), and coating the inside of the nostrils with white lead. However, this summary seems to rely on Ibn Sīnā's regimen for the most part. Following this section, Ibn al-Khaṭīb moves on to his lengthy explanation of dizziness. Here, he compares the stomach of someone riding a ship to a butter churning skin, noting the effect of certain humoural qualities on the process, that there is a difference between people according to the strength of their cardias and brains, and that due to factors and considerations, certain people are more or less susceptible to dizziness.[233] This explanation is also unique and therefore has no parallels in any of the other regimens discussed here.

1.2.14 Regimen for Armies

Regimens for armies are included by al-Ṭabarī and al-Rāzī only, although some of the elements of these can be found in Ibn al-Khaṭīb's regimen as well.[234] In addition to these is Ibn Sīnā's shorter essay on the regimen of armies.[235]

Al-Ṭabarī advises armies according to the season or weather. In wintertime, he instructs to rest close to one another and to the riding animals to utilise the warmth of the breath, sleep in excavated burrows previously warmed up by a fire, putting heating stones around the tents, and drinking honey beverage. This is where al-Ṭabarī shares his experience regarding the people of the mountainous regions of Tabaristan. The second group of advice from al-Ṭabarī pertains to the summertime regimen of armies. He advises setting camp on separate hills, covering the tents with cold trees or shrubs, and consuming *sawīq* mixed with cold water. If the air is thick and foggy, al-Ṭabarī recommends drinking pure wine, eating spicy foods, and consuming more garlic, while on malodorous flatlands fragrant oils are useful. After these, al-Ṭabarī moves on to the issue of the different waters.[236] At a later point in the discussion of water, al-Ṭabarī includes one last section which, although useful for simple travellers, is aimed at armies: he recommends sprinkling the tents of the army with water in which Armenian cucumber (*qiththā* [*sic*] *al-ḥimār*) was boiled, as it repels vermin.[237] Ultimately, al-Ṭabarī's instructions for armies focus on the proper place and way

---

233 Ibn al-Khaṭīb, *al-Wuṣūl*, 132–133.

234 Al-Ṭabarī, *Firdaws al-ḥikma*, 110, 111; al-Rāzī, *al-Manṣūrī*, 295; Ibn al-Khaṭīb, *al-Wuṣūl*, 132. The regimen of al-Rāzī was translated by Frölich. This translation is quoted in Garrison, *Notes on the history of military medicine*, 82. Unfortunately, I was not able to find the articles quoted by Garrison (n. 18 and n. 19) in Langenbeck's Archives of Surgery.

235 Shams al-Dīn, *al-Madhhab al-tarbawī*, 280.

236 Al-Ṭabarī, *Firdaws al-ḥikma*, 110.

237 Al-Ṭabarī, *Firdaws al-ḥikma*, 111.

to set up the camp and sleeping places, in addition to a warming or cooling drink to consume.

Similarly, al-Rāzī starts with instructions on setting up camp in summertime and wintertime. In summertime, he marks out hills, just like al-Ṭabarī, but includes some further instructions: the tents should face the northern winds, they should be set up with some distance between them, and if possible, the riding animals should also be kept away from the tents. In wintertime, he designates depressions sheltered by hills, thickets, or mountains, with the tents facing south or east and set up close to one another, just like the riding animals. Al-Rāzī gives instructions for when sultry, moist, southern airs (eating less, avoiding wine, increasing exercise) or coarse and dry airs (the opposite) are present around the camp. An interesting point he adds is when a lot of souls fall ill in the camp, they should move away from the camp to a place above the winds, not under them. In case of vermin present at the campsite, al-Rāzī refers the reader to his separate chapter on repellents, advising to use the proper repellent for various vermin discussed there. He also notes that bad weeds and trees diffuse pungent or harmful airs, therefore they are to be burned or the camp is to be set up above the wind. His last advice is to examine the foodstuffs and the reason behind illnesses affecting a large portion of the army to oppose and avoid those if necessary.[238]

Ibn al-Khaṭīb includes a chapter in his regimen on choosing the campsite without mentioning the army, writing about the direction houses are to face instead of tents. Nevertheless, his advice is mostly in accordance with al-Rāzī's advice regarding campsite locations and directions of the dwellings, even if it is worded in a different way.[239]

The essay of Ibn Sīnā on the regimen of the military camps is included in the list of the medical works of Ibn Sīnā prepared by Gutas. This list is, however, not separated further into "authentic and pseudepigraphic" works,[240] nor does the editor of Ibn Sīnā's essay supply any information or inquiry regarding this issue.[241] This is especially problematic considering the fact that this essay attributed to Ibn Sīnā follows al-Rāzī's guide for armies almost verbatim. There are only a few differences between them; most or perhaps even all of them are either typos or mistakes due to the typical ways of the corruption of the text in manuscripts. The editor of Ibn Sīnā's essay used two of the three surviving (and known) manuscript copies, and only one of those had Ibn Sīnā's

238 Al-Rāzī, *al-Manṣūrī*, 295.

239 Ibn al-Khaṭīb, *al-Wuṣūl*, 132.

240 Gutas, *Avicenna*, 512.

241 Shams al-Dīn, *al-Madhhab al-tarbawī*, 55.

name in the colophon.[242] Therefore, one must wonder whether a scrutiny of all surviving manuscripts of this essay could prove that this essay is pseudepigraphic, as it would be unlikely that Ibn Sīnā himself copied al-Rāzī so faithfully and decided to circulate the text as his own.

1.2.15 Unique Topics

The more miscellaneous and unique topics are bruising of the skin and injuries due to falling off the mount,[243] preventing splitting of the skin of the feet,[244] lice,[245] and abrasion and wounds caused by riding or the shoes one is wearing.[246] In a way, many parts of Qusṭā ibn Lūqā's regimen for pilgrims can also be considered as unique, since the rest of the regimens do not discuss a lot Qusṭā ibn Lūqā's material (such as his chapters on earache, diseases caused by the changes of weather, and the *dracunculus medinensis*).[247] Ibn Sīnā's chapter on various sings indicating specific diseases also belongs in this category. As Qusṭā ibn Lūqā's regimen is meticulously commented by Bos,[248] in this part I focus on the first four topics mentioned here.

In the opinion of al-Rāzī, if one falls or gets knocked by a riding animal or something else, it is best to perform bloodletting at once on the opposing side, avoid consuming meat and wine, coat the afflicted part of the body, and bandage it with strengthening bandages. If the traveller falls on his head, it is best to perform venesection of his cephalic vein (*qīfāl*), coat his head with a mixture of wine vinegar, rose oil, and three times as much rose water, also drinking from this, giving him barley water to drink, and restricting him for three days until the warm swelling on the outer parts of his brain are dealt with. If the traveller's mind is not confused, then those parts are healthy. If his mind is confused, the treatment requires more bloodletting, pouring more rose oil, rose water, and wine vinegar on his head, and bandaging it with the following preparation: myrtle leaves, flower of pomegranate, and peel of pomegranate are boiled in water and vinegar until these are cooked thoroughly, then this is mixed with some *sukk* (a kind of perfume),[249] aloeswood, calamus (*qaṣab al-dharīra*), vinegar, water, and aged costive wine, all beaten together. Fruit juices and gentle

242 Shams al-Dīn, *al-Madhhab al-tarbawī*, 280, n. 5.
243 Al-Rāzī, *al-Manṣūrī*, 298–300.
244 Al-Rāzī, *al-Manṣūrī*, 297–298.
245 Al-Rāzī, *al-Manṣūrī*, 296; Ibn al-Jazzār, *Ibn al-Jazzār's Zād al-musāfir I–II* (book I chapter 9).
246 Al-Rāzī, *al-Manṣūrī*, 298; Ibn al-Jazzār, *Ibn al-Jazzār's Zād al-musāfir*, 69, 132.
247 Qusṭā ibn Lūqā, *Qusṭā ibn Lūqā's medical regime*, 40–47, 46–53, 72–83.
248 Qusṭā ibn Lūqā, *Qusṭā ibn Lūqā's medical regime*, 85–157.
249 See al-Ṭabarī, *Health regimen*, 160–161 n. 138.

massage to relax the constitution are also recommended, besides some foodstuffs and drinks.[250] Then, al-Rāzī discusses in similar detail the treatment of a fall to the chest or nearby parts of the body, as well as treatment of a severe fall or hit in general.[251] At the end of this chapter, al-Rāzī gives recipes for various remedies against a severe fall and coughing blood, severe fall and bruising, falling followed by fever and a warm swelling, falling or a blow resulting in severe blood loss, and a treatment for minor bruising and weakness.[252] This is the only occasion in this corpus that a regimen contains more recipes instead of the occasional ones scattered in between the texts.

The chapter on how to prevent or treat splitting of the skin of the heel or the feet by al-Rāzī is similar to the skincare sections, therefore footcare might be a proper designation for it. Putting the feet in hot water to loosen them, then sprinkling them with finely pulverised tragacanth followed by a good massage is useful in general against splitting of the skin according to al-Rāzī, while coating the heels with moist pitch or putting a cloth soaked in oil under the feet before putting on shoes are good for preventing such afflictions.[253] Besides this treatment and preventive method, al-Rāzī provides additional ones, some containing additional recipes on how to properly mix certain remedies.[254]

Getting rid of lice is discussed by al-Rāzī and Ibn al-Jazzār, besides al-Majūsī who writes about lice commonly afflicting those travelling on ships. According to al-Rāzī, lice are generated due to the change of waters, lots of fatigue, perspiration, dirt, scarcity of bathing, and scarcity of changing garments, all of which necessarily afflict the traveller.[255] After this statement, al-Rāzī moves on to prevention and treatment. In comparison, Ibn al-Jazzār is of the opinion that "this happens because of a bad and putrid humor which nature expels from the skin and the flesh".[256] While Ibn al-Jazzār does not provide preventive measures, he separates treatment for those who have a cold temperament and those who have a warm temperament as well as for those cases where lice appeared due to dirt. Al-Rāzī recommends taking care about bathing and cleaning oneself whenever it is possible and changing the clothes, wearing cotton if possible.[257] With the exception of the changing of the waters and fatigue, these are all the reasons leading to the generation of lice according to

250 Al-Rāzī, *al-Manṣūrī*, 298–299.
251 Al-Rāzī, *al-Manṣūrī*, 299–300.
252 Al-Rāzī, *al-Manṣūrī*, 300.
253 Al-Rāzī, *al-Manṣūrī*, 298.
254 Al-Rāzī, *al-Manṣūrī*, 298–299.
255 Al-Rāzī, *al-Manṣūrī*, 296.
256 Ibn al-Jazzār, *Ibn al-Jazzār's Zād al-musāfir I–II* (book I, chapter 9, paragraph 1).
257 Al-Rāzī, *al-Manṣūrī*, 296.

al-Rāzī. The treatments al-Rāzī and Ibn al-Jazzār recommend have many similarities. Al-Rāzī recommends putting 'killed' quicksilver (*zi'baq maqtūl*), one mixed into oil, to be put onto a wool necklace and worn around the neck.[258] In comparison, Ibn al-Jazzār recommends preparing ointments for the afflicted body parts prepared from quicksilver killed with ashes of felt, vinegar, and olive oil, or from quicksilver mixed with litharge, vinegar, and olive oil.[259] Al-Rāzī's recipe for an ointment is leaves of chinaberry tree (*azdarākht*) or leaves of oleander (*diflā*) put into oil. Another material to coat the body with for ten days is red arsenic (*zirnīkh aḥmar*), lice-bane (*maywīzaj*), soapwort (*kundus*),[260] and borax with vinegar left on the body for a while and then washed off with warm water.[261] A quite similar ointment of Ibn al-Jazzār contains lice-bane, borax, and arsenic mixed with oil and vinegar which he recommends for those who have a cold temperament.[262] Additionally, al-Rāzī also advises to fumigate the clothes with soapwort, lupine (*turmus*), leaves of chinaberry tree, or costus (*qusṭ*), or anointing oneself with powdered quicksilver or soapwort mixed into an oil.[263] Besides other ointments and treatments which do not have a parallel in al-Rāzī's chapter on lice, Ibn al-Jazzār recommends pulverised red arsenic mixed with olive oil to anoint the body with.

The last unique topic to be discussed in this chapter is abrasions and wounds caused either by riding or by the shoes. For any part of the body that became abraded, al-Rāzī advises treatment as soon as the traveller rests. This means sprinkling the afflicted part with cold water to cool, clean, and refresh it. If the part is still hot, then it is to be covered with a cotton cloth soaked in cooled rose water, changing this dressing when it warms up. In case of a burning sensation and pain, the skin is cured with liniment of white lead. For blisters caused by the tightness of the shoes al-Rāzī advises taking the shoes off, sprinkling the blisters with cold water or finely pulverised pomegranate flowers, and coating them with lyceum (*ḥuḍaḍ*),[264] acacia Senegal (*aqāqiyā*), Armenian bole, or gallnuts (*ʿafṣ*) rubbed in water.[265] Ibn al-Jazzār also discusses wounds caused by pressure of the shoes and offers treatments for it, depending on whether the wound is accompanied by an inflammation or not. If there is inflammation, he recommends a poultice of the lung of a ram, lamb, or fox; if there

258 Al-Rāzī, *al-Manṣūrī*, 296.
259 Ibn al-Jazzār, *Ibn al-Jazzār's Zād al-musāfir I–II* (book I, chapter 9, paragraph 1).
260 Dietrich, *Dioscurides triumphans*, II/308–310.
261 Al-Rāzī, *al-Manṣūrī*, 296.
262 Ibn al-Jazzār, *Ibn al-Jazzār's Zād al-musāfir I–II* (book I, chapter 9, paragraph 2).
263 Al-Rāzī, *al-Manṣūrī*, 296.
264 Dietrich, *Dioscurides triumphans*, II/155–160.
265 Al-Rāzī, *al-Manṣūrī*, 298.

is no inflammation, his first remedy is sprinkling the wound with the burnt and pulverised bottom part of the shoe, and his second remedy is quite similar to that of al-Rāzī, as it is burnt and pounded gallnut, pomegranate flower, pomegranate peels, sumac (*summāq*), or acacia Senegal.[266] Additionally, Ibn al-Jazzār advises what to do if someone stumbles and the toes are affected by stumbling.[267] Bos points out that the first two remedies of Ibn al-Jazzār (lung poultice, pulverised shoe leather) are quite similar to those of Paul of Aegina.[268] This suggest that either al-Rāzī was not consulting Paul of Aegina's text for this chapter, or he decided not to include these two remedies. Since one of al-Rāzī's sources is Paul of Aegina, it can be assumed that al-Rāzī knew about Paul of Aegina's discussion of this topic, which favours the second assumption.

1.2.16 Further Observations Based on the Topics of Travel Regimens

While the above sections took under scrutiny each of the various topics discussed by travel regimens separately and therefore allowed for a closer study of aspects and elements of the discussion of certain topics, there are some general remarks to be made as well as observations to be stressed which appear in most of the thematic discussions but might, at first reading, not be adequately pronounced.

The most striking observation is likely the fact that Qusṭā ibn Lūqā's treatise indeed does not seem to be an integral part of the tradition in the sense that his division of topics to be included in travel regimens is clearly disregarded by later physicians. In addition to the difference of topics, Qusṭā's approach to dealing with these is also different from that of the other physicians writing their travel regimens. These aspects combined explain the lack of passages identified as being copied or used by later physicians.

Similarly to Qusṭā's treatise, Ibn al-Jazzār's *Zād al-musāfir* also seems underrepresented at first. This is, for the most part, due to it being a medical compendium of diseases *a capite ad calcem* and not a travel regimen, as its title might misleadingly suggest. Nevertheless, there are still a few passages shared, at least to some degree, between Ibn al-Jazzār's relevant chapters and, most notably, al-Rāzī's regimen.

On the grounds of the above scrutiny, the relationship of the source texts is as follows. There are many passages attesting to the fact that al-Majūsī's regimen was used by Ibn Sīnā, Ḥājjī Bāshā, and Ibn al-Quff, even if to varying

266 Bos renders *aqāqiyā* as gum Senegal: Ibn al-Jazzār, *Ibn al-Jazzār's Zād al-musāfir*, 132.

267 Ibn al-Jazzār, *Ibn al-Jazzār's Zād al-musāfir*, 69, 132.

268 Ibn al-Jazzār, *Ibn al-Jazzār's Zād al-musāfir*, 132 n. 320–321.

degrees. Al-Rāzī's regimen seems to have influenced Ibn Sīnā, Ḥājjī Bāshā, and maybe even Ibn al-Quff, although these influences are far less obvious than the copied and reworked passages of al-Majūsī found in other physicians' works. Ibn Sīnā's regimen was used by Ḥājjī Bāshā and most likely by Ibn al-Khaṭīb as well. Besides these relationships, there is a section of Ibn al-Quff's and Ḥājjī Bāshā's texts which might indicate a relationship between those two texts. It is striking that al-Ṭabarī's name does not appear in this list; it seems that his text was not consulted by later physicians when they compiled their regimens, or at least not with the intent to reuse parts of the text.

It is important to point out that despite the connections between the texts listed in the above paragraph, each and every physician's regimen contains novelties. Besides the constantly varying arrangement, inclusion, and omission of topics, upon closer reading we can also find at least one but usually more elements in all the texts which lack an antecedent in earlier travel regimens. This stands true even in the case of Ḥājjī Bāshā, who is most often pointed out as having copied or reused sections from his predecessors throughout the thematic analysis of the regimens.

As the majority of the travel regimens scrutinised are contained in encyclopaedias, the question of their usability without their contexts—i.e. the whole encyclopaedias—might arise. While there is no single regimen which covers all of the possible topics, it can be said that the topics they include are mostly discussed in such a way that they can be useful even without the rest of the encyclopaedias (assuming, of course, a general knowledge of medical theory). The most notable examples of interconnectedness between the regimens and the other parts of the encyclopaedias can be found in Ibn Sīnā's and, to a smaller extent, al-Rāzī's regimens, as these refer their readers to other chapters of their encyclopaedias for discussion of certain topics. When such issues are mentioned, it is agreed upon that treating certain afflictions do require a physician (fevers which do not improve) or a surgeon (serious affliction of the limbs).

Generally speaking, the regimens focus on prevention and aim to provide general knowledge on the proper regimen to follow during travels. As such regimens are part of the practical side of medicine, explanations of the theoretical background of afflictions and treatments are scarce. Some examples for such can be found in al-Rāzī's guide and in al-Majūsī's text to a smaller degree. As for treatments, the regimens focus on changing the regimen of the six non-naturals appropriately; while variants of a recipe related to quenching the thirst appears in some regimens, we do not find references to previously prepared compound medicaments or using single medicaments together in a way that their combining would require the knowledge or skills of a pharmacist.

In summary, the medical tradition of *tadbīr al-musāfirīn* of the 9–15th centuries is an ever-changing and evolving mass of information realised by each physician in a different manner both in terms of their selection and their structuring of the material that they include in their regimens, in addition to enriching it by additional details. The above scrutiny proves that studying either the whole tradition or parts of it yield both particular and general results and will hopefully prompt further inquiries based on the same sources as well as through the inclusion of new source material.

1.2.17 A Remark on Misleading Titles

The list of the texts belonging to the corpus of medieval Arabic travel regimens demonstrates a straightforward terminology. The term 'travel regimen' consistently appears as *tadbīr al-musāfir*, 'regimen of the traveller' or with the plural form, *tadbīr al-musāfirīn*, 'regimen of the travellers'. In the case of encyclopaedic works, the titles of the relevant chapters testify to this terminology, similarly to the shorter treatises' titles. As for the longer treatises, while there is some variation in their titles, the chapter headings and the texts use the same phrasing. Even in this case, the titles seem to contain some form of the *s.f.r* root consistently. Still, the appearance of some form of the *s.f.r* root in a title does not necessarily guarantee a travel regimen.

One such example is 'Ubayd Allāh ibn Jibrīl's (d. 450s/1058–1066) *Kitāb tadhkirat al-ḥāḍir wa-zād al-musāfir* ('The book of the reminder of the sedentary and provision of the traveller'). 'Ubayd Allāh, a friend of Ibn Buṭlān (d. ca. 458/1065),[269] was "not only celebrated for his skill as a practitioner but also familiar with all aspects of medical theory".[270] He was likely born in Baghdad but moved to and settled in Mayyāfāriqīn later, where he worked in the Fāriqī hospital.[271] According to Ibn Abī Uṣaybi'a, he authored ten works on various medical topics, the *Kitāb tadhkirat al-ḥāḍir wa-zād al-musāfir* being one of them. While it has no known, extant manuscripts, 'Ubayd Allāh composed an abridgement of it under the title *al-Rawḍa al-ṭibbiyya* ('Medical garden') at the request of Abū al-Ḥasan Muḥammad ibn 'Alī.[272] As this treatise offers concise explanations for 50 medico-philosophical terms,[273] it becomes evident that

269 On his life, see Schacht, *Ibn Buṭlān*.

270 LHOM, 8.6.

271 'Ubayd Allāh ibn Bukhtīshū', *Kitāb taḥrīm dafn al-aḥyā'*, 1–4.

272 For its edition, see Paul Sbath, *Ar-Raoudat at-tibbiyya (Le jardin medical) par Ubaîd-Allah Ben Gibraîl Ben Bakhtichoû, chrétien décédé en 1058*, Cairo: H. Friedrich & Co., 1927 [reprinted: Piscataway, NJ: Gorgias Press, 2010]. On who Abū al-Ḥasan Muḥammad ibn 'Alī might be, see LHOM, 8.6., n. 5.

273 On these, see Ullmann, *Die Medizin*, 110; Meyerhof, *An Arabic compendium*.

the original work must be on medical theory rather than practical medicine, to which travel regimens belong. Therefore, the *Kitāb tadhkirat al-ḥāḍir wa-zād al-musāfir* is a fortunate case, as we still have some knowledge pertaining to the original work, due to its abridgement. If we were to find a title alone without any additional information, it could only be included in a list of dubious titles.

Another case is Ibn al-Jazzār's (d. 369/979–980)[274] *Zād al-musāfir wa-qūṭ al-ḥāḍir* ('Provisions for the traveller and nourishment for the sedentary'), a medical handbook on different diseases discussed *a capite ad calcem* in a concise form. The whole work is edited,[275] but Bos argues it is not a proper critical edition for many reasons.[276] His editions with English translations are available of the 1st and 2nd books,[277] the 6th book[278] and the 7th book in two parts,[279] the second part including the critical edition of a Hebrew translation as well. Bos gives detailed descriptions of the manuscripts used in the editions.[280] Although the *Zād al-musāfir* does not contain chapters dedicated specifically to the concerns of a traveller, it does deal with specific issues bearing importance during travel as well, for example, the 1st book's chapters 9–10 on head lice and headache, chapter 13 on dizziness and vertigo, chapter 24 on spasms (*kuzāz*); the 2nd book's chapter 6 on dimness of the eye; the 3rd book's chapter 14 on swoon

---

274 On his life and works, see Ibn al-Jazzār, *Ibn al-Jazzār on sexual diseases*, 5–7; ʿAbd al-Wahhāb, *Kitāb al-ʿumr*, II/738; Ullmann, *Die Medizin*, 147–149; GAS III/304–307; GAL I/274; GAL S I/424.

275 Bibliographical details: *Zād al-musāfir wa-qūt al-ḥāḍir* [Books 1–7], eds. Muḥammad Suwaysī, al-Rāḍī al-Jāzī, Tunis: al-Dār al-ʿArabiyya li-l-Kitāb, 1986–1999.

276 See Ibn al-Jazzār, *Ibn al-Jazzār's Zād al-musāfir*, 2–3.

277 Bibliographical details: *Ibn al-Jazzār's Zād al-musāfir wa-qūt al-ḥāḍir, Provisions for the Traveller and Nourishment for the Sedentary, Books I and II: Diseases of the Head and the Face*, ed., transl. Gerrit Bos—Fabian Käs, Leiden–Boston: Brill, 2022.

278 Bibliographical details: *Ibn al-Jazzār on sexual diseases and their treatment, A critical edition of Zād al-musāfir wa-qūt al-ḥāḍir, Provisions for the traveller and nourishment for the sedentary, Book 6*, ed., transl. Gerrit Bos, London–New York: Routledge, 2010 (1997).

279 Bibliographical details: *Ibn al-Jazzār on fevers, A critical edition of Zād al-musāfir wa-qūt al-ḥāḍir, Provisions for the traveller and nourishment for the sedentary, Book 7, Chapters 1–6*, ed., transl. Gerrit Bos, London–New York: Routledge, 2011 (2000) [Pormann concludes in his review of this work that "this is a disappointing edition with an often unreliable translation of an important medical text", while also noting its merits: Pormann, *Review of Ibn al-Jazzār on fevers*, 69.]; *Ibn al-Jazzār's Zād al-musāfir wa-qūt al-ḥāḍir, Provisions for the traveller and nourishment for the sedentary, Book 7* (7–30), ed., transl. Gerrit Bos, Leiden–Boston: Brill, 2015.

280 For the list of manuscripts see GAS III/305–306 (2.—*Zād al-musāfir wa-qūt al-ḥāḍir*); GAL I/274; GAL S I/424; as well as in the edition and translation of Books I–II by Bos and Käs.

(*ghashy*); the 4th book's chapter 6 on thirst and chapter 10 on nausea;[281] the 7th book's chapters 9–12 on poisons, viper bites, stings by wasps, bees, and scorpions, chapter 14 on fatigue and pain, and chapter 29 on wounds caused by the pressure of the shoes. Still, this does not make the *Zād al-musāfir* a travel regimen, despite what especially its Greek and Latin titles (*Ἐφόδια τοῦ ἀποδημοῦντος* and *Viaticum peregrinantis*) would suggest. Instead, on closer inspection of its title, as well as that of ʿUbayd Allāh ibn Jibrīl's work, we see the rhetorical device of merismus in action.[282] In both cases, the encyclopaedias written for the sedentary and the traveller according to the titles indicate that both works are meant for everybody.[283]

1.2.18 The Place of Travel Regimens in Encyclopaedias

Based on the corpus of travel regimens, it seems that there are more encyclopaedias that include such a regimen than there are self-contained treatises dedicated to the topic. Although the scale might tip in favour of the latter as more treatises and their manuscripts will hopefully be (re-)discovered and edited, the occurrence of travel regimens in encyclopaedias deserve some further thought, as some observations regarding the inclusion of regimens and their position in the whole work can be made.

Travel regimens are always situated in the sections of encyclopaedias dedicated to the preservation of health (*ḥifẓ al-ṣiḥḥa*), which is a subject within the practical part of medicine. An obvious consequence of this fact is that in the case of encyclopaedias which are dedicated to the theoretical part of medicine, travel regimens alongside all other regimens for preserving health are absent. A straightforward example of this is Ibn Rushd's (d. 595/1198)[284] *Kitāb al-kulliyyāt fī al-ṭibb*; while the sixth book of the work is on the preservation of health, the approach is highly theoretical, in accordance with the concept and method of the whole work. The book that complements the theoretical approach of the *Kulliyyāt* is Ibn Zuhr's (d. 557/1162)[285] *Kitāb al-taysīr fī al-mudāwāt wa-al-tadbīr*,

281 The list of these chapters is based on Ibn al-Jazzār, *Ibn al-Jazzār's Zād al-musāfir I–II*.

282 I would like to thank my anonymous reviewer for bringing this to my attention.

283 For an example of a similar phenomenon, albeit in a different context, see Pormann, Peter E., "Chapter 5, Avicenna on medical practice, epistemology, and the physiology of the inner senses", in Peter Adamson (ed.), *Interpreting Avicenna, Critical essays*, Cambridge: Cambridge University Press, 2013, 91–108.

284 On his life and works, see Arnaldez, *Ibn Rushd*.

285 On his life and works, see Álvarez Millán, *Zuhr, Banū*, 147–150. On the *Kitāb al-taysīr*, see Azar, *The sage of Seville*, 36–42. On the relationship of Ibn Rushd and Ibn Zuhr (and therefore on the connection of the two works), besides their biographies, see Azar, *The sage of Seville*, 75–82.

which focuses on the symptoms and treatments of diseases, rather than the preservation of health.

As for the preservation of health, the parts of encyclopaedias (as well as monographs) discussing it are focused on the six non-naturals (air, movement and rest, eating and drinking, sleeping and wakefulness, excretion and retention, and mental movements) but the proper regimen of these is unique to each and every person based on their physiology. While there is an abundance of medical material on the preservation of health written in Arabic, some detailed and comprehensive, some specific,[286] what is of special importance regarding the encyclopaedias under partial scrutiny here is the categories created by the physicians which form the basis for discussions of the proper regimens, even though not all of them are discussed in each encyclopaedia. In some cases, we find general or specific advice on all the six non-naturals. Sections on regimens tailored to the properties of the seasons are commonly included, as are special regimens according to the various temperaments. Perhaps even more prevalent is the discussion of regimens according to age groups, starting from childbirth and on to the regimen of the elderly. This is where one can find chapters dedicated to the care of pregnant women or for those in childbed, occasionally for people recuperating from diseases, and other specific or 'miscellaneous' categories. This is also where travel regimens are generally placed by the authors. Travel regimens are routinely included after the discussion of regimens according to the seasons, temperaments, and age groups, but their position amongst the additional regimens varies from author to author.

In al-Ṭabarī's *Firdaws al-ḥikma*, the earliest encyclopaedic source discussed here, the only regimen besides those for the seasons is the one for travellers. The fourth treatise of the *Kitāb al-Manṣūrī* of al-Rāzī is dedicated to the preservation of health. Focusing on the six non-naturals and touching on toothcare, eyecare, preserving the hearing, and safeguarding against contagious diseases, it includes regimens according to the seasons, for pregnant women and childbirth, for women in childbed, for the newborn, for the wetnurse, and then simply for 'the rest of the people' (*sā'ir al-insān* [*sic*!]; weaned children, young people, grown-up people, and the elderly). In contrast to this, the sixth treatise of this encyclopaedia is wholly dedicated to the regimen of travellers. Contrary to these distinguished positions, al-Majūsī and Ibn Sīnā included their travel regimens at the very end of their sections on the preservation of health. However, we find that in the next encyclopaedic source, written some 200 years

286 See for example Ullmann, *Die Medizin*, 190–192, 193–203; Ullmann, *Islamic medicine*, 97–103; Pormann—Savage-Smith, *Medieval Islamic medicine*, 49–51, 135–138.

after Ibn Sīnā, Ibn al-Quff promotes his travel regimen to the beginning of his 'miscellaneous' regimens right after discussing temperaments and age groups. As for Ibn al-Khaṭīb's *Kitāb al-wuṣūl*, a cursory look at the contents is misleading. He discusses three regimens, those for children, for the elderly, and for the travellers, respectively. While this way his travel regimen comes at the very end, it is far more detailed than his second regimen, and it is also important to point out that while he omits almost all of the usual main categories (including only some of the regimens for specific age groups), he still includes a regimen for travellers. Ḥājjī Bāshā's *Shifāʾ al-aqsām* betrays a similar arrangement, albeit his regimens before that of the travellers cover all the main categories in addition to many specialised ones.

Based on these considerations, it seems that travel regimens formed a highly valued part of an encyclopaedia's section on the preservation of health in the 9th and 10th centuries, and while they fall behind other regimens by the end of the 10th century, their importance is still sufficient to warrant inclusion until the 13th century, from which time they enjoy a modest revival. The periods in which shorter or longer treatises were dedicated to the discussion of travel regimens corroborate this observation in general; however, Ibn Mandawayh's lost treatise might indicate a slightly later decline in popularity, while Ibn al-Amshāṭī's treatise entitled *al-Isfār ʿan ḥikam al-asfār* from the 15th century attests a renewal of interest in the topic.

2 The Author, Ibn al-Amshāṭī

In the manuscripts of the travel regimen entitled *al-Isfār ʿan ḥikam al-asfār*, the author is referred to as al-shaykh al-imām al-ʿallāma Muẓaffar al-Dīn Maḥmūd al-ʿAntābī, known as al-Amshāṭī. One of these manuscripts also contains a short biography of the author, which names al-Sakhāwī's *al-Ḍawʾ al-lāmiʿ* and some other unnamed work(s) as its source material.[287]

While there are a number of short entries on the author, Ibn al-Amshāṭī, in the standard reference works and we can find a handful of relevant biographical sources as well, these present various problems. Nevertheless, it is possible to resolve most of these and present an in-depth biography and the author's literary output.[288]

---

287 For this biography, see section *3.1.2 MS Mosul, Madrasat Yaḥyā Bāshā 175/9*.

288 I would like to thank Máté Horváth and Mónika Schönléber for their invaluable comments on an earlier version of this chapter.

2.1 *Sources*

Brockelmann wrote a short entry on Ibn al-Amshāṭī in his GAL. From this, we learn that Muẓaffar al-Dīn Abū al-Thanāʾ Maḥmūd ibn Aḥmad al-ʿAyntābī al-Amshāṭī was born around 812/1407 [*sic*] and died in Rabīʿ II 902/December 1496 in Cairo. He studied *fiqh*, medicine, and military science, utilising his knowledge as a cannon master in many campaigns. Brockelmann's sources are al-Sakhāwī's *al-Ḍawʾ al-lāmiʿ* and al-Shawkānī's *al-Badr al-ṭāliʿ*. He lists manuscripts for four of Ibn al-Amshāṭī's works (*al-Qawl al-sadīd, al-Isfār, Taʾsīs al-ṣiḥḥa*, and a *Mūjaz* commentary).[289] Notably, 812 AH corresponds to 1409 AD, while 1407 AD would match 810 AH, an alternate birth date. Although Brockelmann does not mention this second date, it is the most likely cause for the discrepancy in the birth dates he gives.

Ḥājjī Khalīfa records a significant fact in his *Kashf al-ẓunūn* in the entry for the *Mūjaz al-Qānūn*. He writes: "And one of its commentaries is *al-Munjaz*. It is an elaborate commentary in two volumes by the chief physician (*raʾīs al-aṭibbāʾ*) Maḥmūd ibn Aḥmad al-Amshāṭī, the Hanafi, born in the year 810 [AH]."[290] Here, in addition to the alternate birth date, we find a piece of crucial information: according to Ḥājjī Khalīfa, Ibn al-Amshāṭī was chief physician. However, if we turn to the entry for the *Lamḥa*, another medical work on which Ibn al-Amshāṭī commented, we find Ḥājjī Khalīfa stating: "Muẓaffar al-Dīn Maḥmūd al-ʿAyntābī, known as Ibn al-Amshāṭī, commented on it and named it *Taʾsīs al-ṣiḥḥa*."[291] While Ḥājjī Khalīfa omits to bring up the chief physicianship here, he includes it again in the entry on Ibn al-Amshāṭī in the *Sullam al-wuṣūl*,[292] his biographical dictionary. As he adds that "al-Suyūṭī mentioned him in his *Aʿyān al-aʿyān*," we can quickly locate the source for this critical detail.

As for the works of al-Baghdādī supplementing the data found in the *Kashf al-ẓunūn*, both contain entries on Ibn al-Amshāṭī and his works. In his biographical dictionary, the *Hadiyyat al-ʿārifīn*, under Ibn al-Amshāṭī, he states: "Muẓaffar al-Dīn Abū al-Thanāʾ Maḥmūd ibn Aḥmad ibn al-Ḥasan ibn Ismāʿīl ibn Yaʿqūb, the Cairene, the Hanafi, known as Ibn al-Amshāṭī, was born in 815 [AH] and died in 902 [AH]."[293] Since none of the sources gives the date 815 AH, it is perhaps a typo for 810 AH. Four of his works are listed here, namely: *Taʾsīs al-ṣiḥḥa*, a commentary on *al-Niqāya*, *al-Qawl al-sadīd*, and the *Munjaz*. In

289 GAL II/100, GAL S II/93.
290 Ḥājjī Khalīfa, *Kashf*, II/1900.
291 Ḥājjī Khalīfa, *Kashf*, II/1561.
292 Ḥājjī Khalīfa, *Sullam*, III/305 (no. 4839).
293 Al-Baghdādī, *Hadiyyat*, II/411.

al-Baghdādī's bibliographical supplement to the *Kashf al-ẓunūn*, the *Īḍāḥ al-maknūn*, we find short entries on only two of Ibn al-Amshāṭī's works, *al-Kifāya Sharḥ al-Niqāya*[294] and *al-Qawl al-sadīd*.[295] Interestingly, al-Baghdādī remains silent on the issue of chief physicianship as well as the rest of Ibn al-Amshāṭī's works.

Regarding modern Arabic biographical dictionaries, both al-Ziriklī and Kaḥḥāla have entries on the author.[296] In his *al-Aʿlām*, al-Ziriklī presents his entry under the name Ibn al-Amshāṭī. He gives the exact dates as Brockelmann. For the author's name, al-Ziriklī gives Maḥmūd ibn Aḥmad ibn Ḥasan ibn Ismāʿīl, Muẓaffar al-Dīn, Abū al-Thanāʾ al-ʿAynī (al-ʿAyntābī) by origin, the Cairene, the Hanafi, known as Ibn al-Amshāṭī. As for his life, al-Ziriklī summarises the accounts given in his primary sources in a few short phrases and then lists the same four works as Brockelmann. Lastly, he quotes al-Sakhāwī regarding his friendship with Ibn al-Amshāṭī, then explains that al-Amshāṭī was Ibn al-Amshāṭī's maternal grandfather, who was a comb trader. Al-Ziriklī references al-Shawkānī's *al-Badr al-ṭāliʿ*, al-Sakhāwī's *al-Ḍawʾ al-lāmiʿ*, two catalogue entries,[297] and both of Brockelmann's entries.[298]

In Kaḥḥāla's *Muʿjam al-muʾallifīn*, there are two entries for the author. One is under the name Maḥmūd al-Amshāṭī (no. 16,521). Here, Kaḥḥāla gives the same dates of birth and death but provides the alternate birth date 810/1407 in a footnote. For the full name, he offers Maḥmūd ibn Aḥmad ibn Ḥasan ibn Ismāʿīl ibn Yaʿqūb ibn Ismāʿīl al-gh.t.ā.b.y [*sic*; doubtless a typo for al-ʿA(y)ntābī] by origin, the Cairene, the Hanafi, known as Ibn al-Amshāṭī (Muẓaffar al-Dīn). Besides the same dates of birth and death (with a typo of the former in the main text), there is a summary of Ibn al-Amshāṭī's life quite similar to al-Ziriklī's entry and the list of the same four works. Kaḥḥāla's sources are al-Shawkānī's *al-Badr al-ṭāliʿ*, al-Sakhāwī's *al-Ḍawʾ al-lāmiʿ*, Ḥājjī Khalīfa's *Kashf al-ẓunūn*, al-Baghdādī's *Īḍāḥ al-maknūn* and *Hadiyyat al-ʿārifīn*, al-Ziriklī's *al-Aʿlām*, and Bockelmann's Supplement entry.[299] Kaḥḥāla's second

294 Al-Baghdādī, *Īḍāḥ*, II/371.

295 Al-Baghdādī, *Īḍāḥ*, II/249.

296 For a study of their approaches to earlier sources, see Bray, *Literary approaches*, 239–243.

297 *Al-Fihris al-tamhīdī*, 535 (MS Cairo, Dār al-Kutub, ṭibb 126: *al-Munjaz sharḥ al-Mūjaz li-Ibn al-Nafīs al-juzʾ al-awwal yashtamilu ʿalā matn al-juzʾ al-ʿilmī wa-al-naẓarī li-Maḥmūd bin Aḥmad al-Amshāṭī*); Hitti, *Garrett*, 348 (no. 1110, MS Princeton, Garrett 570H: *Taʾsīs al-ṣiḥḥa bi-Sharḥ al-Lamḥa*).

298 Al-Ziriklī, *al-Aʿlām*, VII/163.

299 Kaḥḥāla, *Muʿjam* (1993), III/794. The exact same entry can be found in the earlier edition as well, with the typo in the name but without the typo for the date of birth: see Kaḥḥāla, *Muʿjam* (1957), XII/145.

entry is for Maḥmūd al-ʿAyntābī (no. 16,534), augmenting the previous entry[300] with more elements of his name and completing the list of his four works.[301]

While the individual purposes of the works mentioned above differ significantly, I would like to point out some noteworthy issues before moving on to the primary sources. Firstly, there is no complete list of Ibn al-Amshāṭī's works in any of the accounts mentioned. The case of al-Baghdādī is also intriguing, as he lists four works in his short biographical entry while only two of the four are accounted for in his register of titles. Secondly, only the same two biographical works are cited as sources in all of the reference works discussed above. The exception is Ḥājjī Khalīfa, who references al-Suyūṭī. If we broaden the scope of the search for information on Ibn al-Amshāṭī, we find that Behrens-Abouseif mentions a certain al-Amshāṭī when discussing master calligraphers, citing al-Sakhāwī's *al-Ḍawʾ al-lāmiʿ* and his *Dhayl ʿalā Rafʿ al-iṣr*.[302] This al-Amshāṭī is, however, the brother of our author. Thirdly, the case of chief physicianship is intriguing, to say the least. Ḥājjī Khalīfa is the only author to record that Ibn al-Amshāṭī was chief physician, most likely relying on al-Suyūṭī here. As being appointed to this position was quite an achievement,[303] it seems genuinely peculiar that this fact is not present in all of the accounts of Ibn al-Amshāṭī's life.

The sources mentioned in the above accounts are Shams al-Dīn Muḥammad al-Sakhāwī's (830–902/1427–1497) *al-Ḍawʾ al-lāmiʿ*, Jalāl al-Dīn al-Suyūṭī's (843–911/1445–1505) *Aʿyān al-aʿyān*, and Muḥammad al-Shawkānī's (1173–1255/1759–1839) *al-Badr al-ṭāliʿ*. The rich historiographical production of the 15th century, however, compels one to try and locate additional contemporary accounts of the author's life besides those of al-Sakhāwī's and al-Suyūṭī's. Despite the generous abundance of source material, probing the works of the most prominent historians of the century has not yielded much new information, as we will see shortly.[304]

---

300 Kaḥḥāla, *Muʿjam* (1957), XII/188.

301 Kaḥḥāla, *Muʿjam* (1993), III/797.

302 Behrens-Abouseif, *The book*, 118. I would like to thank Peter Nagy for bringing this reference to my attention.

303 Regarding what this position meant, see Pormann—Savage-Smith, *Medieval Islamic medicine*, 87–88; Chipman, *The world of pharmacy*, 125, referencing Doris Behrens-Abouseif, *Fatḥ Allāh and Abū Zakariyya, Physicians under the Mamluks* (Cairo: Institut français d'archéologie orientale, 1987), citing al-Qalqashandī's *Ṣubḥ al-aʿshā*.

304 Additionally, I consulted Najm al-Dīn al-Ghazzī's (d. 1061/1651) *al-Kawākib al-sāʾira* (2 vols., ed. Khalīl al-Manṣūr, Beirut: Dār al-Kutub al-ʿIlmiyya, 1997). Unfortunately, he does not record Ibn al-Amshāṭī in the first *ṭabaqa* of his book consisting of those who died between 901–933 AH. While I did not consult ʿAbd al-Wahhāb al-Shaʿrānī's (d. 973/1565) works, he

The relevant parts of the works of Taqī al-Dīn Aḥmad al-Maqrīzī (766–845/1364–1442), one of the foremost historians of the period,[305] are still too early for our author's life. The same can be said about his famous rival, Badr al-Dīn al-ʿAynī (762–855/1361–1451),[306] even though it would be quite interesting to read Badr al-Dīn al-ʿAynī's account of someone with whom he shares the al-ʿAynī or al-ʿAyntābī *nisba*. The case remains the same for the works of the last of the famous trio, Shihāb al-Dīn Ibn Ḥajar al-ʿAsqalānī (773–852/1372–1449).[307] As for Taqī al-Dīn Ibn Qāḍī Shuhba (779–851/1377–1448), besides his dates of birth and death, the scope of his *Dhayl* also disqualifies him as a likely source.[308] Jamāl al-Dīn Ibn Taghrībirdī's (812–874/1409–1470)[309] *al-Manhal* contains biographies from 1248 to the 1450s, his *al-Nujūm al-zāhira* continues up to 1467, and his *Hawādith al-duhūr* covers the years 1441–1469. These dates rule out finding our author's short biographical note in the list of those deceased during the year 1496, and there is no passing mention of him in these works. ʿAlī ibn Dāwūd al-Jawharī al-Ṣayrafī's (819–900/1416–1494)[310] *Nuzhat al-nufūs wa-al-abdān* covers the years 1384–1475, while his other historical work, *Inbāʾ al-haṣr* deals with a much shorter period, 1468–1473 and parts of 1480–1481. There is no passing mention of our author in either of the works, even though the second one mentions our author's brother, Shams al-Amshāṭī, many times. A fellow physician, ʿAbd al-Bāsiṭ ibn Khalīl al-Malaṭī (844–920/1440–1515),[311] son of Khalīl ibn Shāhīn (d. 872/1468), mentions Shams al-Amshāṭī in the *Nayl al-amal* a few times and reports his death as well. The major work of Muḥammad ibn Aḥmad Ibn Iyās al-Ḥanafī (852–874/1448–1524),[312] the *Badāʾiʿ al-zuhūr* also mentions Shams al-Amshāṭī but not our author.

However, the biographical account written by al-Sakhāwī on Ibn al-Amshāṭī provides a clue: Ibn al-Amshāṭī travelled with al-Biqāʿī, who said that our author was born at the end of 810 AH, corresponding to early 1408. Addition-

---

does not mention Ibn al-Amshāṭī according to Jean-Claude Garcin's *Index des Tabaqāt de Shaʿrāni (pour la fin du IXe et le début du Xe s. H.)* (in: *Annales Islamologiques* 6 (1966), 31–94), however, Garcin lists Ibn al-Sāʿigh, Ibn al-Amshāṭī's protégé (as a Hanafite doctor who died around 930/1523–1524, on p. 90; more on him later).

305 See vol. 7, no. 2 of the *Mamlūk Studies Review* devoted to him.

306 On his life, see Marmon, *al-ʿAynī, Badr al-Dīn*.

307 On his life, see Rosenthal, *Ibn Hadjar al-ʿAskalānī*. On the rivalries of the three, see Broadbridge, *Academic rivalry*.

308 See Reisman, *A holograph MS*.

309 On his life, see Popper, *Abu 'l-Maḥāsin*.

310 See Massoud, *The chronicles*, 133–134.

311 See Massoud, *The chronicles*, 67.

312 On his life, see Brinner, *Ibn Iyās*.

ally, al-Suyūṭī quotes from al-Biqāʿī's *"Muʿjam"* an anecdote related by Ibn al-Amshāṭī to al-Biqāʿī.[313] Therefore, the relevant works of Burhān al-Dīn Ibrāhīm ibn ʿUmar ibn Ḥasan al-Biqāʿī (809–885/1407–1480)[314] likely hold some further details about Ibn al-Amshāṭī. However, al-Biqāʿī's biographical dictionary, *ʿUnwān al-zamān bi-tarājim al-shuyūkh wa-al-aqrān* regrettably does not mention our author or his brother. While it does contain an autobiography with some details on his travels,[315] it still does not mention Ibn al-Amshāṭī. A later abridgement of the *ʿUnwān al-zamān* compiled by al-Biqāʿī himself under the title *ʿUnwān al-ʿunwān* lists the names and dates of birth and death of the teachers, peers, and students of al-Biqāʿī. Here we find a short entry on Ibn al-Amshāṭī containing his name and date and place of birth.[316] Al-Biqāʿī's chronicle, *Iẓhār al-ʿaṣr li-asrār ahl al-ʿaṣr* covers the years 855–870/1451–1467. The parts comprising the years 855–865 AH are available in edition; the rest is preserved in manuscript form only. In the edited parts, Shams al-Amshāṭī is mentioned twice and Ibn al-Amshāṭī also appears once.[317]

To summarise, it seems that we are, for the most part, left with the same three sources for Maḥmūd Ibn al-Amshāṭī's life, i. e. al-Sakhāwī's *al-Ḍawʾ al-lāmiʿ*,[318] al-Suyūṭī's *Aʿyān al-aʿyān*[319] on account of Ḥājjī Khalīfa's *Sullam*[320] as the source for the chief physicianship, and al-Shawkānī's *al-Badr al-ṭāliʿ* as the earliest mention of a date of death.[321] However, the entry in al-Biqāʿī's *ʿUnwān al-ʿunwān*[322] must also be added to this list as a fourth source, as it is the origin of an alternate birth date, even if it does not contain any other information. Al-Sakhāwī's account is by far the most detailed, but it naturally cannot give a date of death, nor does it contain any information regarding the chief physicianship. Regrettably, biographies of the brother, Muḥammad,[323] do not contain much additional information on Maḥmūd himself.

---

313 Al-Ṣuyūṭī, *Naẓm*, 174.

314 On his life, see Saleh, *al-Biqāʿī*, as well as the material listed in the following footnote.

315 Al-Biqāʿī, *ʿUnwān al-zamān*, II/61–85. Studies on various events recorded in this autobiography from different points of view are: Goudie, *How to make it in Cairo*; Goudie, *Al-Biqāʿī's self-reflection*; Saleh, *In defense of the Bible*, 7–20; Guo, *Al-Biqāʿī's chronicle*; Guo, *Tales of a medieval Cairene harem*.

316 I would like to thank Kenneth Goudie for bringing this entry to my attention.

317 Al-Biqāʿī, *Iẓhār*, I/285 (Maḥmūd Ibn al-Amshāṭī), III/75 (Muḥammad Shams al-Amshāṭī), III/372 (Muḥammad Shams al-Amshāṭī).

318 Al-Sakhāwī, *al-Ḍawʾ*, X/128–129 (no. 541).

319 Al-Ṣuyūṭī, *Naẓm*, 174 (no. 189).

320 Ḥājjī Khalīfa, *Sullam*, III/305 (no. 4839).

321 Al-Shawkānī, *Badr*, II/292–293 (no. 536).

322 Al-Biqāʿī, *ʿUnwān al-ʿunwān*, 346 (no. 814).

323 A non-exhaustive list of his biographies and mentions: al-Sakhāwī, *al-Ḍawʾ*, VI/301–304

2.2 *Biography*

For the reasons discussed above concerning the source material, the following biography of Ibn al-Amshāṭī is based primarily on al-Sakhāwī's account, with additional information from other accounts as well as from biographies of others. To resolve the problems pointed out with regard to the data present in the reference works and the sources, the biography is separated into six parts. The first of these is dedicated to Ibn al-Amshāṭī's family relations and his name. In the second part, I propose a resolution of the multiple birth dates recorded for Ibn al-Amshāṭī. The third part focuses on his studies. Here, wherever it was possible, I tried to identify his teachers and contemporaries by referring to their biographies in al-Sakhāwī's *al-Ḍawʾ*, in the hope that it would facilitate further research on them. The fourth part of this biography focuses on Ibn al-Amshāṭī's travels and the more practical skills he acquired. The fifth part is dedicated to his teaching activities and the positions that he held. The last, sixth part is devoted to his last years and death, besides offering a glimpse of the praise of his character in the biographical accounts.

2.2.1 Family

Maḥmūd ibn Aḥmad ibn Ḥasan ibn Ismāʿīl ibn Yaʿqūb ibn Ismāʿīl Muẓaffar al-Dīn Abū al-Thanāʾ al-ʿAyntābī [= from Gaziantep] by origin, the Cairene, the Hanafi, was the son of the imām Shihāb al-Dīn and full brother of Shams al-Dīn Muḥammad al-Kajkāwī. He was known as Ibn al-Amshāṭī. This *nasab* can be traced back to Maḥmūd's and Muḥammad's maternal grandfather, Shams al-Dīn or al-Shams Muḥammad ibn Sulaymān ibn Mūsā, who was a comb trader (the Arabic word for comb being *misht̩/musht̩*, pl. *amshāṭ*). Their mother was called Firdaws.[324] Unfortunately, the sources remain silent on which of the two brothers was older, for which I presently offer a resolution. Their father died in 819/1416–1417, so they grew up under the care of their grandfather, the comb trader.[325] Turning back to Maḥmūd Ibn al-Amshāṭī, the sources do not mention marriages or offspring, but their possibility cannot be ruled out solely on this basis.

(no. 1004); al-Sakhāwī, *al-Dhayl*, 205–219; al-Sakhāwī, *Wajīz al-kalām*, III/913 (no. 2067, obituary); al-Malaṭī, *Nayl al-amal*, IV/284, VII/48, 76, 94, 137, 270 (obituary); al-Ṣayrafī, *Inbāʾ al-haṣr*, 156,251, 284, 320, 324, 360, 361, 362, 448, 491, 492, 493, 503, 512, 517.

324 Recorded in the biography of Muḥammad in al-Sakhāwī, *al-Ḍawʾ*, VI/301.

325 Recorded in the biography of Muḥammad in al-Sakhāwī, *al-Dhayl*, 205.

2.2.2 Date of Birth

While all sources agree that Ibn al-Amshāṭī was born in Cairo, they record two different birth dates: 810/1407–1408 and 812/1409–1410. The first one is based on the account of al-Biqāʿī, and it is repeated by al-Suyūṭī; the second one can be found in al-Sakhāwī's report, repeated by al-Shawkānī. According to al-Sakhāwī, Ibn al-Amshāṭī's brother, al-Shams Muḥammad al-Kajkāwī was born on 26 Dhū al-Ḥijja or Dhū al-Qaʿda 811/12 May or April 1409, as he read it in Muḥammad's handwriting,[326] while ʿAbd al-Bāsiṭ al-Malaṭī writes that Muḥammad was born in 812/1409–1410.[327] Suppose we evaluate ʿAbd al-Bāsiṭ's 812 as an inaccurate version of the very end of 811 and accept April/May 1409 as the correct date of birth for Muḥammad. In that case, there could have been enough time for Muḥammad's mother, Firdaws, to become pregnant and give birth to Maḥmūd still in 812 (from late May 1409 to early May 1410). However, if 810 (from June 1407 to late May 1408) is the correct birth date of Maḥmūd, it would mean more time in between the two pregnancies (even up to a year, instead of a maximum of three months). Although both scenarios are biologically possible, 810 and the end of 811 are more probable. Therefore, I would suggest that 810/1407–1408 is the more likely birth date of Maḥmūd Ibn al-Amshāṭī.

2.2.3 Studies

Al-Sakhāwī gives a detailed account of Ibn al-Amshāṭī's studies.[328] He memorised (*ḥafaẓa*) the Quran, Ṣadr al-Sharīʿa al-Thānī's (d. 747/1346) *Niqāya fī al-fiqh*, and Ibn Ḥājib's (d. 646/1249) *Kāfiya*. He versified (*naẓama*) parts of Ibn Ḥajar al-ʿAsqalānī's (d. 852/1449)[329] *Nuzhat al-naẓar* and Fakhr al-Dīn al-Khujandī's (fl. beginning of 8th/14th c.) *al-Talwīḥ fī al-ṭibb*. He studied *fiqh*, jurisprudence under (*ishtaghala fī al-fiqh ʿalā*) Ibn al-Dīrī (d. 867/1463),[330] al-Amīn al-Aqṣarāʾī (d. 880/1475),[331] al-Shumunnī (d. 872/1468),[332] and al-Badr Ibn ʿUbayd Allāh (d. 875/1471).[333] He studied (*akhadha fī*) *naḥw*, grammar and other subjects as well from al-Amīn al-Aqṣarāʾī.[334] As for medicine, he studied (*akhadha*)

326 Al-Sakhāwī, *al-Ḍawʾ*, VI/301; al-Sakhāwī, *al-Dhayl*, 205.
327 Al-Malaṭī, *Nayl al-amal*, VII/270.
328 Al-Sakhāwī, *al-Ḍawʾ*, X/128.
329 Al-Shawkānī explicitly mentions Ibn Ḥajar: see al-Shawkānī, *al-Badr*, II/293.
330 For his biography, see al-Sakhāwī, *al-Ḍawʾ*, III/249–253.
331 For his biography, see al-Sakhāwī, *al-Ḍawʾ*, X/240–243.
332 For his biography, see al-Sakhāwī, *al-Ḍawʾ*, II/174–178.
333 For his biography, see al-Sakhāwī, *al-Ḍawʾ*, X/138–140.
334 Al-Shawkānī gives al-Shumunnī as Ibn al-Amshāṭī's *naḥw* teacher, which is most probably

under al-Shumunnī and al-Sharaf ibn al-Khashshāb (d. 873/1468–1469),[335] as well as under Salām Allāh (d. 886 or 887/1481–1483)[336] in Mecca. He learned from him the *qirāʾa*, Qurʾān recitation of al-Khaṭīb Abū al-Faḍl al-Nuwayrī[337] in the Shamsiyya. In Mecca, he also studied from (*samiʿa ʿalā*) al-Taqī ibn Fahd (d. 871/1466–1467)[338] and Abū al-Fatḥ al-Marāghī (d. 859/1454–1455).[339] He learned (*akhadha*) *mīqāt*, timekeeping from al-Shams al-Maḥallī.[340] He studied (*samiʿa ʿalā*) from al-Shams al-Shāmī (d. 831/1428)[341] the *Dhayl mashyakhat al-Qalānisī* written by al-ʿIrāqī (d. 806/1404).[342] From al-Shāmī's biography, we can gather that he learned this work from Abū al-Ḥaram al-Qalānisī (d. 765/1364)[343] himself. As for Ibn al-Amshāṭī's next teacher, he studied under al-Badr Ḥusayn al-Būṣīrī (d. 838/1434–1435)[344] the *Sunan* of al-Dāraquṭnī (d. 385/995) as a classmate of al-Sunbāṭī.[345] Al-Sakhāwī writes that Ibn al-Amshāṭī studied from "our shaykh", undoubtedly referring to Ibn Ḥajar al-ʿAsqalānī, and that he received *ijāza*s from a number of his teachers. Even though Ibn al-Amshāṭī is not a figure well-known to us today, the list of his teachers and fellow students undeniably places him in the centre of the network of the learned late Mamluk Cairene elite.

---

an error: al-Shawkānī, *al-Badr*, II/293. Al-Sakhāwī lists Ibn al-Amshāṭī's *fiqh* teachers, then writes that he learned *naḥw* from the second one and others. Al-Shawkānī does the same but mentions only two of Ibn al-Amshāṭī's *fiqh* teachers, so the phrase 'second one' as the *naḥw* teacher ends up referring to al-Shumunnī, therefore it is most likely a mistake which occurred during the process of copying and abridging the account of al-Sakhāwī.

335 For his biography, see al-Sakhāwī, *al-Ḍawʾ*, VI/284–286.

336 For his biography, see al-Sakhāwī, *al-Ḍawʾ*, III/257–258.

337 Either the younger or older Muḥammad Abū al-Faḍl al-Nuwayrī, as the brothers followed their father and one another as *khaṭīb*s of Mecca. See al-Sakhāwī, *al-Ḍawʾ*, VII/44–45 (no. 93) and al-Sakhāwī, *al-Ḍawʾ*, VII/45 (no. 94).

338 On the Ibn Fahd family, see Meloy, *Ibn Fahd*.

339 For his biography, see al-Sakhāwī, *al-Ḍawʾ*, VII/161–162; al-Suyūṭī, *Naẓm*, 139–140.

340 Maybe he is Muḥammad ibn ʿAlī ibn Ismaʿīl ibn Riḍwān al-Shams al-Maḥallī, then al-Azharī, al-Khaṭīb. See al-Sakhāwī, *al-Ḍawʾ*, VIII/171 (no. 418). Another candidate is Aḥmad ibn Muḥammad ibn ʿAlī ibn Ismāʿīl al-Shihāb, called Barakāt al-Shams al-Maḥallī by origin, the Meccan, the Shafiite, known as al-Khaṭīb. See Sakhāwī, *al-Ḍawʾ*, II/146 (no. 412).

341 For his biography, see al-Sakhāwī, *al-Ḍawʾ*, VII/14.

342 For his biography, see al-Sakhāwī, *al-Ḍawʾ*, IV/171–178.

343 For his biography, see al-ʿAsqalānī, *al-Durar*, IV/235.

344 For his biography, see al-Sakhāwī, *al-Ḍawʾ*, III/150.

345 Al-Sakhāwī writes only al-Sunbāṭī. For the biography of Muḥammad ibn Muḥammad ibn ʿAbd al-Laṭīf al-Sunbāṭī (d. 1457), who studied from al-Shams al-Būṣīrī, see al-Sakhāwī, *al-Ḍawʾ*, IX/113–114. Perhaps a more likely candidate is ʿAbd al-ʿAzīz ibn Yūsuf ibn ʿAbd al-Ghaffār al-Sunbātī (d. 1475) who studied from al-Shams al-Būṣīrī and al-Būṣīrī, see al-Sakhāwī, *al-Ḍawʾ*, IV/237–239.

2.2.4 Travels and 'Practical' Skills

Ibn al-Amshāṭī travelled to Damascus many times and attended paraenetic sessions of Abū Shiʿr (d. 844/1441).[346] He also performed the pilgrimage many times and lived in Mecca for studying or teaching (*jāwara*);[347] we can pinpoint at least two such periods. Al-Sakhāwī records that Salām Allāh resided in Mecca for the first time shortly before 850/1446, and this was when Ibn al-Amshāṭī studied medicine from him.[348] According to manuscript evidence, Ibn al-Amshāṭī finished penning a partial copy of one of his works in Mecca on 5 Jumādā II 887/22 July 1482,[349] and his *mujāwir*-period in the same year, 887/1482–1483, inspired him to write another one of his works.[350] Ibn al-Amshāṭī visited al-Ṭāʾif accompanying al-Biqāʿī. As mentioned above, al-Biqāʿī's *ʿUnwān al-zamān* contains a short autobiography written in 841/1437. While most of his travels recorded in this autobiography are dated, he does not mention travelling to al-Ṭāʾif. It might be that this particular journey took place after 841/1437. Another explanation for its omission is the possibility that it would be taken for granted that one would visit this town after the pilgrimage (which al-Biqāʿī does not date) rather than as another separate journey from Cairo.

Ibn al-Amshāṭī was stationed in some frontier towns or ports (*thughūr*)[351] and travelled to participate in *jihād*. This *jihād* could very well refer to the campaigns to Cyprus and Rhodes (in which al-Biqāʿī participated as well and wrote *al-Isfār ʿan ashraf al-asfār wa-al-ikhbār bi-aẓraf al-akhbār* or *al-Isfār ʿan ashridat al-asfār*, an eyewitness account of his experience, lost today).[352] If so, it might be a logical assumption that Ibn al-Amshāṭī was stationed in the frontier ports of Cilicia. However, as ships from Būlāq, Beirut, and Tripoli sailed to Cyprus and Rhodes in campaigns in the 1430s and 1440s,[353] pinpointing the exact possibilities based on the data provided by al-Sakhāwī (the life span of

346 For his biography, see al-Sakhāwī, *al-Ḍawʾ*, IV/82–83.

347 See Ende, *Mudjāwir*.

348 Al-Sakhāwī, *al-Ḍawʾ*, III/257.

349 MS Istanbul, Feyzullah Efendi 848, f. 123:2–3.

350 MS Mashhad, Āstān-e Qods-e Rażavī 6339, f. 1ᵛ:4–6; MS Istanbul, Süleymaniye Kütüphanesi, Shahīd ʿAlī 2006, f. 1ᵛ:8–9.

351 See Bosworth—Latham, *al-Thughūr*.

352 Goudie, *How to make it in Cairo*, 221. On al-Biqāʿī's *jihāds*, see also Guo, *Al-Biqāʿī's chronicle*, 122, 125, Saleh, *In defense of the Bible*, 12–13, al-Biqāʿī, *ʿUnwān al-zamān*, II/67. A glimpse of al-Biqāʿī's personal account of naval campaigns is preserved in Ibn Ḥajar al-ʿAsqalānī's *Inbā al-ghumr* and is available in an annotated translation: Frenkel, Yehoshua, *Al-Biqāʿī's naval war-report*, in Stephan Conermann (ed.), *History and society during the Mamluk period (1250–1517)*, *Studies of the Annemarie Schimmel Research College I*, Göttingen: V&R Unipress–Bonn University Press, 2014, 9–19.

353 See Fuess, *Rotting ships*, 53–56.

Ibn al-Amshāṭī, plus the terms *thughūr* and *jihād*) would be an ambitious, if not impossible undertaking.[354] Ibn al-Amshāṭī devoted attention to swimming, bookbinding, and archery. He was treating patients, fencing, shooting cannons, and worked in naphtha and perhaps ointment production.

2.2.5 Teaching and Positions

Ibn al-Amshāṭī took up the leadership of numerous schools (*madrasa*). As for medicine, he also taught it and composed works on it and instructed a group of students. According to al-Sakhāwī, he visited the sick, the leading officials (*ruʾasāʾ*), and others in modesty, with the aim of doing pious deeds.

Ibn al-Amshāṭī taught *fiqh* in the Zimāmiyya *madrasa*[355] in the *Suwayqat al-ṣāḥib*[356] quarter after al-Shams al-Rāzī (d. 870/1465).[357] Ibn al-Amshāṭī took over two positions from his brother who died in 885/1480. One of these is the imamate of the Ṣāliḥiyya *madrasa*.[358] The other one is another teaching position of *fiqh* at a certain *dars Baklamish* in the Muʾayyadiyya. This *dars*, 'class' or 'lecture' is only mentioned on two occasions by al-Sakhāwī: in the biography of Ibn al-Amshāṭī and in the biography of Ibn al-Amshāṭī's brother.[359] Due to lack of additional sources, the most that can be said is that this was a class endowed by a certain Baklamish which took place in the Muʾayyadiyya.[360] Additionally, Ibn al-Amshāṭī taught *fiqh* in the old Ẓāhiriyya *madrasa*[361] after Saʿd al-Dīn al-Kamākhī (d. 886/1481).[362] He taught medicine in the Ibn Ṭūlūn mosque and the Manṣūriyya[363] after al-Sharaf ibn al-Khashshāb's death in 873/1468–1469 as a deputy of (*niyābatan ʿan*) Ibn al-Khashshāb's son, then in his own right.

---

354 For a comparison and analysis of the *thughūr* in the 14th–15th centuries, see Dekkiche, *Crossing the line*, 268–273.

355 Founded in 797/1394–1395 by the amīr Zayn al-Dīn Muqbil al-Rūmī. For the description of the *madrasa*, see al-Maqrīzī, *al-Khiṭaṭ*, IV/584–585.

356 For the description of the market, see al-Maqrīzī, *al-Khiṭaṭ*, III/244–245.

357 For his biography, see al-Sakhāwī, *al-Ḍawʾ*, X/99.

358 For the description of the *madrasa*, see al-Maqrīzī, *al-Khiṭaṭ*, IV/485–490. On the position of *imām*, prayer leader, see Petry, *The civilian elite*, 258–259.

359 In the biography of Ibn al-Amshāṭī: al-Sakhāwī, *al-Ḍawʾ*, X/128. In the biographies of Ibn al-Amshāṭī's brother: al-Sakhāwī, *al-Ḍawʾ*, VI/302, al-Sakhāwī, *Dhayl*, 209, 219.

360 On the various endowed classes that took place in mosques, see Berkey, *The transmission*, 50–56.

361 For the description of the *madrasa*, see al-Maqrīzī, *al-Khiṭaṭ*, IV/505–512.

362 For his biography, see al-Sakhāwī, *al-Ḍawʾ*, I/160–161.

363 For the description of the *madrasa*, see al-Maqrīzī, *al-Khiṭaṭ*, IV/513–515. For the description of the hospital, see al-Maqrīzī, *al-Khiṭaṭ*, IV/692–707. As there was a specific place for the chief physician in the hospital to teach (al-Maqrīzī, *al-Khiṭaṭ*, IV/696), and al-Ṣuyūṭī writes that Ibn al-Amshāṭī was chief physician, the designation 'al-Manṣūriyya' might refer to the hospital rather than to the *madrasa* in this case.

He also substituted (*nāba*) Saʿd ibn al-Dīrī (d. 867/1463), *shaykh* of the Mu'ayyadiyya[364] and those after him in judgeship.[365] Therefore, it seems that Ibn al-Amshāṭī was mostly active in the former Fatimid centre of Cairo, since the above *madrasas* are situated in the walled part of the city (almost exclusively in the *Bayna al-Qaṣrayn* area), with the notable exception of the Ibn Ṭūlūn mosque.[366] Later, at an unspecified date, Ibn al-Amshāṭī abandoned all the professions and positions mentioned above, except for those related to medicine.

Unfortunately, there is no reference to Ibn al-Amshāṭī's position as chief physician, *ra'īs al-aṭibbā'*, other than al-Ṣuyūṭī's short account.[367] When recounting the events of 9 Muḥarram 857/20 January 1453, al-Biqāʿī refers to the then 46–47 years old Ibn al-Amshāṭī as *ḥanafī qāḍī* and physician (*mutaṭabbib*).[368] Thus, if Ibn al-Amshāṭī was named chief physician, this presents a plausible *terminus post quem*.

2.2.6 His Character, Last Years, and Death

Al-Sakhāwī dedicates a fairly extensive part of his biographical account to praising the character of Ibn al-Amshāṭī, emphasising his modesty, righteousness, charm, his desire to do good and pious deeds, and so on. As an example of his interest in the friendship of those with distinguished merits, al-Sakhāwī writes that he had a firm belief in the *imām* of the Kāmiliyya *madrasa*[369] and Ibn al-Ghamrī.[370]

When Ibn al-Amshāṭī's brother died in 885/1480, he inherited his brother's fortune. Once in Ibn al-Amshāṭī's possession, he set it aside for some projects apart from the ones they had previously managed together, like construction of a cistern near the *khānqāh* of Siryāqūs. He commissioned a *turba* as well.

According to al-Sakhāwī, Ibn al-Amshāṭī was one of his oldest friends, listening to his newest works once a week. The biographer even compiled his *al-Ibti-*

364 For his biography, see al-Sakhāwī, *al-Ḍaw'*, III/249–253. Al-Biqāʿī writes that Saʿd ibn al-Dīrī became shaykh of the Mu'ayyadiyya in 827/1423–1424 after his father until his own death, see al-Biqāʿī, *ʿUnwān*, III/26.

365 On the office of *nā'ib qāḍī*, deputy judge, see Petry, *The civilian elite*, 228–229.

366 On the "urban centers" of 15th-century Cairo, amongst them the *Bayna al-Qaṣrayn* area, see Petry, *The civilian elite*, 131–138.

367 Al-Ṣuyūṭī, *Naẓm*, 174.

368 Al-Biqāʿī, *Iẓhār*, I/285.

369 For the description of the *madrasa*, see al-Maqrīzī, *al-Khiṭaṭ*, IV/494–496.

370 Probably Abū al-ʿAbbās al-Ghamrī, son of Muḥammad al-Ghamrī (d. 1445). Unfortunately, al-Sakhāwī does not give his date of birth or death, only that he was young when his father died. For his biography, see al-Sakhāwī, *al-Ḍaw'*, II/161–162.

hāj bi-adhkār al-musāfir al-ḥājj for his friend's sake. Even when Ibn al-Amshāṭī was becoming frail, he kept visiting monthly. Al-Sakhāwī recounts hearing Ibn al-Amshāṭī saying that on a cloudy day in his youth, he saw, without a doubt, a man walking in the clouds. This is the same anecdote told by Ibn al-Amshāṭī to al-Biqāʿī, according to al-Suyūṭī's entry.[371] Al-Sakhāwī's account ends with the statement that, as of 899 AH (1493–1494), Ibn al-Amshāṭī was confined to his house, as he had become too weak to move. He forsook most of his positions, such as teaching at the Ẓāhiriyya, in favour of his student, al-ʿallāma al-Shihāb ibn al-Ṣāʾigh (born 854/1450–1451).[372] From al-Shihāb ibn al-Ṣāʾigh's biography, we can gather that he was not only a student of Ibn al-Amshāṭī but also a relative, being the son of Shams al-Amshāṭī's brother-in-law. Based on the biographical accounts, it seems that Ibn al-Amshāṭī probably left several other positions to be filled by this young relative.

The biography included in the Mosul manuscript gives Ibn al-Amshāṭī's date and place of death as 902 (1496–1497), Cairo. As the manuscript's year of copying is 1568, it would be interesting to know whether there is indeed an additional biographical account of Ibn al-Amshāṭī's life, or else some 70 years after his death, the author or copyist of the biography was able to gather this information some other way.[373] This is an especially intriguing question if we consider the evidence of a listening certificate of another manuscript: a reading of Ibn al-Amshāṭī's *Taʾsīs al-ṣiḥḥa* commenced in 1025/1617 in the Dār al-Shifāʾ of Cairo and the scribe of the certificate referenced al-Sakhāwī for the date of birth and (a lack of) date of death for Ibn al-Amshāṭī.[374] Al-Shawkānī, four centuries later, gives the date of death as Rabīʿ I 902/November–December 1496 with the additional detail that the burial took place in Cairo.[375]

2.3 *Oeuvre*

To reconstruct the literary output of Ibn al-Amshāṭī, al-Sakhāwī's account is the most detailed and thus used as a starting point. Al-Shawkānī mentions only three commentaries rather briefly[376] and al-Ṣuyūṭī's and al-Biqāʿī's short accounts do not touch on this issue at all. However, even the list provided by al-Sakhāwī requires supplementation.

---

371 Al-Ṣuyūṭī, *Naẓm*, 174.

372 Al-Sakhāwī, *al-Ḍaw'*, X/129. For his biography, see al-Sakhāwī, *al-Ḍaw'*, I/239.

373 See section 3.1.2 *MS Mosul, Madrasat Yaḥyā Bāshā 175/9* for a detailed description of the Mosul manuscript and the text of this biography.

374 MS Princeton, Princeton University Library, Garrett 570H, ff. 293r:27–293v:2.

375 Al-Shawkānī, *al-Badr*, II/293.

376 Al-Shawkānī, *al-Badr*, II/293.

Although in most cases the information regarding the works of Ibn al-Amshāṭī are rather limited, they can be grouped into four categories. The first is a commentary on jurisprudence (*fiqh*), the second is two medical commentaries, the third is two additional works on medicine, and the fourth is a work on the buying of slaves, the only one of Ibn al-Amshāṭī's works available in an edition up to now. Without looking at the exact titles, this brief categorical enumeration already shows that the oeuvre of Ibn al-Amshāṭī reflects what his late-life choices attest to, namely that he was a physician first and foremost.

The list below follows the order of the above categories. In the hope of facilitating further research, I attempted to list as many of the surviving manuscript copes of the works as possible, also mentioning the names of the copyists and dates of copying if recorded in a catalogue.

Based on these lists, there are (at least) 38 manuscripts of Ibn al-Amshāṭī's six works with dates of copying ranging from 870/1465 to 1143/1730–1731 which attest his popularity and a continuous interest in his works lasting for approximately two and a half centuries.

2.3.1 *Al-Kifāya*

Among Ibn al-Amshāṭī's works, the sources record only one which is not on medicine, being a commentary of Ṣadr al-Sharīʿa al-Thānī's *al-Niqāya fī al-fiqh*[377] which Ibn al-Amshāṭī memorised during his education. It is entitled *al-Kifāya sharḥ al-Niqāya*[378] or *al-Kifāya fī tawḍīḥ al-Niqāya*.[379] Al-Sakhāwī notes that Ibn al-Amshāṭī borrowed material from his teacher al-Shumunnī's commentary for his own book. Al-Shumunnī allowed him (*adhina lahu*) to use it for teaching and giving legal opinions.[380]

Ibn al-Amshāṭī references and praises his teacher's said commentary in the preface of the *Kifāya* and writes that he intended to abridge it with some additional commentaries to examine and clarify the problems, meanings, and riddles of the *Niqāya*, 'following the clearest methods'.[381] Based on MS Istanbul, Feyzullah Efendi 848, it seems that the commentary is in two volumes (*juzʾ*) and Ibn al-Amshāṭī penned a copy of the first volume on 5 Jumādā II 887/22 July 1482 in Mecca.[382]

377 Being a commentary on his grandfather Burhān/Tāj al-Sharīʿa al-Maḥbūbī's (d. 673/1274–1275) *Wiqāyat al-riwāya fī masāʾil al-Hidāya*, which is a commentary on Burhān al-Dīn al-Marghīnānī's (d. 593/1197) *al-Hidāya*.

378 Al-Baghdādī, *Īḍāḥ*, II/371.

379 MS Istanbul, Feyzullah Efendi 848, f. 1ᵛ:15.

380 Al-Sakhāwī, *al-Ḍawʾ*, X/129.

381 MS Istanbul, Feyzullah Efendi 848, f. 1ᵛ:8–14.

382 MS Istanbul, Feyzullah Efendi 848, f. 123:2–3.

Manuscripts:
- MS Istanbul, Millet Kütüphanesi, Feyzullah Efendi 848 (ʿAbd al-Raḥmān ibn al-Marḥūm ʿAlī al-Damayjamūnī al-Mālikī al-Azharī, 1st part 6 Shaʿbān 1071/6 April 1661, intended for (*bi-rasm*) *al-sayyid al-ḥasīb al-nasīb* al-Sayyid Yaḥyā *nāẓir al-maqām al-burhānī* (f. 123ʳ), 2nd part with the name of the same copyist but without a date (f. 330ᵛ)); this manuscript seems to be a copy of a holograph based on f. 123ʳ:1: *nuqilat hādhihi al-nuskha min khaṭṭ muʾallifihi*, 'this copy was transcribed from the writing of its author' and f. 330ᵛ:9–10: *intahā mā wujida bi-khaṭṭ muʾallifihi fī hādhā al-maḥall*, 'the extant writing of its author ends here'. The text continues on ff. 331ʳ–362ᵛ but stops mid-sentence at the end of the page.
- MS Cairo, Dār al-Kutub, [fiqh al-imām Abī Ḥanīfa?] 398[383]

2.3.2 *Al-Munjaz*

Ibn al-Amshāṭī wrote a commentary on *al-Mūjaz fī al-ṭibb*. Although the *Mūjaz*, an abridgement of Ibn Sīnā's *Qānūn*, is routinely attributed to Ibn al-Nafīs (d. 687/1288), Nahyan Fancy raised various points showing why this is doubtful.[384] As for Ibn al-Amshāṭī's work, it is "a nice commentary in two volumes" that learned men wrote from his dictation and the people circulated a copy of it amongst themselves,[385] named *al-Munjaz*. Ḥājjī Khalīfa had a copy of it and writes that it "demonstrates his proficiency in the profession"[386] and also records the gist of the origins of this work.[387]

In the preface of the work, Ibn al-Amshāṭī praises the *Mūjaz* which he attributes to Ibn al-Nafīs and then writes that he wanted to comment on the section of the *Kulliyyāt*, being the first book of the *Qānūn*, and explain the meaning of the single and compound remedies by overcoming various terminological difficulties. He intended to combine it with his work entitled *Taʾsīs al-ṣiḥḥa bi-sharḥ al-Lamḥa* to connect the two areas of medicine. However, when he finished, he received an order from his full brother, the Ḥanafī chief judge, to finish commenting upon the whole *Mūjaz*. Ibn al-Amshāṭī proceeded in this 'following the best methods'.[388] Based on MS Tunis, Dār al-Kutub al-Waṭaniyya 6713, Ibn al-Amshāṭī finished the commentary on 16 Muḥarram 878/16 June 1473.[389]

---

383 *Fihris Dār al-Kutub 1921*, I/457.
384 Fancy, *Science and religion*, 116–120.
385 Al-Sakhāwī, *al-Ḍawʾ*, X/129.
386 Ḥājjī Khalīfa, *Sullam*, III/305.
387 Ḥājjī Khalīfa, *Kashf*, II/1900.
388 MS Istanbul, Feyzullah Efendi 1319, f. 2ᵛ:14–24.
389 Ibn al-Amshāṭī, *al-Qawl al-sadīd*, 23.

Manuscripts:[390]

- MS Tunis, Dār al-Kutub al-Waṭaniyya 6713 (Muḥammad ibn abī al-Fatḥ Muḥammad al-Ṣūfī, 17 Rabīʿ II 892/12 April 1487)[391]
- MS Istanbul, Süleymaniye Kütüphanesi, Fatih 3581 (Muḥammad ibn ʿAbd al-Raḥmān al-Shāmī, 891/1486[392] and 918/1512–1513)[393]
- MS Istanbul, Millet Kütüphanesi, Feyzullah Efendi 1319 (Aḥmad ibn Muḥammad, 938/1531–1532);[394] this manuscript seems to be a copy of a copy made of a holograph draft based on f. 329ᵛ:23–25: *qāla al-muṣannif raḥimahu wa-kāna al-farāgh min naql hādhā al-kitāb min muswaddatihi ʿalā yad muʾallifihi al-ʿabd al-faqīr ilā Allāh taʿālā Maḥmūd bin Aḥmad al-ʿAyntābī* [poorly dotted] *fī rābiʿ al-Qaʿda al-ḥarām sanat thamān wa-sabʿīn wa-thamānī miʾa*, 'its author said, [God] have mercy on him, copying this book from its draft by the hand of its author was finished [by] Maḥmūd ibn Aḥmad al-ʿAyntābī on 4 Dhū al-Qaʿda 878 [23 March 1474]'.
- MS Cairo, Dār al-Kutub, ṭibb 126 (before 987/1579–1580)[395]
- MS Dublin, Chester Beatty Library, Ar 4027 (undated, 10th/16th c.);[396] the title page, f. 2ʳ specifies that this is volume two of the *Munjaz* and on f. 297ʳ:6–8 we find that Ibn al-Amshāṭī finished copying this book from its draft (*muswadda/musawwada*) on 4 Dhū al-Qaʿda 878/23 March 1474.
- MS Rabat, al-Khizāna al-Ḥasaniyya 238 (Yūsuf ibn Muḥammad ibn Yūsuf, known as al-Wakīl al-Malawī al-Shāfiʿī, 4 Ramaḍān 1093/6 September 1682)[397]
- MS Edirne, Selimiye Camii, Selimiye 4714 (1096/1684–1685)[398]
- MS Paris, Bibliothèque nationale de France, Arabe 2930 (1126/1714–1715);[399] volume two of the *Munjaz*.
- MS Istanbul, Süleymaniye Kütüphanesi, Ḥājī Bashīr Āghā 508 (Aḥmad ibn al-Ḥusayn, 1143/1730–1731)[400]

---

390 Brockelmann lists Erg. 69,100/101, Āṣaf III, 404, 780 (GAL S I/825) and Haddad lists a manuscript in Beirut (Haddad, *An illustrated Arabic medical manuscript*, 251 (n. 8)) which I was unable to verify.

391 Ibn al-Amshāṭī, *al-Qawl al-sadīd*, 22–23.

392 İhsanoğlu, *Fihris*, 103–104.

393 Haddad, *An illustrated Arabic medical manuscript*, 250 (n. 1).

394 İhsanoğlu, *Fihris*, 104.

395 Al-Munajjid, *Maṣādir jadīda*, 251 (no. 31); *al-Fihris al-tamhīdī*, 535; Haddad, *An illustrated Arabic medical manuscript*, 250 (n. 4).

396 Arberry, *Chester Beatty*, V/9–10.

397 Al-Khaṭṭābī, *Fahāris*, 147–149 (no. 143).

398 İhsanoğlu, *Fihris*, 104.

399 Slane, *Catalogue*, 523.

400 İhsanoğlu, *Fihris*, 104.

- MS Cairo, Dār al-Kutub, ṭibb taymūr 194[401]
- MS Cairo, al-ʿAbdaliyya 3500, 3501[402]
- MS Sami I. Haddad Memorial Library, 79/510/883Am/… /74a[403]

2.3.3 *Taʾsīs al-ṣiḥḥa bi-sharḥ al-Lamḥa*

Ibn al-Amshāṭī's other medical commentary is of Abū al-Saʿd ibn Abī al-Surūr al-Sāwī al-ʿAfīf al-Isrāʾīlī's (d. after 689/1290)[404] *al-Lamḥa al-ʿafīfa fī al-ṭibb*. It is named *Taʾsīs al-ṣiḥḥa*. Besides citing its title and part of its incipit, Ḥājjī Khalīfa notes that the commentary is interspersed with the original text.[405]

According to the preface of the work, the *Lamḥa* was so well-known that not memorising it prevented one from prescribing remedies. Furthermore, as a book without an equal amongst abridgements with its brevity but rich terminology, it cannot do without a commentary. As Ibn al-Amshāṭī did not know about such a work, he decided to comment upon the *Lamḥa*, drawing on a number of books.[406] Then he proceeds to detail his methods, one of them being that he mixes the original text in red ink into the commentary, and also 'following the best methods'.[407]

Manuscripts:[408]

- MS Princeton, Princeton University Library, Garrett 570H (Abū al-Wafāʾ Muḥammad ibn Ismāʿīl, 18 Rabīʿ II 870/8 December 1465); copied for Shams al-Dīn al-Qūṣūnī, collated with a copy dated 881/1476–1477, with a reading statement (by Abū al-Ṣalāḥ Madyan ibn ʿAbd al-Raḥmān [al-Qūṣūnī], in the Dār al-Shifāʾ in Miṣr, dated beginning of Rabīʿ al-Awwal 1020/May 1611 to 26 Dhū al-Ḥijja 1025/4 January 1617)[409]

---

401 Al-Munajjid, *Maṣādir jadīda*, 251 (no. 31).

402 Al-Munajjid, *Maṣādir jadīda*, 251 (no. 31).

403 Biesterfeldt—Haddad, *Fihris*, 117–118 (no. 79), Haddad, *An illustrated Arabic medical manuscript*. The manuscript does not appear in Serikoff, *Arabic medical manuscripts* (see both its *Appendix 1, Concordance of manuscripts described in the present catalogue* on pp. 493–494 and its *Appendix 2, List of manuscripts which were not purchased by the Wellcome Library* on pp. 495–496).

404 Al-Sakhāwī, *al-Ḍawʾ*, X/129 names him as Ibn Amīn al-Dawla.

405 Ḥājjī Khalīfa, *Kashf*, II/1561.

406 Listed in Savage-Smith, *A new catalogue*, 355.

407 MS Princeton, Garrett 570H, ff. 1^v:7–2^r:11, MS Paris, BnF Arabe 3025 ff. 2^v:9–3^v:7.

408 Borckelmann lists Gotha 1970 (GAL S II/93) but MS Gotha, orient A. 1970/1 is rather the *Lamḥa*. Cf. Pertsch, *Die arabischen Handschriften*, IV/13 (no. 1970/1).

409 Hitti, *Garrett*, 348 (no. 1110); https://catalog.princeton.edu/catalog/9950819503506421. I would like to thank one of my anonymous reviewers for bringing this entry of the new online Princeton catalogue to my attention.

- MS Istanbul, Beyazıt Devlet Kütüphanesi, Bayazid ʿUmūmī 4212 (956/1549–1550)[410]
- MS Istanbul, Beyazıt Devlet Kütüphanesi, Walī al-Dīn Efendi 2511 (Aḥmad ibn ʿUbayd Allāh ibn Kamāl, 959/1551–1552)[411]
- MS Aleppo, Aḥmadiyya 1264 (26 Rabīʿ I 963/8 February 1556)[412]
- MS Istanbul, Süleymaniye Kütüphanesi, Bagdadli Vehbi 1400 (Zayn al-Dīn al-Jazarī, 26 Rajab 963/5 June 1556)[413]
- MS Oxford, Bodleian Library, Huntington 169 (1st part Sharaf al-Dīn Yaḥyā al-Azharī ibn Nūr al-Dīn ʿAlī al-Kutubī ibn Badr al-Dīn Muḥammad ibn Nūr al-Dīn ʿAlī ibn Sulaymān ibn Hāshim ibn Shams al-Dīn Muḥammad, 1 Rabī I 964/1 February 1557, 2nd part Muḥammad Abū al-Naṣr al-Manūfī al-Ḥanafī)[414]
- MS Paris, Bibliothèque nationale de France, Arabe 3025 (17th c.); 1st part[415]
- MS Paris, Bibliothèque nationale de France, Arabe 3026 (17th c.); 2nd part[416]
- MS Cairo, Dār al-Kutub, ṭibb 497 (Yūsuf ibn ʿAbd Allāh, 1123/1711–1712)[417]
- MS Rampur, Raza Library, 4016 aʾṭ-Ṭib / 4556 M. (12th/18th c.)[418]
- MS Rampur, Raza Library, 4017 aʾṭ-Ṭib / 407 D. (12th/18th c.)[419]
- MS Mashhad, Āstān-i Quds-i Rażawī 24496 (12th SH c./1721–1821)[420]
- MS Istanbul, Beyazıt Devlet Kütüphanesi, Walī al-Dīn Efendi 2512 (2nd part of the work, Aḥmad ibn Aḥmad ibn Muḥammad al-Qānūnī)[421]
- MS Cairo, Maktabat al-Azhar, 7402/72[422]

There is also a *muntakhab* of the work: MS Qum, Marʿashī Najafī 12078/2 (11th SH c./1621–1721).[423]

2.3.4 *Al-Isfār ʿan ḥikam al-asfār*

As for Ibn al-Amshāṭī's other medical works, al-Sakhāwī states that formerly, Ibn al-Amshāṭī used to work for Ibn al-Bārizī who is the recipient of the advice

410 İhsanoğlu, *Fihris*, 17.
411 İhsanoğlu, *Fihris*, 17.
412 Qaṭāya, *Makhṭūṭāt al-ṭibb*, 130–133.
413 İhsanoğlu, *Fihris*, 17.
414 Savage-Smith, *A new catalogue*, 355–358 (no. 79).
415 Slane, *Catalogue*, 538.
416 Slane, *Catalogue*, 538.
417 *The contributions*, 101.
418 ʿArshī, *Catalogue*, V/300–301.
419 ʿArshī, *Catalogue*, V/302–303.
420 Dirāyatī, *Fihristagān*, VI/826.
421 İhsanoğlu, *Fihris*, 17.
422 Al-Munajjid, *Maṣādir jadīda*, 251 (no. 30).
423 Dirāyatī, *Fihristagān*, VI/826–827.

in his *Kurrāsa yuḥtāju ilayhā fī al-safar* ('A booklet needed during the journey').[424] Although the sources do not mention its actual title, this is the treatise *al-Isfār 'an ḥikam al-asfār*.[425] While the fact that a supposed close friend does not mention the treatise by its precise title can seem confusing at first, it might indicate that it was not only al-Sakhāwī sharing his works in progress with Ibn al-Amshāṭī but also the other way around.

As Ibn al-Amshāṭī explains in the preface of the work, he intended to compile a book for his patron that would substitute carrying various books on medicine in which he shows how to preserve health when travelling. This appears to be the only work of Ibn al-Amshāṭī written explicitly for a patron. It is arranged into an introduction, eight chapters on various topics of travel regimens, and an epilogue in two chapters, the first on simple drugs and the second on compound drugs the traveller should bring with himself.

Manuscripts:
- MS Cairo, Dār al-Kutub, majāmīʿ 210/16[426]
- MS Mosul, Madrasat Yahyā Bāshā 175/9;[427] Muḥammad ibn ʿAlī ibn Muḥammad ibn ʿUmar al-Qaltī al-Azharī, 16 Rabīʿ I 976/9 September 1568.
- MS Tarīm, Maktabat al-Aḥqāf, majmūʿat Āl Yaḥyā, 123 majāmīʿ (123/11) (Abū al-Ṣalāḥ Muḥammad al-Ḥanafī, 1083/1672, Egypt)[428]

2.3.5 *Taʾsīs al-itqān wa-al-matāna fī ʿilal al-kulā wa-al-mathāna*

The short biography on the title page of the Mosul manuscript gives one additional title, *Taʾsīs al-itqān wa-al-matāna fī ʿilal al-kulā wa-al-mathāna* ('The foundation of proficiency and hardiness regarding the illnesses of the kidney and the bladder'). However, this is not mentioned in any of the sources or the literature utilised in this chapter, even though there are at least two surviving manuscript copies of the work.

According to its preface, Ibn al-Amshāṭī was residing (*jāwara*) in Mecca in 887/1482–1483 where the most prevalent diseases were those of the kidneys and the bladder. Seeing that there was no physician to satisfactorily treat these diseases, Ibn al-Amshāṭī decided to write a book for them to reveal the truth of

424 Al-Sakhāwī, *al-Ḍawʾ*, X/129.

425 Brockelmann uses the title of the Mosul manuscript ("*Al-Isfār fī ḥukm al-asfār*", GAL S II/93) and al-Ziriklī writes that the *Kurrāsa* is perhaps (*laʿallahā*) the treatise *al-Isfār* (al-Ziriklī, *al-Aʿlām*, VII/163).

426 *Fihrist al-kutub al-ʿarabiyya*, VII–1/261; al-Halwaji, *Catalogue*, I/ 154.

427 Al-Jalabī, *Makhṭūṭāt*, 237.

428 Al-ʿAydarūs, *Fihris*, II/1605 (no. 3852).

these afflictions, save them from erroneous treatment, and explain what is useful, 'following in it, by the grace of God, the best methods'.[429]

Being the other medical non-commentary work of Ibn al-Amshāṭī, the structure of the work also deserves some attention. The *Ta'sīs al-itqān* consists of an introduction, two chapters, and an epilogue. The introduction outlines the anatomy of the kidney and the bladder, the first chapter is on the illnesses of the kidney and their treatments, the second chapter is the same for the bladder, and the epilogue is in three chapters on compound medicaments, simple medicaments, and 'occult properties', *khawāṣṣ* and their uses in this matter.[430] The most interesting feature of this structure concerning the *Isfār* is the presence of an epilogue dedicated to the listing of medicaments connected to the topic of the treatise, as this parallel indicates that appending such material to thematic treatises is a systemic decision of Ibn al-Amshāṭī, in all probability based on his views and expertise regarding the usefulness of such additions.

Manuscripts:
- MS Istanbul, Süleymaniye Kütüphanesi, Shahīd ʿAlī 2006 (ʿAbd al-ʿAzīz ibn ʿAlī al-Muqrī, beginning of Shaʿbān 880/end of November 1475);[431] while the date of copying recorded in the catalogue contradicts the information given in the preface of the work, the year of copying is not clearly legible in the manuscript.
- MS Mashhad, Āstān-e Qods-e Rażavī 6339 (Muḥammad ibn Aḥmad al-Asrī, 27 Rabīʿ II 1029/1 April 1620)[432]

2.3.6 *Al-Qawl al-sadīd fī ikhtiyār al-imā' wa-al-ʿabīd*

In addition to the works listed above, one finds mention of one more treatise, named *al-Qawl al-sadīd fī ikhtiyār al-imā' wa-al-ʿabīd*, which Ibn al-Amshāṭī finished writing in 883/1478–1479, according to Ḥājjī Khalīfa.[433] The treatise 'The pertinent remark on selecting female and male slaves' is the only other work of

429 MS Mashhad, Āstān-e Qods-e Rażavī 6339, f. 1v:4–11; MS Istanbul, Süleymaniye Kütüphanesi, Shahīd ʿAlī 2006, f. 1v:5—f. 2r:2.

430 MS Mashhad, Āstān-e Qods-e Rażavī 6339, f. 1v:11–19; MS Istanbul, Süleymaniye Kütüphanesi, Shahīd ʿAlī 2006, f. 2r:3–13.

431 İhsanoğlu, *Fihris*, 17.

432 Dirāyatī, *Fihristagān*, VI/826.

433 Ḥājjī Khalīfa, *Kashf*, II/249. Al-Baghdādī also lists this work (al-Baghdādī, *Hadiyyat*, II/411) as well as Kaḥḥāla (Kaḥḥāla, *Muʿjam* (1993), 794; Kaḥḥāla, *Muʿjam* (1957), 145) and al-Ziriklī (al-Ziriklī, *al-Aʿlām*, VII/163). Brockelmann mentions it as well (GAL S II/93).

Ibn al-Amshāṭī available in a printed edition.[434] It is based on three manuscript copies of the work (marked with asterisks) which are described in the edition.

In the preface of the work, Ibn al-Amshāṭī praises Ibn al-Akfānī's (d. 749/1348)[435] treatise on the buying of slaves. However, he decides to compose another treatise on the topic to aemend Ibn al-Akfānī's with some important and expert useful information from other authorities, 'following in it, with the help of God, the best methods'.[436] According to MS Istanbul, Ayasofya 3361, Ibn al-Amshāṭī finished writing this work on 5 Rabīʿ II 883/6 July 1478.[437]

Manuscripts:
- MS Cairo, Dār al-Kutub, majāmīʿ Muṣṭafā Fāḍil 77/6 (Aḥmad ibn Ḥusayn al-ʿAbbāsī al-Shāfiʿī, 883/1478)[438]
- * MS Istanbul, Süleymaniye Kütüphanesi, Ayasofya 3361 (Muḥammad ibn Abī al-Fatḥ al-Ṣūfī, 895/1489–1490)[439]
- MS Cambridge, Cambridge University Library, Or. 1023/2 (10 Rabīʿ II 964/10 February 1557)[440]
- * MS Gotha, Gotha Research Library, orient. A 1237[441]
- * MS Cairo, Dār al-Kutub, firāsa ṭalaʿat 15[442]

3 *Al-Isfār ʿan ḥikam al-asfār*

Based on the number of surviving manuscript copies of Ibn al-Amshāṭī's work, his travel regimen entitled *al-Isfār ʿan ḥikam al-asfār* was not as widely circulated as his medical commentaries. Regardless, a closer look at the three manuscripts of the *Isfār* shows that the treatise did enjoy interest for at least approximately 200 years after it was written. Moreover, the textual tradition

434 Ibn al-Amshāṭī, Maḥmūd ibn Aḥmad al-ʿAyntābī, *al-Qawl al-sadīd fī ikhtiyār al-imāʾ wa-al-ʿabīd*, ed. Muḥammad ʿĪsā Ṣāliḥiyya, Beirut: Muʾassasat al-Risāla, 1996. For a concise review of the edition in which I pay attention to how the editor treated the text and its wider context, more specifically its genre and its author, see Csorba, *The genre of travel regimens*, 113–115.

435 For his life and works, see Witkam, *Ibn al-Akfānī*; Ullmann, *Medizin*, 178–179.

436 Ibn al-Amshāṭī, *al-Qawl al-sadīd*, 32.

437 Ibn al-Amshāṭī, *al-Qawl al-sadīd*, 25.

438 ʿAbd al-Bāsiṭ, *Fihris*, VII/73–74 (no. 75).

439 Ibn al-Amshāṭī, *al-Qawl al-sadīd*, 24–25.

440 Arberry, *Cambridge*, 6 (no. 31).

441 Ibn al-Amshāṭī, *al-Qawl al-sadīd*, 25–27; Pertsch, *Die arabischen Handschriften*, II/426.

442 Ibn al-Amshāṭī, *al-Qawl al-sadīd*, 28.

preserved in these manuscripts hints at the reasonable possibility that other copies of the text also existed.

Moving on from the manuscripts to the text they contain, the information present in the preface allows for the straightforward identification of Ibn al-Amshāṭī's patron. This, in turn, makes it possible to pinpoint the period in which the *Isfār* was most likely written.

The chapter ends with a concise summary of the contents of the *Isfār* to provide a general overview of the work.

3.1 *Presenting the Manuscripts*

To the best of my knowledge, the treatise *al-Isfār ʿan ḥikam al-asfār* has (at least) three surviving manuscript copies.

These are MS Cairo, Dār al-Kutub, majāmīʿ 210/16, described by the Library's catalogues and the codex majāmīʿ 210 still present and available for consultation in the Library's Nile Corniche branch.

The second is MS Mosul, Madrasat Yaḥyā Bāshā 175/9. A catalogue from 1927 records the contents of the codex and Brockelmann's GAL lists 175/9 as '*Al-Isfār fī ḥukm al-asfār* Mōṣul 237, 175,9'.[443] When double-checking the title in the indices of GAL, instead of this entry, we find a slightly different title in another entry: '*al-Isfār ʿan ḥukm al-asfār* Mōṣul 34, 53,4'[444] listed amongst the works of Abū Saʿd ʿAbd al-Karīm ibn Muḥammad al-Samʿānī (d. 562/1166). The 1927 catalogue gives the additional information that the *Kashf al-ẓunūn* provides the title as *al-Isfār ʿan al-asfār*,[445] but what is worth pointing out is that *majmūʿa* 153 contains nine treatises in total and all the rest are on medicine. Regarding this, Sellheim noted that 'no. 3, *al-Isfār ʿan ḥukm al-asfār* [Mawṣil 34, 53,4] should be deleted because of faulty ascription'.[446] Unfortunately, I was not able to acquire a copy of this manuscript to clear this issue. However, a microfilm copy of 175/9 is available in the Maʿhad al-Makhṭūṭāt al-ʿArabiyya in Cairo. The Maʿhad also possesses copies of some other works of the same codex but not all of them. Sadly, it is a possibility that these codices were not amongst those that were saved from Mosul in which case it is unlikely that we will be able to clarify this matter definitively.

The third surviving manuscript copy of *al-Isfār ʿan ḥikam al-asfār* is MS Tarīm, Maktabat al-Aḥqāf, majmūʿat Āl Yaḥyā, 123 majāmīʿ (123/11). The Library's catalogue describes the treatises contained in the *majmūʿa*, and the

443 GAL S II/93.
444 GAL S I/565.
445 Al-Jalabī, *Makhṭūṭāt*, 34; Ḥājjī Khalīfa, *Kashf*, 1/86.
446 Sellheim, *al-Samʿānī*, 1025.

Maʿhad al-Makhṭūṭāt al-ʿArabiyya has a microfilm copy of 123/11. In this case, I could not locate copies of other treatises from this codex in the Maʿhad's holdings.

In the following, I aim to give a description of the three manuscripts, in the order above (Cairo, Mosul, and Tarīm manuscript). In general, all descriptions follow the same base structure. Firstly, I describe the codices (contents, codicological observations). Then I move on to the specific manuscripts (title, author, date, copyist, dedication, incipit, explicit, colophon, contents, physical description, scribal errors, scripts and hands). As I was able to examine the Cairo manuscript in person, its description is more detailed than the other two. Other than this, the descriptions vary slightly according to unique features of the specific manuscripts. In most cases, I quoted or summarised catalogue entries and texts of library tags wholly or partially, as the information they contain are essential for the descriptions but not all of these are easily accessible. I translated the shorter, list-like descriptions into English, but I quoted the more lengthy and descriptive ones in their original Arabic. When presenting sections of the Arabic texts, a slash (/) indicates ends of lines and the Eastern Arabic number 5 (٥) represents the dividers.

3.1.1 MS Cairo, Dār al-Kutub, majāmīʿ 210/16

3.1.1.1 *Contents of the Codex*

The Khedivial Library's catalogue lists the contents of the whole codex in one entry under its call number.[447] It gives the number of the treatise, its topic/field, title, incipit, explicit, and if known, its author, details of composition and copying besides the folio numbers. The Egyptian National Library's catalogue of its collections, indispensable as it is, does not give any index to ease locating the contents of whole collections. Rather, one must find the titles individually in the alphabetical list of the four volumes. Thanks to the Khedivial Library's catalogue, the titles to be located were known. While their entries contain much additional information, they seem to accommodate many mistakes as well (e.g. measurements, data on *ijāzas*).[448] Table 1 of the Appendix lists the works contained in the codex as well as the information relevant to dating the manuscripts.

---

447 *Fihrist al-kutub al-ʿarabiyya*, VII–1/258–261.

448 The list of the entries in al-Halwaji, *Catalogue*, listed in order of the treatises: 1: II/493–494 (no. 748); 2: II/421–422 (no. 632); 3: III/270–271 (no. 395); 4: I/206–207 (no. 303); 5 [labelled as treatise number 6]: II/108 (no. 150); 6 [labelled as treatise number 7]: II/495 (no. 750); 7 and 8 [labelled as treatise number 8]: I/44–45 (no. 63); 9: I/466–467 (no. 692); 10: II/203 (no. 297); 11: IV/195–196 (no. 291); 12: III/281–282 (no. 411); 13: IV/356 (no. 527); 14: I/129 (no. 188); 15: III/376 (no. 546); 16: I/154 (no. 225).

Seven of the treatises have their dates of copying recorded, ranging from 607 to 882/1210–1478, and the 9th treatise is an autograph with the author's date of death being 1333. Based on the authors, the 14th treatise is from the 13th century, the first two treatises are from the 15th century, as well as the 16th treatise based on its dedication (however, there are no dates of copying to determine whether the manuscripts themselves are from the same century). While this still leaves some treatises without even rough estimates for dating, there is no direct evidence suggesting that the collection contains treatises from after the 15th century.

3.1.1.2 *Description of the Codex*

MS Cairo, Dār al-Kutub, majāmīʿ 210 is a composite volume consisting of 16 different works. During my visit to the Dār al-Kutub in February 2020, I was able to examine the codex. In the following, I give its codicological description.

3.1.1.2.1 Binding

The codex is bound with a Western binding. The book covers measure 19,5×14 cm and are 3 mm thick. The thickness of the closed volume is 5,5 cm. The boards are pasteboards covered with a greyish brown textile, frayed at the long edges of both boards. The spine is covered with a brownish-black leather, extending over the textile-covered boards by 3 cm. This leather cover is worn out as well, frayed at the top, the bottom, and at the joints. The covering material is torn at the top at the joints of the boards and spine (4 cm and 7 cm on the front side and backside, respectively). The call number of the codex is on the spine in gold in two lines (مجاميع / ٢١٠). Both the front and back covers have the stamped impression of the library's stamp on the upper part of the covers over the meeting point of the textile and leather coverings. Its outer border has the text 'Bibliotheque sultanique' (in upper case). The inner part has the Arabic equivalent, although the text is not clearly legible. As the library was named *Dār al-Kutub al-Sulṭāniyya* between 1914–1922, the stamp is a strong indicator that the codex was (last) rebound during this time.

The doublure on the inner side of the boards is a greenish-brown paper. In the end, there is a flyleaf from the same paper with its stub glued to f. 266^{v}. As of now, there are no flyleaves at the front of the textblock. However, another stub from this paper is present in the textblock, glued to f. 11^{r}, indicating that when the volume was (last) rebound, there was a flyleaf at the beginning as well, as expected.

The textblock spine is lined with reused paper with printed French text on it. This lining is torn into smaller sections lengthwise; nevertheless, it completely conceals the stitching of the textblock. The stitching can be seen only on ff. 1–23, as these folios are loose (ff. 1–10 as a quire, f. 11 completely loose, ff. 12–22 as a quire, f. 23 completely loose). The sewing of these parts seems like it was prepared with three supports.

The textblock itself is attached to the binding only at the end, by three thicker threads secured between the board on the back and its cover. On the front, the stubs of these threads can be seen in between the front board and its cover. These observations support the previous assumption about the sewing of the textblock.

The primary endbands are covered by secondary endbands of a simple pattern of yellow and red threads alternating.

3.1.1.2.2 Textblock

The textblock[449] has a modern foliation of Hindu-Arabic numerals written by pencil on the middle top part of the rectos. There are some exceptions where certain folios have text on these parts. F. 1 is numbered on the verso. The foliation was originally erroneous, as the number 25 was written twice, leading to misnumbered pages until page number 50. Then, this foliation was corrected by the same hand either by writing on top of the erroneous form or by crossing it out and then writing the correct number. As a result, there is a discrepancy of one folio number between the numbers given in the Khedivial Library's catalogue and the numbers present in the volume now in case of the second, third, fourth, and fifth works of the volume.

A closer observation of the textblock reveals that it is quite difficult to deduce information on the history of this composite volume. Since the basic features and measures of the textblock generally change for each work it contains, these are summarised in the following table. The sizes of the textblocks are given in centimetres. While the textblock measurements are varying, they were trimmed, as suggested by many cases where parts of the marginalia are cut off. Measurements of the written areas and numbers of lines vary with each work, occasionally even in the same work. Therefore, these data are not summarised in the table. In general, the inks used throughout the texts seem to be a solid black, with a few exceptions of more translucent, greyish blacks or browns. Reds are sometimes used for chapter headings, keywords, overlining, and dividers. The hands change with each work, occasionally even within a given work in case of notes and certificates. The page layouts are generally the same, the main texts occupy the middle of the pages in a justified block, except for some title pages, colophons, certificates, and poetry. As for the writing support, it is generally a creamy white, varnished paper, with no visible fibres.

---

449 I use the term 'textblock' in the following sense: "The textblock is the body of the codex, made up of quires (gatherings) that receive the text and that can later be sewn and attached to protective covers." Gacek, *Arabic manuscripts*, 265.

No.	ff.	Textblock	Ink	*Misṭara*	Catchwords
1.	1^r–11^v	18×13,5	black, red	n	slanted
2.	12^v–22^v	18×13,5	black	ruling ?	horizontal
3.	23^r–47^v	18×13,5	black, red	n	45°
4.	48^r–52^v	17,5×13	black	ruling ?	horizontal
5.	53^r–57^v	17,5×13	black, red	y	horizontal
6.	58^r–63^v	18×13	black	n	–
7.	64^r–67^v	18×13	black, red	y	occasional
8.	68^r–76^r	18×13	black, red	n	45°
9.	77^r–103^v	18×13	greyish black	n	–
10.	104^r–138^v	18×13	black, red	y	slanted
11.	139^r–186^v	17,5×13	brown	y	–
12.	187^r–204^v	18×13	black	n	45°
13.	205^r–242^r	18×13	brownish black, red	n	45°
14.	242^v–244^v	17×12,5	greyish black	n	–
15.	245^r–253^v	17×12,5	black, red	n	horizontal
16.	254^r–269^v	17,5×12,5 / 18,5×12,5	black, red	y	horizontal

There are some unique features not presented in the above table. Nos. 1–2 have the same yellow discolouration on the outer bottom corners, probably from flipping the pages there. Nos. 3–8 have traces of soaking on the top, which seem quite similar as if soaking happened at the same time. The support of no. 4 is a brown paper with visible fibres, with additional traces of soaking on the side and bottom, as well as traces of bookworms. No. 5 has different traces of bookworms and heavy yellow discolouration on the upper outer corners of the paper. The paper of no. 7 is visibly less varnished. Its catchword on f. 66^v does not match the text of the following folio (a certificate begins there). No. 8 has manmade, clean, straight, and small holes punched through all its folios on the top and bottom near the spine. No. 9 is less varnished with heavy stains of soaking from the top down to the bottom of the folios. No. 10 is less varnished as well, with a lot of discoloured yellow dots, smaller and occasional stains of soaking, and visible fibres. The support of no. 11 is a warm pink-tinted paper with some traces of bookworms, its folios punched through similarly to no. 8, however, only at the bottom. Most probably, it was previously in a type II binding, as the traces of a flap are visible on ff. 139–141 and f. 155 as well. There are unfoliated, smaller bifolia inserted between ff. 159–160 and ff. 171–172 (the latter is not tinted). After no. 12, there is a smaller, unfoliated, empty folio, from a visibly different paper.[450] The support of no. 15 is a brown paper. No. 16 has a creamy white, varnished paper, but with traces of fibres. It has two different textblock sizes: ff. 254–263 measure 17,5×12,5 cm, while ff. 264–269 measure 18,5×12,5 cm. Ff. 264–266 are creased. I was not allowed to use a light sheet for the examination of papers. Therefore, I could not determine whether the group of works with identical textblock sizes and similarly looking papers indeed have the same type of paper.

Due to the modern binding, the quires are not apparent. In the cases where the textblock sizes change, it is visible that approximately half a centimetre of paper width is lost due to the binding, which in some cases results in the ends of lines or catchwords being difficult to read (especially in no. 13). There are only a few cases where the stitching in the middle of the quires is visible. Quire signatures are not present in the volume; the only exception seems to be no. 9, where there is a Hindu-Arabic number two on the upper left corner of f. 86ʳ and a Hindu-Arabic number three on the top left corner of f. 96ʳ. Therefore, I have dispensed with trying to determine the formula of the quires.

3.1.1.2.3 Description of MS Cairo, Dār al-Kutub, majāmīʿ 210/16

I was provided with a digital copy of the manuscript in the form of 31 JPG files of different sizes (2409–3182×3401/4107 pixels; 72 dpi). All images are watermarked with the logo of Dār al-Kutub. The edges of the paper or the bindings rarely appear on the photos. During my visit to the Dār al-Kutub in February 2020, I was able to examine the manuscript itself while examining the codex.

The manuscript is described in the Khedivial Library's catalogue[451] and in the Egyptian National Library's catalogue[452] as well. The first description suggests that this work is a commentary of the text before it in the codex, which is not the case. The second description treats the incipit with some liberty and there seem to be some typos in both the text and the measurements.

3.1.1.2.4 Title, Author, Date, and Dedication

MS Cairo, Dār al-Kutub, majāmīʿ 210/16 (ff. 254ᵛ–269ᵛ) bears the title *al-Isfār ʿan ḥikam al-asfār* (f. 255ʳ, the word '*ḥikam*' being vocalised). The manuscript is not dated. No name of author, scribe, copyist, or owner is recorded in the manuscript; the only reference to these is in the colophon (f. 269ᵛ: *ghafara Allāh*

450 This inserted folio is not accounted for in any of the foliations or catalogues, therefore I avoided devising a new, 'corrected' foliation with a shift in all consecutive folio numbers.

451 *Fihrist al-kutub al-ʿarabiyya*, VII–1/261.

452 Al-Halwaji, *Catalogue*, I/ 154.

li-kātibihi wa-li-ṣāḥibihi wa-li-muṣannifihi wa-li-man qara'a la-hum). It is dedicated to a patron (f. 45v, *al-Kamālī Abū al-Maʿāl Muḥammad al-Juhanī al-Bārizī al-Shāfiʿī*).[453]

3.1.1.2.5 Incipit (f. 254v)[454]

الحمد لله الذي امر بالاسفار ه للتفكر والاعتبار ه وأداء فرايض الحج / والاعتمار ه وجعل
فى الطب من الاسرار ه ما يحفظ الصحة ويبري من / الاضرار ه وصلى الله على سيدنا محمد
اعبده ورسوله الشافي من المضار ه/ ⟦...⟧ وعلى اله واصحابه الاخيار ه ما طرد الليل النهار ه
وأضاء / فجر وانار وبعد

3.1.1.2.6 Explicit (f. 269v)

واما ما يحتاج اليه من السنونات فسنون / يجلو الاسنان زبد البحر محرق ورماد الصدف ورماد
اصل / القصب الفارسي وزراوند مدحرج اجزا سويه وسنون يشتد / اللثه والاسنان قرن ايل
محرق ملح اندراني محرق هليلج اصفر / ورد من كل واحد جزو جلنار نصف جزو ∴

3.1.1.2.7 Colophon (f. 269v)

∴ وهذا / ما اردنا عمله قد كمل ه نسال الله تعالى ان يجعله من صالح العمل ه / ه منقذا من
الاوصاب والعلل ه مبريًا من كل امر حلل ه / ه والحمد لله رب العالمين وصلى الله على سيدنا
ه / ∴ محمد واله وصحبه وسلم ∴ / غفر الله لكاتبه ولصاحبه / ولمصنفه ولمن / قرا لهم ودعا /
بالمغفره / ولجميع / المسلمين / اجمعين ///

The colophon begins in the last line of the explicit, with spacing between the triple dividers. To the right of the colophon's triangle is the stamp of the Khedivial Library (*al-Kutubkhāna al-Khidīwiyya al-Miṣriyya*) in blue ink. To the left of the colophon's triangle is a librarian's note on the number of pages (*ʿadad awrāqihi* ٢٦٩) underlined and signed. It is written over the same faded note that was recorded by the person who wrote the folio numbers in pencil.

453 For more details on the patron and an approximate dating of the treatise itself, see subchapter 3.2 *Dating the Work*.

454 In the cases of the incipit, explicit, and colophon, I attempted to provide a typographical reproduction or diplomatic transcript of the text of the manuscript.

3.1.1.2.8 Contents

The treatise begins with a *basmala* and *ṣalwala*, which are followed by the incipit (f. 245^{v}). The preface proper is on ff. 254^{v}–255^{r}. On f. 255^{r}, there is a list of the chapters with their titles. The treatise is arranged into a short introduction, eight chapters, and an epilogue. The introduction is on the reasons for compilation (ff. 255^{r}–255^{v}). The 1st chapter is on some general issues of travelling (ff. 255^{v}–257^{r}); the 2nd chapter is on travelling in hot weather (ff. 257^{r}–257^{v}); the 3rd chapter is on burning winds (ff. 257^{v}–258^{v}); the 4th chapter is on travelling during winter (ff. 258^{v}–259^{v}); the 5th chapter is on the preservation of limbs (ff. 259^{v}–261^{r}); the 6th chapter is on the preservation of complexion (ff. 261^{r}–261^{v}); the 7th chapter is about water (ff. 261^{v}–263^{r}); the 8th chapter is on travelling on the sea (ff. 263^{r}–263^{v}). The epilogue is divided into two chapters: the 1st is on simple medicaments, hot and cold (ff. 263^{v}–264^{r}); the 2nd is on compound medicaments, listed in 13 categories (ff. 264^{r}–269^{v}). The treatise ends with the colophon on f. 269^{v}.

3.1.1.2.9 Physical Description

The writing surface is a creamy white, varnished, non-watermarked paper with some visible, browner fibres. The chain lines are horizontal, grouped in threes, with 1 cm between each of them. The distance between two groups is 4,3 cm. The number of laid lines in 2 cm is 17–18. These data put this paper in type 3/3 according to the rough typology of non-watermarked papers provided by Humbert.[455]

The textblock measures 17,5×12,5 cm for ff. 254–263 and 18,5×12,5 cm for ff. 264–269. Despite the different sizes, both parts were trimmed, as both have marginalia with parts of their texts cut off. At the meeting point between the two parts, an additional 0,5 cm width can be measured, which is lost due to the current binding of the codex. F. 254 is torn at the crease at the bottom up to the lowest stitching. It folded upon itself on the verso side. There is a brownish yellow thread sticking out between f. 257 and f. 258. Ff. 264–266 have creases as if they were crumpled together. There is a round yellow discolouration on f. 266 (over the written area, lines 7–10, close to the spine). Towards its middle, on the recto side, the ink is slightly paler black. The stub of the greenish-brown

455 This type of paper was present from the 11th to the 15th century in most places of the Islamic world, becoming frequent in the 14th century, and almost exclusive in the 15th century. Unfortunately, this does not facilitate accurate dating of the paper. However, it is worth noting that similar measurements are present in most of the 15th century manuscripts of this paper type in Humbert's corpus (Tableau IV, Type 3/3). Humbert, *Papiers*, 21–22, 33–38.

end flyleaf is glued to f. 266^{v}. F. 269 is glued to f. 267^{r} with a stub. The modern binding makes it quite impossible to give a formula for the quires. Only these last details show that the penultimate quire ends with f. 266, while the last quire is a singulion (ff. 267–268) with a single folio (f. 269) attached to its beginning with a stub.

The written area from the bottom of the first line to the bottom of the last line is 11 × 9 cm. The written area is a justified block in the middle of the pages. The number of lines per page is 17. A *misṭara* (11 × 9 cm) was used for preparing the written area. The first lines of pages are written on top of the upper line of the *misṭara*. On f. 63^{v}, one line is left empty between the 8th chapter and the epilogue. For justification of the text, superscription is used in many cases, though the justification is somewhat sloppy. The manuscript was not foliated. Page numbers were added later, on the middle top of the recto pages by pencil. Catchwords appear on all the verso pages, written horizontally below the last line separately. They are the first word of the next folio (f. 254^{v}, 255^{v}, 256^{v}, 257^{v}, 258^{v}, 267^{v}), with the preceding *wa-* (f. 264^{v}, 265^{v}, 266^{v}, 268^{v}), *aw-* (f. 260^{v}), *min* (f. 259^{v}), *fa-innahu* (f. 261^{v}), or *an* (f. 262^{v}). The catchword on f. 263^{v} is the only exception, being *bizr al-mulū* for *bizr al-mulūkhiyya*. The text was written with solid black ink. Chapter headings, keywords, and the dividers (inverted commas on ff. 254^{v}–255^{r} and f. 269^{v}; three inverted commas in a triangle shape on f. 269^{v}) are written with a deep red ink. In some cases, keywords are in black ink but marked with red overlines. While the reds seem the same with some slight variation (maybe different batches prepared with the same pigment), there are two instances when the red is rather orangey (f. 257^{v}:16, *wa-idhā kāna*; insertion above f. 268^{r}:9, *mā*).

3.1.1.2.10 Scribal Errors

A curved line between the words indicates places of omission. The insertions are inscribed on the margin mostly horizontally, or in an approximately 45-degree angle upside down (f. 255^{v}, 266^{v}), and once vertically (f. 264^{r}). Omitted words are also inserted above the line (f. 257^{v}, 263^{v}, 268^{r} twice). Occasionally, parts of the marginalia are cut off, but it is obvious that all the insertions end with the abbreviation *ṣād-ḥā*ʾ for *ṣaḥḥa*, with one exception (f. 265^{v}). In one case, the correction of cacographic error is done by repeating the word in the margin with the abbreviation *bā*ʾ for *bayān*(*uhu*) (f. 256^{v}). There are examples of writing the affected letter in small above or below the main letter shape (f. 256^{v}, 262^{r}, 268^{r}, 269^{r}). The third method is writing the abbreviation *ṣād-ḥā*ʾ similarly to the shape of the Eastern-Arabic numeral 4 (٤) under the affected letter while writing on top of the original letter to try to conceal and correct the cacographic error (f. 254^{v}, 255^{r}, 256^{v}, 257^{v}, 258^{v}, 259^{v} twice, 260^{v}, 261^{r}, 264^{r}, 265^{r}, 266^{v},

268^{r} [three more corrections are not marked], 269^{r}). Cancellations are made by crossing out the main letter shapes with a continuous line (f. 255^{r} twice, 256^{r}, 256^{r}). In some cases, whole words are scraped off the paper (f. 254^{v}, 262^{r}, 262^{v}). Scraping off certain letters and diacritical marks to correct the text is common (f. 254^{v} twice, 255^{r}, 255^{v}, 256^{r}, 257^{r}, 258^{v}, 259^{r}, 262^{r}, 263^{r}, 264^{r}, 264^{v} twice, 265^{r}, 266^{r}, 266^{v} twice). In many cases, this was employed to correct the conjugation of verbs and change masculine forms to feminine and vice versa (f. 255^{v} twice, 257^{r}, 258^{v} twice, 261^{r} twice, 262^{r} twice, 262^{v}, 263^{r}, 265^{v} thrice). In one case, the two dots of the infixum *tāʾ* of stem VIII were removed (263^{r}); the stem I form of the verb was used in the other two manuscripts. On f. 267^{v}, two red dots were placed above a word and then removed, probably sponged up while the ink was still wet.

3.1.1.2.11 Scripts and Hands

The script of the main text is a serifless, legible *naskh*. The words are slightly descending onto the baseline. The letter *alif* in its joined form is slanted to the right above the x-line. The *lām-alif* ligature does not have a visible loop. The counters of the letters *ʿayn, ghayn, fāʾ, qāf, mīm, hāʾ* (in final connected position), *wāw*, and *tāʾ marbūṭa* are generally not present. The catchwords, interlinear insertions, and corrections of cacographic errors are made by the same hand. He is probably the *kātib* referred to in the colophon. In the marginalia, a second hand can be observed: it is a serifless, legible *naskh* as well, but the letter-shapes are slenderer. Joined *alif*s are vertical. The *lām-alif* ligature has a triangular-shaped loop. The bodies of *ʿayn* and *ghayn* not in first positions are triangular and counterless, but the other counters are present. The *alif maqṣūra* in the preposition *fī* is characteristically different as well. This second hand is responsible for most of the cancellations and addenda (f. 255^{r} [two cancellations and marginalia], 255^{v}, 256^{r} [cancellation], 257^{r}, 257^{v}, 258^{v}, 261^{r}, 263^{r}, 264^{r}, 266^{v}, 268^{r}, 269^{r}). On f. 255^{r}, where the second hand corrected the table of contents, it is also obvious that he did not only make cancellations in the main text and added marginalia, but also inserted two prepositions into the main text. Also, certain vocalizations seem to be from this second hand (f. 258^{r}, 264^{v}, 265^{v}). However, a few marginalia and cancellations of single words are from the main hand (f. 256^{r} [cancellation], 256^{v} [correction of cacographic error], 261^{v}, 264^{v}, 265^{r} [cancellation], 265^{v}, 266^{v} [cancellation], 267^{r} [cancellation], 268^{v} [two cancellations]).

Diacritical pointing is used throughout the main text and the marginalia as well. The preposition *fī* is mostly written with *alif maqṣūra*. The *tāʾ marbūṭa* has its dots almost all the time. Conjugation of third-weak verbs is not consistent. Scraping off diacritical marks mentioned in the previous section is frequently employed to correct conjugation, mostly for alternating the *yāʾ* and *tāʾ* imperfect prefixes. In some cases, the letter *sīn* has three subscript dots (f. 256^{v}, 257^{r}, 257^{v}, 258^{v}, 263^{r} marginalia, 265^{r}, 268^{r}); however, the same words can be found in the text written with dotless *sīns*. Dots are occasionally missing from verbal prefixes and *yāʾ* letters in medial or end positions. Diacritical points are missing systematically only once in a short sentence (f. 261^{v}). Vocalization is rarely present (f. 254^{v}, 255^{r} twice, 258^{r} twice, 260^{v}, 261^{v}, 265^{v}, 268^{r}). The letter *hamza* only appears in a few cases (written on the line, on *alif* chairs, or dotted *yāʾ* chairs), mostly toward the beginning of the text. Generally, it is omitted or replaced by *yāʾ* in medial positions. However, *hamza* is written peculiarly on top of a *wāw* chair in one case on f. 256^{r} (line 16: *fī buṭʾihā*, في بطؤها).

3.1.2 MS Mosul, Madrasat Yaḥyā Bāshā 175/9

3.1.2.1 *Contents and Description of the Codex*

A catalogue of the manuscripts of Mosul from 1927 does not give any kind of physical description, but it lists the treatises contained in the codex as follows:[456]

> **١٧٥** مجموعة. فيها: «١» الاقراباذين على ترتيب العلل، لنفيس الدين بن عوض السمرقندي. «٢» كتاب الاغذية والاشربة. «٣» كتاب اطعمة المرضى. «٤» رسالة في الادوية المستعملة عند الصيادلة. «٥» الادوية المسهلة. «٦» كتاب الادوية المركبة. وهذه الكتب الخمسة الاخيرة تدعى بالخمسة النجيبية نسبة لنجيب الدين السمرقندي. «٧» كمال الفرحة في دفع السموم وحفظ الصحة، لشمس الدين محمد القوصوني. «٨» مقالة في الحمام، للقوصوني ايضاً. «٩» كتاب الاسفار عن حكم الاسفار، لمظفر الدين محمود العنتابي المعروف بالامشاطي. «١٠» مقالة في دفع السموم لموسى بن عبد الله الاسرائيلي. «١١» كفاية الاريب عن مشاورة الطبيب، للشيخ سري الدين احمد.

The author of the catalogue, al-Jalabī had read this collection and wrote an article three years later correcting a mistake in the catalogue entry. Initially, he attributed both the 7th and 8th treatise to the same author; however, they were written by a father and his son, respectively. He also quoted the biography of the son, present in the manuscript under the title of the 8th treatise.[457] In

456 Al-Jalabī, *Makhṭūṭāt*, 237.

457 Al-Jalabī, *Man huwa al-Qūṣūnī*.

another article, al-Jalabī quoted two more biographies which were recorded in the manuscript by the same hand: one for the author of the 9th treatise, and one for the author of the 11th treatise.[458]

Other than the catalogue and the two articles mentioned above, I have not found further descriptions of this codex; therefore, I am not in the position to give a proper codicological description of it.

Despite this, some characteristics can be observed due to the following. Besides the 9th treatise, the Maʿhad al-Makhṭūṭāt al-ʿArabiyya prepared microfilm copies of the 7th and 8th treatises as well under the call numbers al-ṭibb 693 and al-ṭibb 762, respectively. Both are foliated on the upper left corner of the recto sides with Hindu-Arabic numerals. This foliation was seemingly prepared with the same ink as that of the main texts. However, it is not always clearly visible, due to apparent trimming of the textblocks or creases. As for the 7th treatise, its f. 10ʳ has *al-thānī* written above the numeral (slightly trimmed, but legible). F. 20ʳ most definitely had its quire signature (being *al-thālith*), even though it is not visible on the manuscript due to trimming, for f. 10ʳ of the 8th treatise has *al-rābiʿ*. Unfortunately, this treatise is comprised of only 14 folios; therefore, no further observations can be made regarding the quire signatures. While the same foliation is present on the 9th treatise as well, none of its nine folios has visible quire signatures. Nevertheless, paired with the similarities of the textblocks and scripts, this might indicate that at least these three treatises (with either the current 6th treatise or an entirely different work) formed a codicological unit before ending up as part of MS Mosul, Madrasat Yaḥyā Bāshā 175. Since the 11th treatise has its own short biography, it might be that this proposed previous codicological unit contained treatises 10 and 11 as well. Regardless of the above speculations, the codex as a whole is a quite practical medical collection with six of its treatises on pharmacology and dietetics, two on poisons and antidotes, and the rest also on practical matters.

3.1.2.2 *Description of MS Mosul, Madrasat Yaḥyā Bāshā 175/9*

I was provided with a digital copy of the microfilm copy of the manuscript in the form of 13 JPG files of different sizes (2880 × 4736 pixels for the cover; 5176–5696 × 4864–4992 pixels for 2–2 pages; 5288 × 4864 pixels for the back; 200 dpi). The microfilm copy was made by the Maʿhad al-Makhṭūṭāt al-ʿArabiyya with the call number al-ṭibb 317. During my visit to the Institute, I was able to consult the microfilm copy in addition to the digital images.

---

458 Al-Jalabī, *Maḥmūd al-ʿAntābī al-Amshāṭī*.

3.1.2.2.1 Description on the Library Tag

The information on the library tags is as follows:[459]

Library: Madrasat Yaḥyā Bāshā al-Jalīlī—al-Mawṣil No. of film: 33 [+34]
No. of book: 8
Title of book: Majmūʿa fī al-ṭibb (containing 11 treatises)
Topic: medicine
Author: numerous authors
Date of copying:—
No. of leaves:—[257]
Size: 24,5 × 15 cm

3.1.2.2.2 Title, Author, and Date

MS Mosul, Madrasat Yaḥyā Bāshā 175/9 (ff. 1ʳ–9ʳ) bears the title *Kitāb al-isfār ʿan ḥukm al-asfār* (f. 1ʳ, vocalized). The name of the author is given immediately after the title: al-shaykh al-imām al-ʿallāma Muẓaffar al-Dīn Maḥmūd al-ʿAntābī, known as al-Amshāṭī. The name of the copyist is given in the colophon (f. 9ʳ): Muḥammad ibn ʿAlī ibn Muḥammad ibn ʿUmar al-Qaltī al-Azharī. The date of copying is given in the colophon as well: 16 Rabīʿ I 976 (9 September 1568).

3.1.2.2.3 Title Page (f. 1ʳ)[460]

كتَاب الإسْفَار عن حُكْمِ الأَسْفار / للشيْخ الامام العَلّامة مُظَفّر الدين مّحْمُود / العنتَابِي المعْرُوف بالأمشَاطي / تغمدَهُ الله تعين برحمَته /

مولفه محمود بن احمد ں حسن بن اسمعيل ں يعقوب ں اسمعيل الشيخ مظفر الدين ں الامام شهاب الدين الامشاطى / العنتابي الحنفى القاهرى اخو قاضى القضاه بمصر محمد الامشاطى الحنفى ولد فى حدود سنه اثني عشر / وثمانمايه وكان فقيها طبيبا فاضلا متفننا فى جميع العلوم درس وافتى وحدث والف شرحا / على النقايه فى الفقه وشرحا على الموجز (فى الطب) لابن النفيس حسنا جامعا حافلا في مجلدين كبيرين وشرحا / على اللمحه فى الطب ايضا لابن امين الدوله وكتب عدّه رسايل فى الطب منها تاسيس الاتقان / والمتانه فى علل الكلى والمثانه ومنها القول السديد فى اختيار الاماء العبيد / ومنها رساله في ما يحتاج اليه المسافر كتبها لابن البارزى

459 The data in square brackets is given only on the tag at the end.

460 In the cases of the title page, incipit, explicit, and colophon, I attempted to provide a typographical reproduction or diplomatic transcript of the text of the manuscript.

وكان صالحا خيرا حسن الاعتقاد / ذكر انه راي وهو دون البلوغ رجلا يمشى فى الغمام لا شك فى ذلك وكان على طرتقه حسنه / وعمر واسن فنزل عن وظائفه واقبل على الله تعالى وعمل عدة من الخيرات والآثار الي / توفى سنه اثنتين وتعمام بالقاهره رحمه الله تعالى نقلت ذلك من الضو وغيره ///

3.1.2.2.4 Incipit (f. 1v)

الحَمْدُ لِلَّهِ ە الَّذِي امَر بالاسْفار ە للتفكّر وَالاعتبار / واذاء فرايض الحج والاعتمار ە وجهَاد المتمردين مِن ە/ الْكُفّار ە وجَعَلَ فِي الطّبّ مِنَ الاسْرَار ە ما يخفظ / الصّحة ويبْرى الاضرار ە واشهد ان لا اله الا الله ە/ وَحْده لا شرِّيكَ له النّافِع الضّار ە واشهَدُ ان سَيّدنا / محمدًا عَبْده المختَار ە ورَسُولهُ الشَافِي مِن الاضرار / المضار ە الهادِيُءِ الي المنافِع وَالمباد ە صَلى الله عَلَيْهِ / وَعَلى آله الاخيَار ە وازواجه الاطهار ە وإصحابه ە/ الاجيَار ە ما طرد الليل النهار ە وَاضَآ الفجر وَانار ە/ وبَعْدُ ...

3.1.2.2.5 Explicit (f. 9r)

واَمّا ما يحتاج اليه من / السنونات فسنون بجلو الاسنان زبد البحر محرق ورماد الصّدف ورماد / اصل القصب الفارسي وَرراوند مدحرج اجزا سوية وسنون تشد اللثه / والاسنان قرن ايل محرق ملح اندرانى محرق هليلج اصفر ورد من كل واحد / جز مجُلّناد نصف جزء

3.1.2.2.6 Colophon (f. 9r)

ە هَذا اخر مَا اردنا عمَله ە تم الكّاب ە بعون / الملك الوهاب ە والله اعلم بالصّواب ە واليه المرجع والماب ە / ە على يد اقل عباد الله واحوجهم الى عفوه وغفرانه ە / ە محمد بن على بن محمد بن عمر القلتى الازهرى عفى الله ذنوبه ە/ ە وستر عيوبه وعفى عنه وسامحه ە / ە ولمانحه ولجميع المسامين ە / ە في سادس عسر ە / ە ربع الاول ە / سنه / ە ٩٧٦ ە///

The colophon begins in the last line of the explicit.

3.1.2.2.7 Contents

The treatise begins with the title and author's name. The actual text of the treatise is preceded by a short biography of the author (f. 1r). After this part, the manuscript follows the same structure as MS Cairo, Dār al-Kutub, majāmīʿ

210/16. On f. 1^{v}, the text begins with the *basmala*, which is followed by the incipit. The preface continues after the incipit, but with some changes compared to the Cairo manuscript's text (ff. 1^{v}–2^{r}). After this part, on f. 2^{r}, the chapters with their contents or titles are listed. The introduction is on ff. 2^{r}–2^{v}. The 1st chapter is on ff. 2^{v}–3^{r}; the 2nd chapter is on ff. 3^{r}–3^{v}; the 3rd chapter is on ff. 3^{v}–4^{r}; the 4th chapter is on ff. 4^{r}–4^{v}; the 5th chapter is on ff. 4^{v}–5^{r}; the 6th chapter is on f. 5^{r}; the 7th chapter is on ff. 5^{r}–6^{r}; the 8th chapter is on f. 6^{r}. The epilogue's 1st chapter is on ff. 6^{r}–6^{v}; its 2nd chapter is on ff. 6^{v}–9^{r}. The treatise ends with the colophon on f. 9^{r}.

3.1.2.2.8 Physical Description

It seems that the lower right corner of the manuscript got soaked, leaving a mark on the folios up to ten lines from the bottom vertically and to the middle of the lines horizontally. However, the text remained legible even on the copy. The number of lines per page is 31. The title page and first page have 14 lines, while the last page has 34 lines. The justification of the text block is quite neat. There are only a few cases of superscription, mostly in the biographical section. The manuscript was foliated on the upper left corners of the recto sides with Hindu-Arabic numerals. Catchwords appear on all the verso pages, written in an approximately 45° angle below the last line separately. They are the first word of the next folio (f. 1^{v}, 4^{v}, 5^{v}, 6^{v}, 7^{v}, 8^{v}), with the preceding *wa-* (f. 2^{v}, 3^{v}). The catchwords on f. 2^{v}, 3^{v}, and 4^{v} stained the following recto pages. The text was written most probably in black ink. Chapter headings, keywords, and the dividers (full circles on ff. 1^{v}–2^{r}, full and hollow circles on f. 9^{r}) are most probably in red ink. In the digital copy, these parts are greyer and blurrier compared to the darkness and sharpness of the supposed black ink. In some cases, keywords are overlined. The title and author's name on f. 1^{r} also show on f. 1^{v}, while the dividers and the red *wa-baʿdu* (especially the part "*aʿdu*") show on f. 1^{r}, and these parts also left faint marks on f. 2^{r}.

3.1.2.2.9 Scribal Errors

There are only a few scribal errors I was able to locate on the copy of the manuscript. Place of omission is indicated once by an inverted caret between the words with its extended arm pointing towards the margin. The insertion is inscribed on the margin horizontally, with the abbreviation *ṣād-ḥāʾ* for *ṣaḥḥa* under the inserted word (f. 2^{v}). The numeral 2 (٢) is used once on f. 5^{r} for a one-word gloss. A cacographic error is corrected by writing the abbreviation *ṣād-ḥāʾ* in a shape similar to the Eastern-Arabic numeral 4 (٤) under the affected letter while writing the correct form above the letter shape (f. 7^{v}).

3.1.2.2.10 Scripts and Hands

The script of the short biography is a serifless, legible *nastaʿlīq*. The words are descending onto the baseline. The isolated *alif*s are either straight and vertical or slanted to the right with left-foot hairlines. The *lām-alif* ligature does not have a visible loop. The counters are visible only in the letterforms of *ṭāʾ-ẓāʾ*, *ṣād-ḍād*, and isolated *hāʾ*. Horizontal lines are somewhat elongated. The bowls of the letterforms are pronounced, and the descenders are elongated, almost reaching to the ascender lines of the next lines. The title of the biography is a more decorative, partially seriffed *naskh* with some variation in each of its four lines regarding the lettershapes.

The script of the main text is a serifless, legible *naskh*. The words are sitting neatly on the baseline. The letter *alif* is straight and vertical in isolated positions but slightly slanted to the right above the x-line in its joined form. The *lām-alif* ligatures are neat and somewhat triangular with visible loops, resembling the *al-lām alif al-warrāqiyya*. The counters are visible only in the letterforms of *ṭāʾ-ẓāʾ*, *ṣād-ḍād*, and in some cases in isolated, connected, or final connected forms of *hāʾ* and *tāʾ marbūṭa*. The catchwords, interlinear insertions, and corrections of cacographic errors are made by the same hand. The script on the first page of the main text (f. 1ᵛ) is more spaced out and airy than the rest of the text. Chapter headings are further emphasised by elongation of the horizontal lines. Diacritical pointing is used throughout the text. The preposition *fī* and the *tāʾ marbūṭa* have their dots almost all the time. The preposition *fī* is written in two distinct forms throughout the text by the same hand. Dots are occasionally missing from verbal prefixes. Vocalization is present occasionally throughout the text. The letter *hamza* is omitted or replaced by *yāʾ* in medial positions. It appears once on f. 6ʳ.

3.1.3 MS Tarīm, Maktabat al-Aḥqāf, majmūʿat Āl Yaḥyā, 123 majāmīʿ (123/11)

3.1.3.1 *Contents and Description of the Codex*

Based on the catalogue of the Maktabat al-Aḥqāf,[461] 123 majāmīʿ contains 12 treatises (nos. 3842–3853).[462] The catalogue gives the number, title, author with the date of death (if known), incipit, explicit, type of script, name of scribe (if known), date and place of copying (if known), whether there are words written in red, number in the collection, number of lines, and finally the measurements. At the end of the entries, all manuscripts are identified as *Maktabat*

461 I would like to thank Kinga Dévényi and Anne Regourd for referring me to this catalogue.
462 Al-ʿAydarūs, *Fihris*, II/1601–1605.

al-Aḥqāf, majmūʿat Āl Yaḥyā, under the number 123, majāmīʿ, Tarīm. In the following, I summarize the treatises of the collection in order based on the catalogue mentioned above, giving only their number, title, and if known, the name of the author, copyist, and date of copying.

No. 3842: *Masʾala li-l-shaykh Aḥmad al-Bājīrīqī fī maʿrifat muddat al-mulūk wa-al-salāṭīn*
Copyist: Yūsuf ibn ʿAlī ibn Muḥammad al-Mallāḥ
No. 3843: *Albūm* [sic] *fī ḥawādith al-Rūm*
Author: ʿAbd al-Raḥmān al-Busṭāmī (d. 858/1454)
No. 3844: *al-Bashāʾir al-ḥātima bi-asbāb ḥusn al-khātima*
Author: ʿAbd Allāh Mīr Ghanī (d. 656/1258)
No. 3845: *Sharḥ al-waraqāt*
Author: Jalāl al-Dīn al-Maḥallī (d. 864/1459)
Copyist: ʿAbd al-Maʿṭī al-Samalāwī
Date of copying: 1077/1666–1667
No. 3846: *Talqīn al-mayyit*
No. 3847: *al-Fawāʾid al-bāriza wa-al-kāmina fī al-niʿm al-ẓāhira wa-al-bāṭina*
Author: Jalāl al-Dīn ʿAbd al-Raḥmān ibn abī Bakr al-Suyūṭī (d. 911/1505)
Copyist: ʿAlāʾ al-Dīn ibn ʿAbd Allāh ibn Kāmil al-Shāfiʿī
Date of copying: 977/1569–1570
No. 3848: *al-Rayḥāna al-aryaḥa li-ʿāqidī al-ankaḥa al-ṣaḥīḥa*
Author: Muḥammad ibn al-Qāḍī ʿAbd al-ʿAzīz al-Minībārī
Copyist: ʿAbd Allāh ibn Muḥammad al-Kāf
Date of copying: 1242/1826–1827
No. 3849: *Arbaʿīn ḥadīthan*
Author: ʿAbd al-Raḥmān ibn Sulaymān al-Ahdal (d. 1250/1835)
Copyist: Muḥammad Ṣāliḥ al-Raʾīs
Date of copying: 1235/1819–1820
No. 3850: *Asʾila fī iʿṭāʾ al-zakāt wa-naqlihā*
No. 3851: *Sharḥ al-dāʾira*
Author: Abū al-Ḥasan ʿAlī al-Shādhalī (d. 656/1258)
No. 3852: *al-Isfār ʿan ḥikam al-asfār*
Author: Maḥmūd al-ʿAntābī al-Amshāṭī (d. 902/1496)
Copysit: Abū al-Ṣalāḥ Muḥammad al-Ḥanafī
Date of copying: 1083/1672, in Egypt
No. 3853: *Ḥall al-rumūz wa-mafātīḥ al-kunūz*
Author: ʿAbd al-Salām ibn Muḥammad ibn Ghānim al-Maqdisī (d. 678/1279)

As for the authors, the given dates of deaths range from 656 to 1250/1258–1834. The dates of copying range from 977 to 1242/1569–1826. Due to the presence of 19th century treatises in this collection, as well as the slightly varying measurements in general, it is right to assume that MS Tarīm, Maktabat al-Aḥqāf, majmūʿat Āl Yaḥyā, 123 majāmīʿ is a composite volume with 12 treatises on various topics, which were bound together not earlier than 1826. It is a possibility that the codex was (re)bound when it was microfilmed by the Maʿhad al-Makhṭūṭāt al-ʿArabiyya in 1976.[463] Based on the available data, nothing more can be said about this volume with certainty.

In accordance with the system of shelfmarks of the previous two manuscripts, I will refer to the 11th treatise of this *majmūʿa* as 123/11.

3.1.3.2 *Description of MS Tarīm, Maktabat al-Aḥqāf, majmūʿat Āl Yaḥyā, 123 majāmīʿ (123/11)*

I was provided with a digital copy of the microfilm copy of the manuscript in the form of 13 JPG files of different sizes (2030×1536 pixels for the library tag at the front; 2064×1664 pixels for the library tag at the end; 2064/2080×1664 pixels for the images of the manuscript; 200 dpi). The microfilm copy was made by the Maʿhad al-Makhṭūṭāt al-ʿArabiyya with the call number al-ṭibb 17. During my visit to the Institute, I was able to consult the microfilm copy in addition to the digital images.

3.1.3.2.1 Description on the Library Tag

The information on the identical front and back library tags is as follows:

الإسفار عن حكم الأسفار　　　　ف ٤٣ له ١٥٦

لمظفر الدين محمود　　　　العنتابى الأمشاطى

وهى رسالة فى بيان الحاجة إلى السفر وما ينبغى للمسافر فعله، والسفر فى الحر والشتاء، وحفظ الأطراف واللون وأمور المياه والسفر فى البحر، وما يصطحبه المسافر من الأدوية المفردة والمركبة.

أولها: «الحمد لله الذى أمر بالأسفار، للتفكر والاعتبار.. »

وآخرها: «وأما ما يحتاج إليه من السنونات. وسنون يشد اللثة والأسنان: قرن أيل محرق. وهذا آخر ما أردناه، والله سبحان وتعالى أعلم»

---

463 Van den Boogert, *The manuscript library of Tarīm*, 157.

نسخة كتبت بقلم فارسى، كتبها أبو الصلاح محمد الحنفى سنة ١٠٨٢ هـ بمصر، وبعص [*sic*] كلماتها بالهمزة.

١١ ورقة ضمن مجموعة من ١٠٠–١١٠ ٢٧

سطرا ١٢×٢٠,٥ سم

[مكتبة الأحقاف—مجموعة آل يحي ١٢٣ مجاميع—تريم]

A second tag was put on the library tag with the date of microfilming:

جامعة الدول العربية

المنظمة العربية للتربية والثقافة والعلوم

معهد المخطوطات العربية

صور في يوم الاثنين ٢١ ربيع الأول

١٣٩٦ هـ

الموافق ٢٢ مارس

١٩٧٦ م

3.1.3.2.2 Title, Author, and Date

The 11th treatise of MS Tarīm, Maktabat al-Aḥqāf, majmūʿat Āl Yaḥyā, 123 majāmīʿ (ff. 100r–110r) bears the title *Irshādāt li-man arāda al-safar* (underlined thrice), *Kitāb al-isfār ʿan ḥ.k.m al-asfār* (f. 1r, not vocalized, except for the hamzas) written below the underlining. The name of the author is given immediately after the title: al-ʿallāma Muẓaffar al-Dīn Maḥmūd al-ʿAntābī, known as al-Amshāṭī. The name of the copyist is given in the colophon (f. 110r): Abū al-Ṣalāḥ Muḥammad al-Ḥanafī. The date and place of copying is given in the colophon as well: 17 Jumādā I 1083 (10 September 1672), Egypt.

3.1.3.2.3 Incipit (f. 100v)[464]

الحمد لله الذي امر بالاسفار ه للتفكر والاعتبار ه واداا فرابض الحج والاعتمار ه / وجهاد المتمردن من الكفار ه وجعل في الطب من الاسرار ه ما يحفظ الصحة / ويبري من الاضرار

464 In the cases of the title page, incipit, explicit, and colophon, I attempted to provide a typographical reproduction or diplomatic transcript of the text of the manuscript.

ه واشهد ان لا اله الا الله النافع الضار ه واشهد / ان سيدنا محمدا عبده ورسوله المختار ه الشافي
من المضار ه الهادي الي / المنافع والمسار ه صلي الله عليه وعلي اله الانصار ه وازواجه الاطهار
ه/ واصحابه الاخيار ه ما طرد الليل النهار ه واضا الفجر وانار وبعد /

3.1.3.2.4 Explicit (f. 110^{r})

واما ما يحتاج اليه من السنونات فسنون يجلو الاسنان زبد البحر / محرق ورماد الصدف ورماد
اصل القصب الفارسي ورراوند مدحرج / اجزا سوية وسنون يشد اللثه والاسنان قرن ايل
محرق ملح اندزاني / محرق هلىلج اصفر ورد مس كل واحد حر جلناد نصف جز

3.1.3.2.5 Colophon (f. 110^{r})

وهذا آخر / ما اردناه والله سحانه وتعالى اعلم / تمه الفمر أبو الصلاح محمد / الحنفى / ى ١٧
جمادى الاولى / من شهور سىه ١٠٨٣ ىمصر ///

The colophon begins in the last line of the explicit. The date of copying is written in an approximately 45° angle, the day on the right side, the year on the left side of the copyist's name, shaping a triangle.

3.1.3.2.6 Contents

The treatise begins with a title page with the title and the author's name, as well as many notes (f. 100^{r}). The manuscript follows the same structure as the previous two. On f. 100^{r}, the text begins with the *basmala*, which is followed by the incipit following the text of MS Mosul, Madrasat Yaḥyā Bāshā 175/9 with some changes in the part with the *shahāda*. The preface continues after the incipit (f. 100^{v}). After this part, the chapters with their contents or titles are listed (ff. 100^{v}–101^{r}). The introduction is on f. 101^{r}. The 1st chapter is on ff. 101^{r}–102^{r}; the 2nd chapter is on ff. 102^{r}–102^{v}; the 3rd chapter is on ff. 102^{v}–103^{r}; the 4th chapter is on ff. 103^{r}–103^{v}; the 5th chapter is on ff. 103^{v}–104^{r}; the 6th chapter is on f. 104^{v}; the 7th chapter is on ff. 104^{v}–105^{v}; the 8th chapter is on ff. 105^{v}–106^{r}. The epilogue's 1st chapter is on f. 106^{r}; its 2nd chapter is on ff. 106^{r}–110^{r}. The treatise ends with the colophon on f. 110^{r}.

3.1.3.2.7 Physical Description

Each of the microfilmed images is stained in different patches, making it impossible to make assumptions about the condition of the manuscript. The text, however, remained legible on all folios and areas. F. 104^{v} and f. 105^{r} are the middles of a quire, as the thread clearly shows on the image, so there is a chance that the textblock is a regular quinion. According to the catalogue of Maktabat al-Aḥqāf, the page dimensions are 20,5 × 13 cm.[465] The number of lines per page is 27. The justification of the written area is neat. The chapter headings, as opposed to the main text, are always written in a separate line, aligned to the centre. The manuscript has a modern foliation on the upper left of the recto sides with Hindu-Arabic numerals. Catchwords appear on all the verso sides, written horizontally below the last line separately. They are the first word of the next folio, written by the same hand as the main text. While this is not apparent on the images, as in the case of the Mosul manuscript, some of the words are in red ink according to the catalogue.[466] Keywords are overlined throughout the text.

3.1.3.2.8 Scribal Errors

The text is free of marginalia, and there are only two instances of scribal corrections that I was able to locate. One is an interlinear correction, where the scribe inserted the correct word above the erroneous one with a superscript *ṣād-ḥā*ʾ for *ṣaḥḥa* (f. 103^{r}). The other one is a cancellation by crossing out two words with a single line (f. 109^{v}).

3.1.3.2.9 Scripts and Hands

The script is a serifless, legible *nastaʿlīq*. The words are descending onto the baseline. The isolated alifs are either straight and vertical or slightly slanted to the right. The *lām-alif* ligature does not have a visible loop. The counters are visible only in the letterforms *ṭāʾ-ẓāʾ* and *ṣād-ḍād*, with some exceptions where it is not visible even in these letterforms. Horizontal lines are somewhat elongated. The bowls and descenders of the letterforms are pronounced. The catchwords and the interlinear insertion are made by the same hand. Diacritical pointing is used throughout the text. The preposition *fī* and the *tāʾ marbūṭa* have their dots almost all the time. The preposition *fī* is written in two distinct forms throughout the text. Vocalization is rarely present. The letter *hamza* is omitted, and in medial positions only its chair is present.

3.1.4 The Textual Tradition of the *Isfār*

"Thinking of the stemma one should try to avoid thinking of a tree and its branches. The few disparate textual witnesses that we do have are often noth-

465 Al-ʿAydarūs, *Fihris*, II/1605.
466 Al-ʿAydarūs, *Fihris*, II/1605.

ing more than a small pile of twigs and branches, of which we will probably never know where in the tree(s) of transmission they had their place."[467] This is how Witkam starts his article in which he recounts his practical experience in editing Arabic texts, stemmatology, and Islamic manuscripts. In this article, he focuses on the course of his editing of a text with sixty-six manuscripts. However, in an earlier article, he gave some other examples and scenarios as well, where he did not "reject the principles of stemmatization", but concluded that "it is hardly ever possible to establish in practice a carefree and unstrained stemma".[468] In the case of *al-Isfār ʿan ḥikam al-asfār*, there are three manuscripts at our disposal. This number certainly spares many problems resulting from having an abundance of copies as well as those coming from editing unique manuscripts. Despite this, it still has its pitfall. Namely, it would be quite convenient to arrange the manuscripts in chronological order and link them together, as a cursory study of the variant readings could support this decision. Such a stemma, however, could be misleading. Even with an only potential connection of the manuscripts and inclusion of hypothetical versions, it would be unlikely to include possibly surviving, but not yet discovered copies, neither those lost to us in their correct place in the 'tree'. Instead of producing such a stemma full of uncertainties, I aim to compare them based on the descriptions above and the variant readings. In order to make the text less cumbersome, hereinafter I reference the three manuscripts in a shortened form: (MS) C for MS Cairo, Dār al-Kutub, majāmīʿ 210/16; (MS) M for MS Mosul, Madrasat Yaḥyā Bāshā 175/9; and (MS) T for of MS Tarīm, Maktabat al-Aḥqāf, majmūʿat Āl Yaḥyā, 123 majāmīʿ (123/11).

Even though a chronological order might be misleading, as mentioned above, the first things to consider are the data on copying. While we have such data on M (16 Rabīʿ I 976/9 September 1568) and T (17 Jumādā I 1083/10 September 1672; Egypt), for C, we have no relating information in the colophon or other places of the manuscript.

As noted in the description, nothing indicates that the codex of C contains treatises copied after the 15th century. Based on the dedication of the work, I infer in sub-chapter *3.2 Dating the Work* that the most probable period the treatise was written is 842–850/1438–1447. I presume that C is an early copy of the treatise copied in the 15th century. This presumption is supported by some observations of the text of C. Firstly, the characteristics of the paper seem to correspond to those of the 15th century. Secondly, it has the simplest prefaces

467 Witkam, *The philologist's stone*, 34.
468 Witkam, *Establishing*, 98.

of the three manuscripts. As the other two texts have whole rhythmic units inserted into the *sajʿ* and on more occasions break up a rhythmic unit of C into more units, this is not a case where the principle of *difficilior lectio potior* would be applicable by default. A simpler preface, however, would provide the perfect opportunity for later copyists to amend it and shape it more to the needs and liking of their commissioners. It could be a possibility that the text of C is an earlier version preserved in a later copy. However, the corrections present in the manuscript make this implausible. Thirdly, there is a distinct second hand responsible for the majority of cancellations and addenda. Only a few marginalia and single-word cancellations are made by the main hand of the text, while the second one made the more significant changes. A conspicuous feature of these is the chapter titles. These are corrected by the second hand both in the table of contents and in the actual text. The substantial changes of the epilogue are also made by the second hand. This would suggest that C might be an early copy of the text, maybe even a quite neatly composed draft or scholarly copy which was re-read and corrected after composition. Lastly, a unique feature of C is providing the correct spelling or meaning of foreign words on three occasions, all omitted by M and T. These are for *qayrūṭī* (as vocalised in the manuscript) and *dūgh* in chapter 1 (see in the edition: 124:3–4; 124:8) and *kāghad* in chapter 5 (134:7). On the other hand, both M and T have the spelling and explanation of *būlīmūs* in chapter 4 (130:3–4). Even with this exception, the principle of *difficilior lectio potior* can be applied here, especially since the treatise is dedicated to the head of the chancery, a layman. While some explanation of technical terms can be a welcome addition in such a case, if physicians had commissioned M and T, such information might have been superfluous. (Since the codex of M comprises medical treatises, at least one of the two manuscripts might indeed have been prepared for a physician.)

While the observations above could suggest a reasonably straightforward stemma, other clues indicate that the copyists of M and T might have had a slightly different version of the text at their disposal. M and T both omit the text of C in some cases where an involuntary scribal mistake is not likely. Such examples can be found in 126:20 and 134:7. They also simplify the text ending chapter 8 (144:15–16); while they have a simple God almighty knows best, C has a more lengthy praising formula separating the actual chapters from the prologue on simple and compound medicaments. In 126:20 and 136:1, both M and T supplement the text of C with additional information of a medical nature. Despite that these additions are short, it is unlikely that a scribe himself makes such additions or substitutions without the use of another manuscript or notes. The marginal and interlinear notes of C are worth mentioning here as well. In a few cases, C's addenda or corrections made in marginal notes, interlinear notes, or via crossing words out is not reflected in M and T (118:7; 122:10, 146:10) but most of them found their way into both manuscripts (126:1; 128:1; 130:1; 136:16; 140:1; 144:1, 13; 146:1; 150:4; 154:14–15; 160:1, 9, 15, 20). There are also deviations from C on which both M and T agree (122:2, 5, 13; 126:18, 20; 128:10, 12; 130:3, 13, 15; 134:3, 5, 7, 9, 11; 136:1; 138:9; 140:16, 17; 144:2, 8, 8–9; 146:2, 7; 148:1, 4, 14; 150:3, 4, 13; 152:11, 13, 15, 18; 154:8, 18; 156:17; 158:17; 160: 2–3; 162:5, 13, 14). It seems that at some places the scribes of M and T could not make sense of the version(s) they copied from and offered different solutions for certain words (136:3; 140:8; 148:14; 160:5; 162:19).

However, there are also examples indicating that the scribes of M and T had different version(s) as a source to copy from. In case of a liniment recipe, a verb in a marginal note of C is included in M but omitted from T (162:20). In one instance, T includes an erroneously added word also found in M but then this word is crossed out and thus only the correct word found in C remains in T (158:5). T has some shorter insertions as well as omissions in some places not present in C or M (120:7; 124:10–11; 126:21; 128:20; 132:3, 6–7, 10; 138:6, 7; 140:2, 17).

Furthermore, there are two interesting errors in T. The first one is at the end of chapter 4 (132:6–7), where the scribe most probably skipped a line. In a list of plants, after the first word, he copied two plant names, then returned to the beginning of the list, and ended it with the last two plant names already present in the list due to the error. The layout of C (f. 259ᵛ:11–12) could result in such a line-skipping mistake, as the *wa-* for the two repeated plant names aligns perfectly with the *wa-* of the actual second item of the list. As for M (f. 4ᵛ:3–4), the layout is accidentally somewhat similar, but the words do not align as neatly for this error as in C. On another occasion in chapter 7 in 142:9, T skipped another line. Here, the words causing the error are *yushrabu maʿahu*, which appear perfectly aligned in C (f. 262ᵛ:5 and 6). For both line-skipping errors, the layout of C can be pinpointed as the origin of the scribal mistake. In the end, however, this presents only two instances that would obviously link C and T.

Based on the above observations, it seems that the copyists of M and T based their work on a cleaner copy of C, with the reasonable possibility that the copyist of T had C at his disposal as well. Without any further evidence, nothing more can be said about the relationship of the surviving manuscript copies with certainty.

3.2 *Dating the Work*

Of the three surviving manuscript copies of Ibn al-Amshāṭī's *al-Isfār* that we know of, MS Cairo is not dated but the colophons of MS Mosul and MS Tarīm contain dates of copying. These are 16 Rabīʿ I 976/9 September 1568 and 17 Jumādā I 1083/10 September 1672, respectively. The relationship of the textual variants preserved in the three manuscripts indicates that MS Cairo was most likely at the disposal of the scibes of the other two manuscripts, meaning the terminus ante quem for its copying is 976/1568 but codicological evidence of MS Cairo does not contradict a somewhat earlier, 15th-century dating either. While these dates concern only the physical copies of the text, it is also possible to inquire about the dating of the text itself, as a closer look at the *Isfār*'s preface provides some details about the origins of the treatise.[469]

The initia of the manuscript starts with the *basmala* and a *ṣalwala* for Muḥammad, then the text is rendered into a *sajʿ*. In accordance with *ḥusn al-ibtidāʾ*,[470] Ibn al-Amshāṭī praises God for commanding to travel and for making medicine hold secrets which preserve health and cure harms. The initia ends with another *ṣalwala* for Muḥammad, his family, and his companions. The preface proper after the *baʿdiyya* shows the picture of preparing oneself with humbleness and restraint for visiting ritual sites, while anticipating God's forgiveness at the end of times. This is when the patron appears: he is the *imām* whose qualities are praised, then his name and title follow: *al-Muqirr* ('the Safeguarder'), *al-Ashraf* ('the Noblest'), *al-Karīm* ('the Beneficent'), *al-ʿĀlī* ('the Sublime'), *al-Amāmī* ('the Foremost'), *al-ʿĀlamī* ('the Renowned'), *al-ʿAllāmī* ('the Insightful'), *al-Kamālī* ('the Perfect'; shortened form of Kamāl al-Dīn), *Abū al-Maʿāl Muḥammad al-Juhanī al-Bārizī al-Shāfiʿī, nāẓir dawāwīn al-inshāʾ al-sharīf bi-al-diyār al-miṣriyya wa-sāʾir al-mamālik al-islāmiyya* ('the superintendent of the noble chancery of Egypt and the rest of the Muslim countries'). Following this, Ibn al-Amshāṭī elaborates on his reasons and ways of writing this treatise for his patron, the naming of the treatise, and gives the table of contents as well after expressing his hopes that his work will be appreciated.

The phrases *nāẓir dawāwīn al-inshāʾ al-sharīf* and *al-diyār al-miṣriyya wa-sāʾir al-mamālik al-islāmiyya* are strong indications that the patron was a high-ranking official of the Mamluk Sultanate. As the *Ṣubḥ al-aʿshā fī ṣināʿat al-inshāʾ* by al-Qalqashandī (d. 821/1418) is "the culmination of the secretarial manuals and encyclopaedias of the Mamlūk period",[471] it should be the fundamental source when looking for 'the superintendent of the noble chancery'.

469 See the Commentary, chapter 1 *Preface: A Literary Analysis* for a more comprehensive discussion of the preface.

470 Bonebakker, *Ibtidāʾ*, 1006.

471 Bosworth, *al-Ḳalḳashandī*, 510.

In the introductory section, al-Qalqashandī writes about the office of *ṣāḥib al-dīwān* [i.e. *al-inshāʾ*] ('head of the Chancery') at length.[472] Yet in later parts of his work when he gives a detailed description of the administrative office-holders (*arbāb al-waẓāʾif al-dīwāniyya*) and their duties, the *ṣāḥib al-dīwān* is not listed. Still, when writing about the *kātib al-sirr* ('secretary, scribe of the secret'), al-Qalqashandī records that this office was introduced by the sultan Qalāwūn (r. 678–689/1279–1290).[473] Besides the *kātib al-sirr*'s numerous tasks, the *kuttāb al-dast* ('scribes of the pedestal', the higher-ranking scribes) and *kuttāb al-darj* ('secreterial scribes', who prepared the documents for the *kuttāb al-dast*) are in his *dīwān*. This indicates that the *kātib al-sirr* is the *ṣāḥib al-dīwān*, meaning the head of the Chancery. As al-Qalqashandī explains, the latter two designations were used as synonyms: in his time, the superintendent was called *ṣāḥib dīwān al-inshāʾ* in Egypt, and if one wanted to address him in a more exalted way, there were the options of *ṣāḥib dawāwīn al-inshāʾ* (by using *dawāwīn*, the plural form of *dīwān*), *nāẓir dawāwīn al-inshāʾ* (since *nāẓir* is grander than *ṣāḥib*), and even more, *bi-al-diyār al-miṣriyya* and *bi-al-mamālik al-islāmiyya* could be added.[474] All this confirms that the title of *kātib al-sirr* is the one to be looked for when identifying the patron, noting that Ibn al-Amshāṭī used the most exalted designation possible for dedicating his work.

As for the Bārizī *nisba*, the idenfitication is straightforward. The Bārizī family[475] lived in Ḥamā for many generations, where they held several civilian posts besides occupying the judgeship for around 120 years with only one interruption.[476] It was Nāṣir al-Dīn Muḥammad (769–823/1368–1420) who, after various events, ended up in Cairo with ties to none other than the sultan al-Muʾayyad Shaykh (r. 815–824/1412–1421),[477] being his *kātib al-sirr* in addition to holding other posts as well.[478] This Nāṣir al-Dīn Muḥammad had two sons: Shihāb al-Dīn Aḥmad (d. 822/1419), an *amīr* whose funeral was attended by the sultan al-Muʾayyad;[479] and Kamāl al-Dīn Muḥammad, who followed his father as *kātib*

472 Al-Qalqashandī, *Ṣubḥ al-aʿshā*, I/101–129.

473 Al-Qalqashandī, *Ṣubḥ al-aʿshā*, IV/28–29. On the chancery and Qalāwūn, see Northrup, *From slave to sultan*, 239–242.

474 Al-Qalqashandī, *Ṣubḥ al-aʿshā*, I/103.

475 For a comprehensive discussion of the family, see Martel-Thoumian, *Les civils*, 248–266.

476 Hirschler, *The formation*, 106–107, 108.

477 See Holt, *al-Muʾayyad Shaykh*, 271–272; Holt, *The age of the Crusades*, 178–183.

478 Martel-Thoumian, *Les civils*, 250–251; Hirschler, *The formation*, 107–108.

479 Ibn Taghribirdī, *al-Nujūm*, XIV/159; Martel-Thoumian, *Les civils*, 254; Hirschler, *The formation*, 108.

al-sirr and to whom the treatise *al-Isfār ʿan ḥikam al-asfār* is dedicated. One of their sisters, Mughul, married the future sultan Jaqmaq (r. 842–854/1438–1453).[480]

Kamāl al-Dīn Abū al-Maʿālī Muḥammad ibn al-ʿAllāma al-Qāḍī Nāṣir al-Dīn Abī al-Maʿālī Muḥammad ibn al-Qāḍī Kamāl al-Dīn Muḥammad ibn ʿUthmān ibn Muḥammad ibn ʿAbd al-Raḥīm ibn Hibatallāh al-Bārizī al-Ḥamawī al-Juhanī al-Shāfiʿī[481] was born on 11 Dhū al-Ḥijja 796/7 October 1394 in Ḥamā. He grew up under the care of his father, memorizing the Quran. Travelling around the Middle East, they first went to Cairo (809/1406–1407), then returned to Syria, and lived in Ḥamā, Aleppo, and Damascus, in accordance with the posts of the father. Meanwhile, Kamāl al-Dīn pursued studies in the fields of law, grammar, literature, and rhetoric.[482] In 815/1412, they moved to Cairo, where Nāṣir al-Dīn first became *muwaqqiʿ* ('signer'), then filled the post of *kātib al-sirr* from 3 Shawwāl 815/6 January 1413.[483] Due to Kamāl al-Dīn's skills in free prose, poetry, letter writing, and composition, he became his father's deputy.

After his father died, Kamāl al-Dīn paid 40,000 dinars to the sultan to become the new *kātib al-sirr* on 25 Shawwāl 823/2 November 1420.[484] Soon, 17 days after the death of the sultan al-Muʾayyad, on 26 Muḥarram 824/31 January 1421,[485] he left this post and was named *nāẓir al-jaysh* by the *amīr* Ṭaṭar, who was to become sultan al-Ẓāhir Ṭaṭar (r. 29 Shaʿbān 824–824 Dhū al-Ḥijja 824/29 August 1421–30 November 1421).[486] Kamāl al-Dīn lost the post after the death of al-Ẓāhir Ṭaṭar. Between holding offices, he returned to his studies. Later, Barsbāy was enthroned as sultan (r. 8 Rabīʿ II 825–813 Dhū al-Ḥijja 840/31 March 1422–1427 June 1438).[487] He named Kamāl al-Dīn *kātib al-sirr* of

---

480 See Martel-Thoumian, *Les civils*, 255.

481 As recorded by Ibn Taghribirdī. Ibn Taghribirdī, *al-Nujūm*, XIV/13 lists ʿUthmān twice in the genealogy, as opposed to all other sources listing him only once: Ibn Taghribirdī, *al-Manhal*, XI/10; al-Maqrīzī, *Durar*, III/247; al-Sakhāwī, *al-Ḍawʾ*, VIII/236; al-Suyūṭī, *Naẓm*, 168 (the latter two listing Shams al-Dīn Ibrāhīm, also connecting the family to one of the companions of the Prophet).

482 For a detailed list of the works he studied and his teachers, see Ibn Taghribirdī, *al-Nujūm*, XIV/13–14; al-Sakhāwī, *al-Ḍawʾ*, VIII/237.

483 For an account of his life and career, see Martel-Thoumian, *Les civils*, 250–251 and the sources listed by her on p. 262.

484 The sources give different dates: Ibn Taghribirdī, *al-Manhal*, XI/11: 25 Shawwāl 823; Ibn Taghribirdī, *al-Nujūm*, XIV/15: 25 Shawwāl 823; al-Sakhāwī, *al-Ḍawʾ*, VIII/237: Shawwāl 823.

485 Ibn Taghribirdī, *al-Manhal*, XI/11: 26 Muḥarram 824; Ibn Taghribirdī, *al-Nujūm*, XIV/15: Muḥarram 824; al-Sakhāwī, *al-Ḍawʾ*, VIII/237: Muḥarram 824.

486 See Holt, *The age of the Crusades*, 183–184.

487 See Wiet, *Barsbāy*, 1053–1054; Holt, *The age of the Crusades*, 184–189.

Damascus on 7 Rajab 831/22 April 1428. Meanwhile, he was the Damascene shāfiʿī *qāḍī al-quḍāt* as well. After the *kātib al-sirr* of Cairo was removed, Barsbāy recalled Kamāl al-Dīn to Cairo as *kātib al-sirr* on 20 Rabīʿ II 836/14 December 1432.[488] However, he was removed again on 7 Rajab 839/26 January 1436.[489] On 1 Rajab 840/9 January 1437, he returned to Damascus as *qāḍī al-quḍāt* and *khaṭīb* of the Umayyad mosque. After Jaqmaq secured the throne for himself (19 Rabīʿ I 842/9 September 1438),[490] his brother-in-law, Kamāl al-Dīn was called back to Cairo as *kātib al-sirr* once again on 17 Rabīʿ II 842/7 September 1438[491] and remained in this position until his death on 26 Ṣafar 856/18 March 1452.[492] Even Jaqmaq attended his funeral. Kamāl al-Dīn performed the *ḥajj* in 850/1447.[493] According to contemporary sources, he was admired and often portrayed as the embodiment of the ideal *kātib*.[494]

As can be seen, Kamāl al-Dīn Muḥammad filled the position of *kātib al-sirr* of the Sultanate three times: first between 25 Shawwāl 823–826 Muḥarram 824/2 November 1420–31 January 1421; then between 20 Rabīʿ II 836–837 Rajab 839/14 December 1432–26 January 1436; and lastly between 17 Rabīʿ II 842–826 Ṣafar 856/7 September 1438–18 March 1452.

Since the treatise *al-Isfār ʿan ḥikam al-asfār* was dedicated to him as *kātib al-sirr*, it was most probably compiled during one of these three periods. The patron performing the *ḥajj* gives the perfect opportunity for composing such a work for him, a presumption further supported by the theme of travel for religious purposes in the preface of the *Isfār*. This would make the period 17 Rabīʿ II 842–850/7 September 1438–1447 the most convenient timeframe for the writing of the treatise. However, due to the lack of decisive evidence from other sources, a more certain date of composition cannot be determined.

3.3 *Describing the Content*

The brief summary of the contents of Ibn al-Amshāṭī's *al-Isfār ʿan ḥikam al-asfār* below aim to provide a general overview of the work's contents before

488 Ibn Taghribirdī, *al-Manhal*, XI/13; Ibn Taghribirdī, *al-Nujūm*, XIV/15–16.

489 Ibn Taghribirdī, *al-Manhal*, XI/13; Ibn Taghribirdī, *al-Nujūm*, XIV/16.

490 See Sobernheim, *Čaḳmaḳ*, 6; Holt, *The Age of the Crusades*, 189–190.

491 Ibn Taghribirdī, *al-Manhal*, XI/13: Rabīʿ II 842; Ibn Taghribirdī, *al-Nujūm*, XIV/16: 17 Rabīʿ II 842; al-Sakhāwī, *al-Ḍawʾ*, VIII/238: "*fī awwal salṭanat al-Ẓāhir*".

492 Ibn Taghribirdī, *al-Manhal*, XI/15: 16 Ṣafar 856; Ibn Taghribirdī, *al-Nujūm*, XIV/13: 26 Ṣafar 856.

493 Ibn Taghribirdī, *al-Manhal*, XI/14; Ibn Taghribirdī, *al-Nujūm*, XIV/17; al-Sakhāwī, *al-Ḍawʾ*, VIII/239.

494 For the list of his biographies and positions, see Martel-Thoumian, *Les civils*, 262, 264.

moving on to the Arabic text, the English translation, and further analyses of the text. Therefore, it lacks references, comparisons, or preliminary evaluations.

3.3.1 Preface

The initia commences with a *basmala* and a *ṣalwala*. It continues in *sajʿ* with a *ḥamdala*, and then follows the rhetorical concept of 'skilful opening'[495] before ending with another *ṣalwala*.

The middle part starts with the *baʿdiyya*, from where Ibn al-Amshāṭī builds up to the introduction of the patron. After this, Ibn al-Amshāṭī gives his reason and method of compilation for this treatise and expresses the intended purpose of the work. The last item of this middle part of the preface is the title of the treatise.

In the last part of the preface, Ibn al-Amshāṭī turns to God, attempting to secure his favour through praise and appeal. Then, he ends the preface by listing the titles of the treatise's chapters (*faṣl*).

3.3.2 Introduction

In a short but theoretically dense introduction (*muqaddima*), Ibn al-Amshāṭī states that the sudden deviation from the usual circumstances of life can be the cause of dangerous diseases, and the exertion and fatigue of travelling strengthen this effect. He briefly explains the underlying reasons and articulates his approach to the topic; the traveller should know what is useful and harmful to avoid illnesses. In other words, he advocates prophylaxis or prevention.

3.3.3 First Chapter

The first chapter can be divided into three parts of approximately equal lengths discussing preparation for travelling, hunger, and thirst.

In the first part of the first chapter, Ibn al-Amshāṭī lists ten principles to observe for the successful purging (*istifrāgh*) of the body before embarking on a journey. Then, he specifies the means of purification: purgation/diarrhoea (*ishāl*) and bloodletting (*faṣd*). Furthermore, he lists five factors to consider when performing bloodletting. After the issue of purging, Ibn al-Amshāṭī recommends getting used to the various circumstances which are likely to occur during one's travel. He also advises the traveller to bring with himself what eases the anticipated hardships of the journey.

495 Bonebakker, *Ibtidāʾ*, 1006.

In the second part of the chapter, which discusses hunger, Ibn al-Amshāṭī advises eating food prepared from roasted livers, especially if the food was made with oils and fats. He also explains why these foodstuffs work well against hunger, adding some theoretical explanation to the practical list of proper foodstuffs.

In the third part of the chapter on thirst, Ibn al-Amshāṭī advises eating foodstuffs with moistening and cooling effects in addition to those prepared with sour things. Then, he lists useful foodstuffs to consume in the case of hot weather. Ibn al-Amshāṭī completes this list with the recipe of a thirst-quenching pill and also offers two easy to come by substitutes. At the end of this section, he also forbids eating food that causes thirst.

3.3.4 Second Chapter

In this chapter, Ibn al-Amshāṭī discusses travelling in hot weather. He presents a concise theoretical discussion of what happens in this situation and takes note of the usual harms of such travels, then gives practical advice to combat most of these. In the second half of this chapter, he provides detailed instructions for those with dry temperaments. Besides simply presenting instructions, he gives short theoretical explanations to back up his recommendations.

3.3.5 Third Chapter

The object of this chapter is closely related to the previous one, as it discusses the *samūm*, a 'very hot and burning wind'. First come the prophylactic instructions, then approximately two-thirds of the chapter deal with treating the negative effects caused by the *samūm*. Ibn al-Amshāṭī groups his advice into two parts: for those without a fever and for those with affected by fever.

3.3.6 Fourth Chapter

In this chapter, Ibn al-Amshāṭī discusses travelling in winter, in the cold, or to cold places. He explains why cold poses a danger to the body, freezing it or resulting in a kind of hunger, *būlīmūs*. After explaining what this condition is, he lists two more common dangers of travelling in the cold: the limbs falling off and weakening of the vision. Then, he gives general advice. Lastly, he details what to do in case the traveller was affected by the cold.

3.3.7 Fifth Chapter

In the previous chapter, Ibn al-Amshāṭī promises to write ('God Almighty willing') on preserving the limbs in cold weather. In this chapter, he gives some practical preventive measures for the traveller to safeguard his limbs, including the prevention of the weakening of sight. Then he moves on to how to cure the affected limbs. Here, he provides some theoretical background once again. While he notes that this affliction does not necessarily cause ulcers, he nevertheless divides the treatment according to the type of ulcers and the swollenness of the limb. As for the treatment of swollen limbs, he quotes the method of the empiricists (*wa-qāla baʿḍ al-mujarribīn*), then he elaborates on the proper treatment according to the state of the limb.

3.3.8 Sixth Chapter

In this chapter, Ibn al-Amshāṭī provides useful and practical advice on how to preserve the complexion by coating the skin with various substances. He gives a recipe of a cerate for treating fissured skin. Since discolouration of the skin can be caused by excessive heat or cold in addition to washing oneself with costive waters, this chapter offers a thematic link between the previous chapters on travelling in hot or cold weather and the following chapter on waters.

3.3.9 Seventh Chapter

In this chapter, Ibn al-Amshāṭī discusses the various types of water the traveller encounters on his journey. He points out that the constitution needs water more than it needs food; therefore, a change in waters can make the traveller sicker than a change in foodstuffs. In the first part of this chapter, he lists the best and worst kinds of water with their characteristics. In the second part of this chapter, Ibn al-Amshāṭī details the prophylaxis against particular types of water. He states that vaporisation (*taṣʿīd*), distillation (*taqṭīr*), and boiling ward off the possible harms, and he explains why and how these processes work. Then he deals with salty, alumic, and stagnant waters in particular. In the third and last part of this chapter, Ibn al-Amshāṭī recommends two practices to ensure safe consumption of various waters in general.

3.3.10 Eighth Chapter

In the last chapter of the work, Ibn al-Amshāṭī explains why nausea and vomiting occur when travelling on sea. He then gives some practical advice on how to prevent nausea and vomiting and calm and strengthen the stomach. The chapter ends with praising God and a *ṣalwala* for Muḥammad, his family, and his companions.

3.3.11 Epilogue

The epilogue (*khātima*) lists all the medicaments the traveller should bring along in two chapters (*faṣl*).

In the epilogue's first chapter, Ibn al-Amshāṭī lists a total of 74 simple medicaments in two groups, hot (45) and cold (29) ones.

In the second chapter, Ibn al-Amshāṭī lists certain compound medicaments to use for certain ailments, organised according to the type of the medicaments. These are syrups (9), robs (6), electuaries (5), purgative pills (4), suppositories (2), pastilles (3), medicinal powders (3), collyriums and eye remedies (3), oils (13), liniments and powders (2 and 2, respectively), haemostatics (2), and dentifrices (2), for a total of 56 recipes. In some cases, Ibn al-Amshāṭī includes shorter or longer theoretical remarks, additional information, and instructions in addition to the recipe.

Critical Edition and Translation of Ibn al-Amshāṭī's *al-Isfār ʿan ḥikam al-asfār*

1 Editorial Methods

When preparing the critical edition of the treatise, my aim was to produce a readable Arabic text, therefore the only disruption in the main text is the indication of the folios of the manuscripts. Marginalia, interlinear notes, and scribal mistakes and corrections are relegated to the critical apparatus.

All three surviving manuscript copies we know of were used for the critical edition.[1] In the edition, I followed the Cairo manuscript for the initia and the colophon but those of the Mosul and Tarīm manuscripts are reproduced in the apparatus. Differences, additions, and omissions in the manuscripts are always indicated in the apparatus. Occasionally, some elements present only in the Cairo or the Mosul and Tarīm manuscripts are included in the main text; these are also always noted in the apparatus.

The addition or omission of the conjunction *wa-* and the definite article *al-* as well as changing the *al-* to *li-l-* are noted in the apparatus, as well as variant readings of diacritical marks, characters with three diacritical dots, personal suffixes, case endings, and numerals. The exception is the orthography of the *hamza*; the characteristics of the *hamza*s are noted in the description of the manuscripts and the changes in the orthography of *hamza*s in the medial position are not marked in the apparatus.

I reproduced the use of red ink, following the Cairo manuscript, in order to make navigating the text easier for the reader while avoiding the insertion of additional section titles and line breaks in the text. The paragraphs and punctuation marks are my additions. Vocalisation and *hamza*s are rarely present in the manuscripts; however, I supplemented the text with *hamza*s and *shadda*s with the intention of facilitating reading.

2 Translation Methods

When producing the English translation of the original Arabic, my intention was to produce a "precise study translation" as fully as possible.[2] My aim was

1 On their relationship, see section *3.1.4 The Textual Tradition of the Isfār*.
2 See the notes of Hodgson on three different types of translations (re-creative, explanatory,

 | DOI:10.1163/9789004708204_003

not an ornate and lucid English paraphrased version; this means that the English translation can be dull or complicated at times. However, by staying closer to the original Arabic text, the translation I hope manages "to reproduce the information carried by the original work, for the purposes of special study by those who cannot read the original language."[3]

Technical terms and names of *materia medica* are translated consistently. All of these are listed in the glossaries. The ten chapters of the work (eight main chapters and the two chapters of the epilogue) are all designated as *faṣl* in the Arabic, and therefore rendered as 'chapter' in English on all occasions. Other Arabic terms are also translated in the same way throughout the translation and the structure of the original was also observed as much as possible. While this makes the English monotonous at times, especially in the epilogue, this reflects the Arabic original as well. To still produce a readable English, I supplemented the translation with words in square brackets when necessary. In some cases, when the original meaning is not easily reproduced in English, the original is reproduced in transliteration and supplemented with an explanatory note; these terms are also listed in the glossaries and the notes generally provide the reader with the same information as the glossary.

3 Abbreviations and Signs

C	MS Cairo, Dār al-Kutub majāmīʿ 210/16
C^1	marginal note in C
C^2	interlinear note in C
M	MS Mosul, Madrasat Yaḥyā Bāshā 175/9
M^1	marginal note in M
T	MS Tarīm, Maktabat al-Aḥqāf majmūʿat Āl Yaḥyā 123 majāmīʿ (123/11)
T^2	interlinear note in T
|	beginning of next folio; folio number given in the outer margin
+	added
—	omitted
⟦…⟧	deleted by scribe
[…]	editor's additions

and precise study translation): Hodgson, *The venture*, I/67–69. I would like to thank Mónika Schönléber for referring me to this summary.

3 Hodgson, *The venture*, I/68.

C254v, M1v, T100v

بسم الرحمن الرحيم وصلّى الله على سيّدنا محمّد وسلّم.

الحمد لله الذي أمر بالأسفار، للتفكّر والاعتبار، وأداء فرائض الحجّ والاعتمار، وجعل في الطبّ من الأسرار، ما يحفظ الصحّة ويبرئ من الأضرار، وصلّى الله على سيّدنا محمّد عبده ورسوله الشافي من المضارّ، وعلى آله وأصحابه الأخيار، ما طرد الليل النهار، وأضاء الفجر وأنار.

وبعد فلمّا عزم على سير الأبرار، واحتزم لزيارة البيت المختار، من كلّ جبّار، ولزم العجّ بالانتقار، والثجّ والاعتذار، وجوار تلك المشاعر الكبار، بالذلّ والانكسار، رجاء كرم الغفّار، يمحو الذنوب والأوزار، ورفع | الدرجات في دار القرار، خلاصة الأعصار، وإمام أهل الأمصار، عين أعيان ساكني الأقطار، من إذا ذكر جوده استغنى عن السحاب الهمّار، وإذا تُأُمّل علمه استصغر في جنبه البحر الزخّار، وإذا تحدّث عن المجد والسودة علم أنّه القطب الذي عليه المدار، المقرّ الأشرف الكريم العالي الأمامي العالمي العلّامي الكمالي ابو المعالي محمّد الجهني البارزي الشافعي ناظر دواوين الإنشاء الشريفة بالديار المصرية، وسائر الممالك الإسلامية، رجّعه الله بعد بلوغ الأوطار، سالما من الآفات والأخطار، على أجمل الأوصاف وأجلّ الأخطار، وكان من القواعد الكبار، جلب المصالح ودرء المفاسد والمضارّ، وكان من أهمّها حفظ الصحّة M2r

2–4 الحمد ... وأنار] M: الْحَمْدُ لِلّهِ، الَذِي اَمَر بالاسْفار، للتفكّرَ وَالاعتبار واداء فرايض الحج والاعتمار، وجهَاد المتمردين مِن، الْكُفّار، وجَعَلَ فِي الطّبّ مِنَ الاسْرَار، ما يحفظ الصّحة ويبْرى الاضرار، واشهد ان لا اله الا الله، وَحْده لا شرِيكَ له النّافِع الضّار، واشهَدُ ان سَيّدنا محمدًا عَبْده المختَار، ورَسُولهُ الشَافِي مِن الاضرار المضار، الهادِيُءِ الي المنافِع وَالمباد، صَلى الله عَليْهِ وَعَلى آله الاخيَار، وازواجه الاطهار، وإصحابه، الاجيَار، ما طرد الليل النهار، وَاضَآ الفجر وَانار // T: الحمد لله الذي امر بالاسفار، للتفكر والاعتبار، وادا فرابض الحج والاعتمار، وجهاد المتمردن من الكفار، وجعل في الطب من الاسرار، ما يحفظ الصحة ويبري من الاضرار، واشهد ان لا اله الا الله النافع الضار، واشهد ان سيدنا محمدا عبده ورسوله المختار، الشافي من المضار، الهادي الي المنافع والمسار، صلي والله عليه وعلي اله الانصار، وازواجه الاطهار، واصحابه الاخيار، ما طرد الليل النهار، واضا الفجر وانار 3 محمّد] C: محمدا 4 وعلى] C: ، ⟦...⟧ وعلى 5 المختار] C: المحيار 5–6 من ... والاعتذار] C: — 7 ورفع ... القرار] C: — 8 جوده] M: الجود | الهمّار] M: الجهاد 13 جلب] M: حبب 13–118:1 حفظ ... والأخيار] M: حفطه والأخيار T: حفظ الأخيار

In the name of [God,] the Most Gracious, the Most Merciful. May the blessings and peace of God be upon our lord Muḥammad.

Praise be to God, who instructed to travel for pondering and contemplating, and to pursue the religious duties of the pilgrimage and the *ʿumra*;[4] who placed in medicine the secrets which preserve health and cure harms. The blessings of God be upon our lord Muḥammad, his servant and envoy who cures the harms, and upon his family and his outstanding companions, as long as the night chases away the day and the dawn shines and throws light.

When one decides on the travel of the pious [ones] and girds himself for visiting the Chosen House (*al-bayt al-mukhtār*) away from every tyrant, and persists in raising his voice (*al-ʿajj*) with a piercing sound (*intiqār*) and shedding blood (*al-thajj*) and pleading,[5] and [for visiting] the vicinity of those great ritual sites with humbleness and restraint, [then] the anticipation of the Repeatedly Forgiving's generosity abolishes the sins and faults and elevates the stages in the Hereafter[6] at the end of times. The leader[7] of the cities' folk is the most eminent of the dwellers of the lands; when his generosity is mentioned, there is no need for pouring clouds; when his knowledge is regarded, the water-abundant sea seems small besides him; when magnificence and splendour is discussed, it is known that he is the axis of the orbit: the Safeguarder, the Noble, the Beneficent, the Sublime, the Foremost, the Learned, the Scholarly, the Perfect,[8] Abū al-Maʿālī Muḥammad al-Juhanī al-Bārizī al-Shāfiʿī, the Superintendent of the Noble Chancery of Egypt and the rest of the Muslim countries. After [his] wishes are fulfilled, may God turn him away safely from the pests and harms back to the finest qualities and the greatest importance. Obtaining beneficial things and repelling the corrupting and harmful things is [one] of the greatest principles. The most

4 The "lesser pilgrimage" to Mecca. The *ʿumra* can be performed at any time of the year and consists of fewer rituals compared to the *ḥajj*, pilgrimage; however, it is also possible to perform it alongside the *ḥajj* in specific ways. For a detailed analysis of the *ʿumra*, see Chaumont, *ʿUmra*.

5 According to two *ḥadīth*s, sayings of traditions of the Prophet, the Prophet was asked which deeds of the pilgrimage are the greatest, and he anwsered that these are the *ʿajj* (raising of the voice when invoking the *talbiya*, a prayer of the pilgrimage) and the *thajj* (shedding the blood of the sacrificial animals). Ibn Mājah, *Sunan*, III/282 (no. 2924); al-Tirmidhī, *Sunan*, I/343 (no. 827).

6 *Darajāt* and *Dār al-Qarār* in the Arabic: see Afsaruddin, *Garden*, 283, 284 and Hermansen, *Talent*.

7 *Imām* in the Arabic. For more on the meaning of the term, see Aerts, *Imām (technical term)*.

8 *Al-Kamālī* is translated here as 'the Perfect'; it is an abbreviated form of Kamāl al-Dīn.

والأخيار ، والنذور بما لعّله ينفع | لذي البراري والقفار ، حيث لا صاحب ولا جار ، ولا عقاقير C255ʳ ولا عقّار ، رأيت أن أجمع لحضرته الشما ، وحومته العليا ، كتابا أرشد فيه إلى ذلك ، سالكا فيه أجمل المسالك ، فجاء بحمد الله حاويا لأسرار ، كتب هذا الفنّ الكبار ، مغنيا عن حمل تلك الأسفار ، في مفارق الأسفار ، جامعا لانتشار ما تفرّق منها على سبيل الاختصار ، فلذلك سمّيته الإسفار عن حِكَم الأسفار ، والله تعالى المسؤول وهو الكريم الغفّار ، إن يتحفه بالقبول فلا يبتغي له عثار ، ويسعفه بالكمال فلا يحتاج إلى اعتذار ، ويجعله سببا للنجاة من النار ، والفوز بمرافعة الأبرار.

T101ʳ ورتّبته على | مقدّمة وثمانية فصول وخاتمة. المقدّمة في بيان الحاجة إليه. الفصل الأوّل فيما ينبغي للمسافر فعله. الفصل الثاني في أمر السفر في الحرّ. الفصل الثالث فيما يتعلّق من ذلك بالرياح الملتهبة. الفصل الرابع في شأن السفر في الشتاء. الفصل الخامس في حفظ الأطراف. الفصل السادس في حفظ اللون. الفصل السابع في أمور المياه. الفصل الثامن في أحوال المسافر في البحر. الخاتمة فيما ينبغي للمسافر أن يصحبه وفيها فصلان، الأوّل في لأدوية المفردة، الثاني في المركّبة، وبها تمّ جمع فصول الكتاب عشرة.

---

1 لعّله] C^2: صح | حيث] C: حيف 3 لأسرار] M: الأسرار 4 في ... الأسفار] M: — 5 الغفّار] C^2: صح 7 المقدّمة في] C: المقدمة ~~في احوال المسافر~~ في | إليه] C: إلى C^1: وضع هذا الكتاب صح 10 في أمور] M: في حفظ أمور | في أحوال] M: فى حفظ احوال | في ... البحر] C: فى ~~معرفة ما يضره وينفعه~~ فى البحر C^1: احوال المسافر صح

important of these is the preservation of the health and the good things, and offering that which may be beneficial for those of [= travelling in] wastelands and deserts, alas without a companion, a servant, without medicaments, or remedies. I decided to compile a book for His Highness, His Excellency in which I show the way for this, following the best methods. Containing secrets, praise be to God, came the books of this great discipline. Being a substitute for carrying those books on the crossroads of travels and [being] a collection of all which split from it, by means of summarising, I named it *The unveiling of the wisdoms of the books*. God Almighty is the Granter of Wishes; he is the Noble and Repeatedly Forgiving—may He present the book with favourable reception and not desire upon it stumbling, may He grant it completeness so it does not need excuse, may He make it into a reason for redemption from Hell and escape [from Hell] by pleading the pious.

I arranged the book into an introduction, eight chapters, and an epilogue. The introduction is on the need for the compilation of this book. The first chapter is on what is necessary for the traveller to do. The second chapter is about travelling in hot weather. The third chapter is about all that is related to this of the burning winds. The fourth chapter is on the matter of travel during winter. The fifth chapter is on the preservation of the limbs. The sixth chapter is about the preservation of the complexion. The seventh chapter is about the matter of the waters. The eighth chapter is on the conditions of the traveller on the sea. The epilogue is about all the things the traveller should keep in his company in two chapters, the first on simple drugs and the second on compound drugs, with which the book's chapters become complete at ten.

المقدّمة في بيان الحاجة إلى وضع هذا الكتاب

المسافر يخرج عن أمور معتادة له دفعة واحدة والخروج عن المعتاد دفعة واحدة يجلب أمراضا خطرة، | مع أن التعب والنصب يزيدان في ذلك، لأنّهما يسخنان البدن ويذيبان الأخلاط C255v الرديئة، وتنتقل من موضع إلى آخر. فأمّا إن تنصب إلى بعض الأعضاء الرئيسية أو غيرها، فتحدث ورما بحسب كيفية الخلط وكمّيته. وأمّا إن تخالط الأخلاط الجيّدة، فتفسدها وتحدث منها أمراض صعبة. فلذلك وجب على المسافر أن يعرف ما يضرّه | وينفعه ليحرص على مداواة نفسه لأن لا M2v يصيبه شيء من ذلك.

1 في] C: ففي 2 يجلب] M: يحنب 4 الرئيسية] C: الرئسة | فتحدث] CMT: فيحدث 5 تخالط] CM: يخالط | فتفسدها] C: فيفسدها 6 لأن لا] M: لئلا 7 ذلك] T: + وانه الهاوي يفضله

Introduction on the need for compiling this book

The traveller deviates from the things he is accustomed to abruptly, and the sudden withdrawal from the usual things brings along dangerous diseases. Exertion and fatigue encourage this because these warm the body and dissolve the harmful humours so that they move from one place to another. When they then pour into one of the primary organs or non-primary ones, they cause a swelling according to the quality and quantity of the humour. When they mix with good humours, they corrupt them and cause burdensome diseases. For this reason, it is the traveller's duty to know what harms him and what benefits him to strive for treating himself so that none of these affects him.

الفصل الأوّل

ينبغي لمن أراد السفر أن يستفرغ الأخلاط الرديئة من بدنه مع مراعاة للأصول العشرة. أوّلها الامتلاء، فإنّ الاستفراغ مع الخلو ينهك القوّة. الثاني القوّة القوية، لأنّ الاستفراغ مع ضعفها يحلّل الروح. الثالث المزاج الحارّ الرطب، فإنّ المزاج الحارّ اليابس والبارد القليل الدم يمنع، لأنّ كلّ واحد منهما يكون معه الرطوبات الفادية قليلة والاستفراغ يوجب إفراط منها. الرابع الأعراض المناسبة، فإن كان مستعدّا للذرب أو قروح الأمعاء أو تقدّم استفراغ قوي منع منه. الخامس السحنة، فالسمن والقضافة المفرطان مانعان. | T101v السادس السنّ، فإنّ سنّ الشيخوخة والطفولة مانعان لضعف القوّة فيهما. السابع الوقت الشديد الحرّ أو البرد مانع. الثامن البلد، وهو كالوقت. التاسع قلّة عادة الاستفراغ تمنع. العاشر الصناعة إذا كانت كثيرة الاستفراغ | C256r كخدمة الحمّام مانعة بالإسهال والفصد. والعمدة في صواب الحكم بالفصد خمسة: عظم النبض وفور القوّة واكتناز العضل وسنّ الشباب وحمرة اللون.

ثمّ بعد تنقية البدن من الأخلاط يرتاض أكثر من العادة. فإن كان ممن يريد السفر ماشيا ولم يكن له عادة بالمشي، فليرتاض نفسه بالمشي قبل ذلك، ويعودها قليلا قليلا، ويزيد في مقداره على التدريج كلّ يوم حتّى تألّف ذلك ويهون على الطبيعة حمله. وإن كان عازما على السفر راكبا، فيرتاض قبله بالحركات وركوب ما سيعاني ركوبه في السفر. فإن كان يظنّ أن سيصيبه سهر أو جوع أو عطش في سفره، فيعتاد ذلك قليلا قليلا، ويزيد في مقداره على التدريج، فيكون صبورا عليه ولا يثقل على الطبيعة حمله، ويستصحب معه ما يهون عليه ذلك.

أمّا ما يسهل الصبر عن الطعام فالأطعمة المتّخذة من الأكباد المشوية، لأنّ الأكباد بطيئة الهضم وغداوها إذا انهضم كثير محمود ليس بسريع الانحدار. وإذا اتّخذ منها كبب مع لزوجات وشحوم قوية كشحوم البقر مذابة ولوز ودهنه، فإذا تناول منها واحدة، صبر على الجوع زمانا طويلا، لأنّ

2 بدنه] C¹: بالاسهال والفصد بعد صح | مع] C:— | أوّلها] C: وهي 5 معه] MT: مع | منها] MT: قلتها 6 الأمعاء] C: للامعا 7 الشيخوخة] M: الشيوخة 10 بالإسهال والفصد] C: ~~بالاسهال والفصد~~ | الحكم] C: الحلم 12 كان] M¹: كان صح 13 فليرتاض] C: فلير⟦...⟧ض MT: فليرض 15 سيعاني] M: مشا في 16 فيكون] C: فيكو 17 عليه] M:— | ذلك] M: وذلك 18 أمّا] M: و | الأكباد المشوية] M: البا والشهوة 19 كثير] C: كبير M: كثير | كثير محمود] T: كثيرا محمودا و 20–124:1 لأنّ الدهن] C: لأنّ ~~الشحم~~ والدهن

First chapter

It is necessary for the person who wants to travel to purge the harmful humours from his body with the observance of ten principles. [The first principle] is fullness [with harmful humours], for purging with emptiness [of harmful humours] consumes the strength. The second is the potent strength, for with the weakness of strength [purging] loosens the spirit. The third is the warm and moist temperament, for the warm and dry temperament and the cold temperaments which have modest amoutns of blood are prohibited, for each one of these has little superfluous humours, and the purging requires an excess of these. The fourth is the adequate symptoms, for if one is susceptible to diarrhoea, ulcers of the intestines, or developing forceful purging, he is prohibited from it. The fifth is the appearance, for excessive fatness or slimness prohibits it. The sixth is the age, for old age and early childhood prohibit it because of the weakness of the strength in them. The seventh is that very hot or cold times prohibit it. The eight is the country, being the same as the time. The ninth is that rare usage of purging prohibits it. The tenth is the profession; if it is plentiful of purging, like the bathhouse servant, he is prohibited from diarrhea and venesection. The basis of proper decision regarding venesection is five [things]: the intensity of the pulse, bursting of strength, the sturdiness of the muscles, the age of adolescence, and redness of the complexion.

After the purification of the body from the humours, [who wants to travel should] exercise more than it is customary. If he wants to travel on foot and he is not accustomed to walking, he should train himself by means of walking beforehand, getting used to it bit by bit, increasing its quantity gradually each day until he gets accustomed to it and its bearing becomes easy for the constitution. If he decided on travelling mounted, he should train himself beforehand with physical exercises and riding what he will ride during the travel. If he thinks that sleeplessness, hunger, or thirst will fall upon him during his travel, he should habituate himself to it bit by bit, increasing its quantity gradually, so that he will be very enduring against it and bearing it will not be burdensome for the constitution. He should take with him what makes these easy for him to endure.

What helps one to abstain from eating is food made from roasted livers because livers are digested slowly. If food made from it is digested, it is abundant and approvable, and it does not descend fastly. If meatballs are made from it with viscid things and greasy solid fats, like the melted fat of cattle, almond, and its oil, and one meatball is eaten, one endures hunger for a long time, since the oil and the fat, if added to the livers, increase its

الدهن والشحم إذا أضيف إلى الكبود زاد في بطؤها إذا الشحوم مولّدة للبلغم ملطخة للمعدة. ولهذا يؤمر من به الشهوة الكلّية بالأغدية | الدسـمة مثل الأدهان والشحوم والألية. وقيل أنّه من شرب C256v رطلا من دهن البنفسج إذ بثّ فيه قليل من الشمع حتّى صار قيروطيا، بفتح القاف واسكان التحتية وضمّ الراء المهملة ثمّ واو وطاء مهملة، لم يشتهي الطعام عشرة أيّام.

وأمّا ما يمنع من الشرب الكثير فإمّا أن يكون مما يتناول أو مما يمنع المسافر من تناوله.

أمّا الأوّل، فينبغي أن يتناول الأغدية الرطبة المبرّدة، كسويق الشعير بالماء البارد | والسكّر M3r وبقلة الحمقاء بالخلّ والبطّيخ الهندي والقرع والماش وما شاكل ذلك، وكذلك ما اتّخذ بالحصرم والخلّ والدوغ، لفظ فارسي بضمّ المهملة وآخره معجمة، وهو اللبن المخيض. وإن كان الحرّ شديدا فليشرب قبل مسيره لعاب بزر قطونا وبزر البقلة الحمقاء مع شيء من ماء الرمّان المزّ ودهن حبّ القرع، ويمسك | في الفم من حبّ السفرجل أو من الحبّ المسكن للعطش. وهذه صفته: لبّ T102r حبّ القرع ولبّ حبّ القثّاء وبزر البقلة الحمقاء، من كلّ واحد خمسة دراهم، نشا وكثيراء وطباشير، من كلّ واحد درهمين، يدقّ الجميع ناعما ويعجن بلعاب بزر قطونا ويعمل حبّا كبارا مفرطحا ويمسك في الفم. فإن لم يوجد فليمسك في فيه قطعة أسرب أو درهما أطلسا، فإنّ ذلك يسكن العطش ويقلّل الحاجة إلى شرب الماء.

وأمّا الثاني الذي يمنع المسافر من تناوله فالأغدية المعطّشة، مثل السمك المالح والطري والمملّحات والجبن | العتيق والباقلّاء المطبوخ والأشياء الحريفة والحلوة. وإذا شرب الماء بالخلّ C257r كان القليل منه كافيا في تسكين العطش حيث لا يوجد ماء كثير.

---

1 للبلغم] M: البلغم 2 الأدهان] C: الدسـمة 3–4 بفتح ... مهملة] MT: — 4 التحتية] C: التحية 7 بالحصرم] C: الحصر 8 لفظ ... المخيض] MT: — | المخيض] C^1: ب المخيض | شديدا] C: شديد 9 وبزر] C: بز 10 وهذه] CM: هذا 10–11 لبّ ... القرع] T: — 11 حبّ] T: — 12 ناعما] M: + ويعجن ناعما T: وناناعما 13 أطلسا] C: اطلسا C^2: ٢ | فإنّ] M: فكون 14 ويقلّل] M: يقل | الحاجة] C^2: صح

slowness [of digestion], since the fats generate phlegm and blot the stomach. For this, one with carnal appetite is instructed to eat fatty foods, for example, oils, fats, and fatty tails. It is said that who drinks a *raṭl*[9] of oil of violet if there is a little amount of wax dispersed in it until it becomes like *qayrūṭī*,[10] the *qāf* pronounced with a *fatḥa*, the under-dotted [*yā*ʾ] being vowelless, the unpointed *rā*ʾ pronounced with a *ḍamma*, then a *wāw* and an unpointed *ṭā*ʾ, will not feel appetite for food for ten days.

What prevents frequent drinking [fall in two categories:] either things that the traveller should eat or things that he is prohibited from eating.

As for the first [category], he should eat moist and cooling foodstuffs, like barley *sawīq*[11] with cold water and sugar, purslane prepared with vinegar, Indian watermelon, pumpkin, mung bean, and what are similar to these. Likewise, what is prepared with sour grape, vinegar, and *dūgh*, being a Persian word, with the dotless [*dā*ʾ] pronounced with a *ḍamma* and its last [letter] dotted, that is buttermilk. If the weather is really hot, he should drink before his travel mucilage of psyllium seeds and purslane seeds with sour pomegranate juice and pumpkinseed oil, and take in his mouth quince seeds or the thirst-quenching pastille. Its recipe is: kernel of pumpkin seeds, kernel of Armenian cucumber seeds, and purslane seeds, 5 *dirhams* from each one, cornstarch, tragacanth, and chalk, 2 *dirhams* from each one, grind it all finely, knead it with mucilage of psyllium seeds, form flattened pastilles from it, and take it in the mouth. If it is not available, [the traveller is to] take into his mouth a piece of lead or a dirham [which] has no impression, for this quenches thirst and reduces the need for drinking water.

Secondly, the traveller is forbidden to eat foodstuffs which cause thirst, like salty fish or fresh [fish], salted [food], seasoned cheese, cooked fava beans, and acrid and sweet food. If he drinks water with vinegar, a small quality is sufficient for quenching the thirst when there is not a lot of water.

---

9 One *raṭl* is equal to 450 grams. (See the *Glossary, 1 Weights and Measures.*).

10 *Qīrūṭī*, cerate, from the Greek κηρωτή. (Ullmann, *Die Medizin*, 299.) A cream for wounds made of olive oil, wax, and sometimes rose oil.

11 *Sawīq* is a meal of toasted and crushed seeds which can be prepared into a gruel by mixing it with water, sugar, or fats. It is most commonly made from barley or wheat but other seeds or fruits can also be added to it. For additional information and some recipes, see Nasrallah, *Treasure trove*, 475–476, 221–222, 231, 232; Ibn Sayyār al-Warrāq, *Annals*, 126–127.

الفصل الثاني في أمر السفر في الحرّ

السفر في الحرّ مضرّ يحدث أمراضا رديئة. ويؤدّي إلى ضعف القوّة، لأنّ الحرارة محلّلة للرطوبات، وإذا تحلّلت، ضعفت الحرارة الغريزية، إذ هي مركبها، فتضعف القوّة، لأنّ الروح المتولّد عن الحارّ الغريزي، مركبها، وحينئذ ضعفت الحركة واشتدّ العطش. فاستدعت الطبيعة شرب الماء للترطيب والتبريد وتشديد ما يتحلّل من الرطوبات، ويكثر شرب الماء إن وجد إليه سبيل. وذلك سبب لأمراض كثيرة. وإن لم يوجد الماء وكوبد العطش، أدّى إلى ضرر بيّن. وأيضا ربّما أضرّت الشمس بالدماغ فأورث صداعا وحمّى بواسطة اليبس لإفراط التحليل، لاسيّما في المزاج الحارّ اليابس والأبدان القضيفة.

ومن لم يعتد الحركة في الحرّ فإن لم يكن بدّ من السفر فيه فينبغي أن لا يسير في النهار. فإن اضطرّ لذلك فيجب أن يحرص على ستر رأسه ووجهه وصدره بالعمامة أو القلنسوة والمناديل والحباب، لئلّا يصيبه حرّ الشمس، وأن يقلّل استنشاق الهواء الحارّ.

وإذا كان المسافر فيه حال المزاج يابسة، تناول قبل مسيره شيئا من سويق الشعير وشراب
الفواكه، | لأنّ صاحب هذا المزاج يتوفّر الخلط الصفراوي فيه غالبا. فينبغي أن يشغل معدته C257v
بالغذاء، لئلّا ينصب إليها الموادّ فيضربه. وأيضا التحليل يكثر فيه، لأنّ الحرارة الغريزية | تحلّل من T102v
داخل والغريبة من خارج والحركة العنيفة الكثيرة، التي تلازم المسافر، تعيّن على فرط التحليل
وتضعيف القوّة لمّا مرّ. فحينئذ تأمره | باستعمال سويق الشعير، لأنّه غذاء بارد مرطّب، وشراب M3v
الفواكه، فإنّه مبرّد دافع للصفراء. وينبغي إذا تناوله أن يمكث إلى أن ينحدر عن معدته، لأنّه إذا أخذ في السير عقيب تناوله تخضخض في معدته وعلا وطفا إلى فم المعدة ولم يستقرّ في أسفلها، فلم يتمّ هضمه. ويجب أن يصحبه في سفره دهن الورد والبنفسج ليستعمل منهما ساعة بعد ساعة على صدغيه بماء بارد مع اليسير من الخلّ، لأنّ دهن الورد بارد لطيف نافع من الصداع، وأمّا دهن البنفسج فهو بارد رطب مرطّب للدماغ نافع أيضا من الصداع الكائن من الحرارة واليبس.

---

1 في ... الحرّ] C:— C[1]: فى السفر فى الحر صح 3 مركبها] M: مركزها 4 الغريزي] M: العرىر 5 وتشديد] C: ىشديد MT: لشديد | إن] C: ⟦و⟧ان 7 الشمس] C: الشمىس 8 القضيفة] C: العصفة M: الغصيفه 9 يعتد] M: يتعيّد 11 لئلّا] T: لان لا | الشمس] C: الشمىس 12 حال] CMT: حار 14 إليها] C: اليه 16 الشعير] C[2]: صح | لأنّه] M: لان 17 أن] C: ا C[2]: ن 18 وعلا وطفا] MT: وعلى اوطفا 20 بماء ... الخلّ] MT:— | الصداع] MT: + العارض من الحرارة بالما البارد ومع السير من الحل 21 الكائن] M:— | واليبس] T: + والله اعلم

Second chapter on travelling in hot [weather]

Travelling in hot [weather] is harmful, bringing forth malicious diseases. It leads to weakening of the strength, for hotness is dissolving for the fluids, and if they are dissolved, the innate heat is weakened, for it is the fluids' vessel. The strength weakens, for the spirit, originating from the innate heat, is its vessel, and then the movement weakens, and thirst becomes more intense. The constitution demands drinking water for moistening, cooling, and strengthening [that] which was dissolved from the fluids, and drinking water occurs more often if there is a way for it. This is the cause of many diseases. If there is no water, and one suffers thirst, [it] leads to evident harm. The sun possibly harms the brain as well, causing headache and fever through dryness caused by the excessive dissolution, especially in the hot, dry temperament and thin bodies.

If one is not prepared for exercise in hot [weather] and travelling in it is unavoidable, he should not journey during the daytime. If he is forced to do so, he is to strive for covering his head, face, and chest with a turban or hood and kerchieves, so that the heat of the sun does not harm him and inhaling of the hot air is lessened.

If the state of the traveller's temperament is dry, he should consume some barley *sawīq* and fruit syrup before his travel, for yellow bile is generally plentiful in those with this temperament. He is to occupy his stomach with food so that the substances do not flow towards it and cause harm in it. The dissolution is also increased in him, because the innate heat is a dissolvent from the inside, and the external heat [is a dissolvent] from the outside, and the excessive and vehement movement, which is inseparable from the traveller, imposes excessive dissolution and weakening of the strength while he is travelling. Then he is ordered to use barley *sawīq*, for it is a cold and moistening food, and fruit syrup, for it is cooling and repels yellow bile. After consuming it, he should wait until it descends from his stomach, for if he starts travelling after consuming it, it gets shaken in his stomach, and ascends and emerges to the cardia. It will not settle in the bottom [of the stomach] and its digestion will not be complete. He is to take with him on his travel oil of rose and violet to use it hourly on his temples with cold water and some vinegar, for rose oil is cold and gentle, useful against headache, while violet oil is cold and moist, moistening for the brain, also useful against headache caused by heat and dryness.

الفصل الثالث فيـما يتعلّق من ذلك بالرياح الملهبة

ومن خاف السموم، وهي ريح ملتهبة حارّة جدًّا تيبّس الأبدان وتقشفها وإن وصلت إلى داخل أضرّت ضررا بيّنا، فينبغي لمن سافر فيها أن يستر وجهه وأنفه ويصبر على قلّة الاستنشاق والتنفّس، لأنّ استنشاق السموم يؤدّي إلى الهلاك أو إلى | C258r أمراض صعبة. وأن يطعم البصل المنقوع في الدوغ، وإن كان البصل حارًّا ففيه شيء من الرطوبة، والدوغ إذا شرب معه كبّر سورته الحارّة ودفع ضرر السموم. وأن يستنشق دهن الورد أو دهن حبّ القرع، وإنّه يدفع ضرر السموم، لأنّ السموم يورث الحرارة واليبس ودهن حبّ القرع بارد رطب نافع من حرارة الدماغ ويبسه إذا سعط به، وينفع أيضا أصحاب السرسام والماليخوليا إن وضع على رؤوسهم مع شيء من الخلّ.

ومن أصابه شيء من السموم سكب على أطرافه ماء بارد أو غسل وجهه وجعل غذاؤه من البقول الباردة، كالإسفاناخ وبقلة الحمقاء والقرع والخسّ وما شاكل ذلك، ويضع على رأسه الأدهان الباردة والعصارات الباردة، مثل عصارة حيّ العالم ونحوه. واللبن من أجود الأغذية له إن لم يكن به حمّى. فإن كان به حمّى ليست من الحمّيات العفينة فليستعمل الدوغ وليجتنب الجماع ويجب | T103r أن لا يشرب ريّة من الماء، لأنّ القلب يكون حينئذ شديد الجذب للماء البارد لتوفّر الحرارة فيه. فإذا كان المشروب قدر الريّ أو أكثر، لم يكن من المعدة وغيرها من الأعضاء يمانعه عن ذلك إذ الريّ قد حصل لها، فحينذ ينفذ الماء إلى القلب ويطفئ الحرارة الغريزية. وأمّا إذا كان المشروب | C258v أقل من الريّ فإن ماسكة المعدة ينازع جاذبة القلب فلا يصل إليه شيء من الماء إلّا بعد فراغها منه، بل يكتفي المضمضة. وإن لم يكن بدّ من الشرب شرب جرعة بعد أخرى، فإذا سكن ما به من عطش شرب. وينبغي أن يبتدي بشرب دهن ورد وماء ممزوجين ثم يشرب الماء، ويجعل مجلسه منخفضا باردا، ويغسل رجليه بالماء البارد، ويغتدي بغذاء سريع الانهضام، مثل أطراف الجداء والقرع المعمول بماء الحصرم | M4r والخلّ ونحو ذلك.

---

1 فيـما ... الملهبة] C: — C¹: فيما يتعلق مں الرياح الملهبه صح 3 والتنفّس] C: التنفس 5 كبّر] MT: كسر 6 يستنشق دهن] M: ينشق بدهن 10 والخسّ] MT: — 12 ليست] M: لت | العفينة] M: الغضيه | فليستعمل] MT: استعمل 14 من] T: لان 15 ويطفئ] M: ںصفى 16 ماسكة] C: ما⟦يـ⟧سكة 17 المضمضة] C: المضمضمه 18 يبتدي] M: يبدا 19 مجلسه] C: مجلسه T: محله T²: محلسه صح 20 ذلك] T: + والله تعالى اعلم

Third chapter on what pertains to this concerning burning winds

Who is afraid of the *samūm*—which is a very hot and burning wind making the body dry and chapped, and if it gets inside [the body], it causes obvious harm—he who travels in it should cover his face and nose, endure the scarceness of inhaling and breathing, for breathing the *samūm* in leads to death or serious diseases. He should eat onion soaked in *dūgh*, and if the onion was strong, there is some moistness in it, and if the *dūgh* is drunk with it, it strengthens its hotness and repels the harm[ful effect] of the *samūm*. He should inhale rose oil or pumpkin seed oil, as it repels the harm[ful effect] of the *samūm*, for the *samūm* causes hotness and dryness, and the pumpkin seed oil is cold, moist, and useful against hotness and dryness of the brain if inhaled. It also benefits those with *sirsām*[12] and melancholia, if it is put on their heads with some vinegar.

If something befalls a person because of the *samūm*, he is to pour cold water on his limbs or wash his face, prepare his meal from cold herbs, such as spinach, purslane, pumpkin, lettuce, and which is similar to these, and put cold oils and saps on his head, like the sap of houseleek tree and the like, and milk is the best food for him if he has no fever. If he has a fever which is not a putrid one, he is to use *dūgh*, avoid intercourse, and not to drink [even] a draught of water, for the heart is then strongly drawn to cold water because of the abundance of heat in it. If the amount of water is a mouthful or more, nor the stomach or any other organ could prevent it when the draught arrives at it and then the water penetrates the heart and extinguishes the innate heat. If the water is less than a draught, retention by the stomach [of this water] combats the heart's longing [for cold water], and the water only gets to it after it is poured out from it [= stomach], however, it makes it content. If drinking is unavoidable, one should drink gulp after gulp. When his thirst is quenched, he [can] drink. He is to start drinking rose oil and water mixed [together], then to drink water, make his sitting place low and cold, wash his legs with cold water, and eat fastly digestible food, such as the limbs of young goats, pumpkin prepared with sour grape's juice and vinegar, and similar things.

12 Phrenitis, inflammation of (the meninges of) the brain caused by yellow bile. See Dols, *Majnūn*, 57–58.

الفصل الرابع في شأن السفر في الشتاء

السفر في الشتاء والمواضع الباردة عظيم الخطر، لأنّ البرد يطفئ الحرارة الغريزية ويميتها ويحدث الكزاز والتشنّج ويجمد البدن. فإن لم يبلغ ذلك فربّما أوقع في الجوع المسمّى بوليموس، وهي بضمّ الباء الموحّدة وكسر اللام واسكان التحتانية وضمّ الميم وآخره سين مهملة، وهذا النوع من الجوع يسمّي جوع البقر. وهو جوع الأعضاء مع شبع المعدة، فتكون الأعضاء طالبة للغذاء والمعدة عائفة له. وسببه سؤء مزاج بارد، لأنّ البرد الشديد ربّما كان سببا لسوء مزاج بارد يعرض لفم المعدة. والبرد الشديد، ربّما أصاب المسافر فيه سقوط الأطراف، لا سيّما إذا كان المسافر راكبا وأطرافه متدلّية. والنظر إلى الجمد والثلج | يضعف البصر. C259r

وبالجملة، السفر في البرد الشديد والمواضع الباردة صعب خطر. فإن كان لازما فينبغي للمسافر فيه أن يكون مسيره بالنهار وراحته بالليل، فإنّ المسير في النهار يهون نكاية البرد لحصول حرارة الشمس فيه، وأمّا الليل فإنّه يشتدّ فيه البرد جدّا فالأولي بالمسافر أن يستريح فيه ويأوي إلى كنّ يقيه البرد. وينبغي أيضا أن يدهن بدهن البان | والزنبق والزيت أو دهن الغار ونحو ذلك، فإنّه يمنع T103v من وصول البرد إلى الأعضاء داخل البدن لسدّ الدهن المسام. وأن يحفظ الفم والأنف حتّى لا يدخلهما هواء باردا، لا سيّما عند هبوب الهواء البارد، وأن يعتني بحفظ الأطراف، فإنّ البرد إذا استولي عليها حلّت فيها آفة عظيمة، وسنذكر حفظها إن شاء الله تعالى. وأن لا يقصد التدفئ إذا نزل في الحال، بل يندرج في ذلك لتوقّي الخروج من الضدّ إلى الضدّ دفعة واحدة، لأنّه ينهك الأبدان ويضعف القوّة. ولا يستعجل بالاصطلاء أيضا، بل تركه أولى، فإنّ قربانة النار ثمّ تركها والخروج عنها إلى البرد من توارد الحرارة والبرودة على البدن في زمن يسير، وذلك مما يضرّه. فإن كان لا يمكنه الصبر عنه الاصطلاء تدرّج في ذلك. فإن كان عازما على السفر في الحال | وكان الهواء باردا C259v فالواجب تركه، لأنّه يخرج من حرقوي إلى برد مفرط، وذلك مما يوجب ضررا لا يخفى.

---

1 في ... الشتاء] C:— C^1: ى شان السفر ى الشتا صح 2 ويحدث] M: يحدد 3 الكزاز] MT: الكزار | وهي] C:— 4 التحتانية] M: التحتية | سين] M:— 5 فتكون] M: فيكون 6 يعرض] C^2: صح 7 فيه] T:— 10 في النهار] M: بالليل | لحصول] T: حصول 11 الشمس] M: البرد | الليل] C: لليل | فالأولي] M: فالمولي 12 يقيه] M: يقيْة 13 من] MT:— | داخل] C: وداخل | الفم والأنف] T: الانف والفم 15 حفظها] MT: + فيما بعد 17 بل] M: على 18 كان] M: + مما

Fourth chapter on the matter of travelling in winter

Travelling in winter and to cold places is rather dangerous, for the cold quenches the innate heat and suppresses it, causing spasms and convulsion, and freezes the body. If it does not get to that, possibly it leads to the starvation called *būlīmūs*,[13] the one-dotted *bāʾ* with a *ḍamma*, the *lām* with a *kasra*, the under[dotted *yāʾ*] being vowelless, the *mīm* with a *ḍamma*, and its last [letter] is an undotted *sīn*. It is a kind of hunger [also] called as the hunger of the cattle, being the hunger of the organs with the stomach being full. The organs seek nutrition and the stomach feels disgusted towards it. The reason for it is the bad condition of cold temperament, for the severe cold is perhaps the reason behind the fault of cold temperament befalling the cardia. The severe cold probably causes falling off of the limbs of those travelling in it, especially if the traveller is riding and his limbs are dangling. Looking at the ice and snow weakens the vision.

Altogether, travelling in severe cold and to cold places is difficult and dangerous. If it is necessary, the traveller's journey has to be during the daytime and his rest during the night. If [his] travel is in the daytime, he cares little about the harm of the cold, for he gets heat from the sun. As for nighttime, the cold becomes more severe during it. Therefore the traveller is to rest during it and seek shelter at a place that protects him against the cold. He is also to anoint [himself] with oil of Egyptian willow, lily, and olives, or bay laurel oil, and others similar to these, because this prevents the cold from getting to the organs inside the body, for the oil closes up the pores. He should protect the mouth and the nose so that cold air does not enter them, especially when there is cold wind. He is to take care of protecting the limbs because if the cold overcomes them, it causes enormous harm. We will talk about their protection, God Almighty willing. He should not proceed straightaway to warming [himself] if he can do so but advance gradually, to protect himself from going from an opposit to an opposit in one stroke, for this exhausts the bodies and weakens the strength. He should also not hurry with warming himself, but refraining from it is better, for the closeness of the fire, then leaving it and going from beside it to the cold means that hotness and coldness come successively at the body in a short time, and this harms the body. If he can't refrain from this, warming oneself progresses gradually in that [way]. If he is bent on travelling when the air is cold, it is obligatory to leave it because he goes out from [a] burning [hot place] into excessive cold, and this causes evident harm.

---

13 Bulimia, from the Greek βουλιμία, a compound of the words for ox, βοῦς, and hunger, λιμός.

وأمّا إذا أوهنه البرد فينبغي أن يبادر إلى التدفئ والتمريخ بالأدهان الحارّة المسخّنة، مثل دهن السوسن والزنبق والخروع والبابونج ونحو ذلك. وينبغي إذا نزل أن يختار منزلا دافئا، كالأودية والأغوار مستورا عن الريح منحرفا عن ممرّ السيول. وأن يجعل الدوابّ بقرب الفسطاط ليسخن بكثرة النفس. وأن يكثر من الحركة، فإنّها تنعّش الحرارة الغريزية وتقوّيها | وتدفع مضرّة البرد. M4v وأن ينزع أثوابه كلّها إن أمكن، وإلّا فما كان عنها يلاقي البرد أوّلا، ثمّ يلبس غيرها، فإنّه أسرع في التدفئ وهو ظاهر. وينبغي أن يكون غذاؤه حارّا بالقوّة والفعل كثير التوابل الحارّة، كالثوم والجوز والخردل والحلتيت والبصل والفلفل والدار صيبي والدار فلفل والزنجبيل ونحو ذلك. وأن لا يركب خاليا من الغذاء، لأنّ الحرارة يغور في بدنه فرارا من الضدّ. فإن سافر وليس في أحشائه شيء بالغ التحليل في أضعاف القوّة، وحينئذ نأمره بتناول غذاء أحسن له، وأن يصبر إلى أن يستقرّ في أسفل معدته وينحدر عنها لمّا مرّ.

1 والتمريخ] M: التمريخه 3 والأغوار] M: والاعراض | منحرفا ... السيول] M: منه منحر | عن ... السيول] T: — | وأن] M: فاذا 4 تنعّش] C²: صح 6–7 كالثوم ... والزنجبيل] T: كالثوم والدار فلفل والزنجبيل والجوز والخردل والحنتيت والبصل والفلفل والدار صيني والدار فلفل والزنجبيل 8 الغذاء] C: الغداء 9 أضعاف] C²: صح 10 مرّ] T: + والله اعلم

If the cold weakens him, he is to begin warming up and anointing with hot and warming oils, like iris oil, lily oil, castor oil, chamomile oil, and the likes. If he takes lodgings, he is to choose a warm dwelling, like river beds and depressions sheltered from the wind and turned away from the passage of streams. He should put the riding animals in the proximity of the tent to warm with the large quantity of breathing, and do a lot of exercises, for this revives and strengthens the innate heat, and repels the harm of the cold. He is to take off all his garments if it is possible, and if it is not, then first those which suffered the cold, then he should put on something else, for this makes the warming faster, obviously. His food should be warm with strength and effect and rich in warm spices, such as garlic, walnut, mustard seeds, assafetida, onion, pepper, cinnamon, long pepper, ginger, and similar spices. He should not travel without food, because the heat flees deeply into his body from the opposite. If he travels and there is nothing in his intestines ready to dissolve when the strength fades, then we order him to consume food which is best for him and wait for it to move to the pit of his stomach and descend from it when he moves.

C260r T104r

الفصل الخامس في حفظ الأطراف عن تطرّق الفساد إليها | من البرد وعلاجها | إذا حصل فيها

يجب أن يدلك المسافر في البرد أطرافه حتّى تسخن، ثمّ يطليها بالأدهان لحارّة العطرة، مثل دهن البان والسوسن، وإلّا فبالزيت، وخصوصا إذا خلط معه العاقر قرحا والفلفل والحلتيت، أو دهن الياسمين أيضا والثوم يلطخ به الأطراف، والقطران نافع جدّا. وكلّ ذلك مما يمنع تطرّق الفساد إليها. وينبغي أن يجعل بين أصابعه شعر المعز المرعزي وعليها وبر الأرنب أو غيره، ثمّ يلفّ الرجل بالكاغد، بالمعجمة المفتوحة والدال المهملة، وهو الورق فارسي معرّب، ثمّ يلبس عليها الجوارب، وهي اللفائف، ثمّ الخفّ. وأن يحترز أن ينال البصر ضعف من النظر إلى الثلج والجمد، لأنّ شدّة بياضهما يفرّق النور الباصر ويقلّله. ويمنع من ذلك تعليق الخرق السوداء على العين والعمامة السوداء أو لبس الثياب السوداء إن أمكن، وكذلك الخضر والكحلية يقوم مقام السود، فإنّ هذه الألوان تمنع أن يفرّق النور الباصر ويجمعه، والأسود أقواها.

وإذا أخذ الفساد يتطرّق إلى الأطراف من شدّة البرد فعلامته أن صاحبه لا يحسّ الوجع والبرد فيها، ثمّ لا يخلوا إمّا أن يكون البرد أمات الحارّ الغريزي الذي في العضو | وحقن ما كان يتحلّل منه، أو لم يصل الأمر إلى ذلك، بل أضرّ به. C260v

أمّا الأوّل، فإنّ الحرارة والبخار والدم يتوجّه إلى داخل العضو لشدّة البرد وسدّة المسام، وإذا استقرّت هناك أحرقت العضو وعفنت هي وعفنت وأحدثت قروحا. فتعالج بعلاج القروح. وهو إن كانت القرحة نقية جفّفت فقط. وإن كانت عفنة عولجت بالأدوية الحارّة الأكّالة. فإن لم يجع فلا بدّ من الكيّ إن أمكن. وكلّ قرحة لم يتأكّل من وسطها شيء كفي في مداواتها أن تجمع شفتاها وتعصب. وأمّا اللتي لايكون كذلك فإن كان الذاهب منها جلدا، عولجت بالأدوية الخاتمة، كالعفص وقشر الرمّان. أو لحما عولجت بالمنبت، وهو كلّها يجفّف بلا لدغ، مثل شقائق النعمان ومرهم الباسليقون.

---

3 يجب] T:— | أطرافه] MT: + شي | تسخن] C: يسخن M: سخن 4 والسوسن] M: والياس | خلط] M: كانت 5 أيضا والثوم] MT: وايضا الثوم 6 المرعزي] M: المرمن 7 بالمعجمة ... معرّب] MT:— 8 وهي اللفائف] T:— | وهي ... الخفّ] M:— 9 بياضهما] MT: بياضها | يفرّق] C: يعْرق 10 يقوم] M: تقوم | فإنّ] M: فانها 11 أن يفرّق] MT: تفرق 19 وتعصب] C²: صح

Fifth chapter on the guarding of limbs against decay reaching them because of the cold and on their treatment if it befalls them

The traveller has to massage his limbs in the cold until they are warmed up, then coat them with warm and aromatic oils, like oil of Egyptian willow, iris oil, and if not [with these], then with oilve oil, especially if there was pellitory, pepper, and assafetida mixed into it, or jasmine oil as well and garlic to sprinkle the limbs with it, and tar is very useful. All these prevent decay from reaching them. He should put between his fingers the undercoat hair of goats with hare fur or something else on top of it. Then he is to wrap the legs with *kāghad*; the dotted [*ghayn*] with a *fatḥa* and the *dāl* being dotless, that is the Persian word for paper, being Arabized. Then he is to put on stockings on top of it, which are the coverings, then the shoes. He should be wary of the vision getting weak because of looking at the snow and ice, for their sharp whiteness disperses the harsh light. This is lessend and prevented by hanging black rags in front of the eye, and a black turban, or by wearing black garments, if possible. In the same way, green and dark blue can take the place of black, for these colours prevent the dispersion of the harsh light and they collect it. Black is the strongest of them.

When decay starts to get to the limbs due to the harshness of the cold, its symptom is that the affected person does not feel the pain and the cold in it, then it is not devoid of either the cold suppressing the innate heat which is in the organ, and restraining what was dissolving from it, or it does not get to this, but it causes harm.

As for the first [case], the heat, the vapour, and the blood head for the inside of the organ due to the severeness of the cold and the obstruction of the pores. If they dwell there, they burn the organ, and they putrefy and putrefy [*sic*], and cause ulcers. Ulcers are cured by treatment of the ulcers, that is only drying it, if the ulcer is clean, and if it is putrid, it is cured with warm, consuming remedies. If it is not painful, cauterisation is unavoidable, if it is possible. As for an ulcer with nothing being consumed from its middle, it suffices in its treatment to bind its edges together. Those which are not like this, if the skin perished from it, it is to be treated with citatrising medicaments, like gallnuts, pomegranate peel, or [if what perished from it is] flesh, it is cured with [medicaments causing] growth, and these are all drying without hurting, like poppy anemone and basilicon liniment.[14]

14 Ibn al-Amshāṭī provides a recipe for the basilicon liniment which 'grows the flesh, restores the nerved places, and the wounds which do not have warmness in them': see recipe L2.

M5r وأمّا القروح الباطنة فيخلط بمجفّفاتها | أدوية منفدة، كالعسل، وأدوية مخصوصة بالمحلّ. وإذا أراد الاندمال جعل مع قبضها لزوجة، مثل الطين المختوم، ولا تصاب القرحة بماء حارّ في زمن الابتداء ولا في زمن التبريد.

T104v وإن كان الثاني، فلا يخلو، إمّا أن يكون العضو | وارما أو لا. فإن لم يكن فعلاجه بالدلك الجيّد، ثمّ يمرخ بالأدهان الحارّة، كالزيت ونحوه. وإن كان وارما فطريق العلاج فيه أن يوضع العضو في ماء السلجم أو ماء طبخ فيه التين والكرنب أو الرياحين الحارّة أو الشبت والبابونج وما شاكل ذلك C261r مفردة | أو مجموعة. وقال بعض المجرّبين أنّه غمس العضو في ماء بارد فوجد لذلك منفعة، وكأنّ الأذى يندفع عنه، ويوكد ذلك الفاكهة الجامدة إذا وضعت في الماء البارد يخرج الجمد عنها وتزهو ويحسن طعمها.

وإذا أخذ الطرف يكمد فطريق علاجه أن يشرط عميقا ويوضع في الماء الحارّ حتّى يرقا الدم، لئلا يجمد شيء من الدم في فوهات الشرط فينحبس، ثمّ يطلى بالطين الارمني منقوعا في الخلّ وماء الورد ويشدّ يوما وليلة، ثمّ يزال عنه ويعاد الطلي، والقطران نافع أوّلا وآخرا. فإن جاوز الأمر السواد والخضرة وازداد العضو عفونة فيبادر إلى ما يسقط ما تعفّن منه حتّى لا يعفّن الصحيح المجاور له بأن يطبخ أطراف الكرنب والسلق، ثمّ يتّخذ منه خبيصا بالسمن ويوضع على العضو حتّى يسقط منه ما يعفّن، والضماد بورق الخطمى والخبّازي وعنب الثعلب مدقوقة مخلوطة بدهن البنفسج، وهي حارّة، في كلّ يوم مرّتين أو ثلاث، فإنّه يسقط المتعفّن، فإذا سقط يعالج بعلاج القروح.

1 منفدة] MT: متعددة | بالمحلّ] MT: + مثل المرارات في ادوية الات البول 2 أراد] CM: اريد | جعل] M: بجعل 3 التبريد] C: البرد M: التريد T: التزيد 6 السلجم] M: الثلجم M¹: نعلم السلجم | الشبت] M: السهب 7 وكأنّ] CMT: وكان 8 الأذى] T: الاذي 9 ويحسن] M: اويحسن 10 يرقا] M: يرق 13 تعفّن] C²: صح 14 بالسمن] M: بالثخن 15 يعفّن] T: تعفن 16 البنفسج] M: البنصيع | وهي] C: و C²: هي صح | المتعفّن] M: التعفن

Regarding internal ulcers, he is to mix into their drying agents a draining medicament, such as honey, and some medicament specific to the place. If he wants to cicatrise them, he is to produce a stickiness like that of the Lemnian earth by gripping them. Hot water should not distress the ulcer at the beginning, nor during the time of cooling.

If it is the latter and it is not empty, then the organ is either swollen or not. If it is not, its treatment is with a good massage, then with anointing it with warm oils, such as olive oil and the likes. If it is swollen, the way of its treatment is to put the organ in the water of rapeseed, or in water in which fig and cabbage were boiled, or hot aromatic plants, or dill and chamomile, or what resembles these singly or together. One of the empiricists said that he immersed the organ in cold water and found that this was useful for repelling the pain. He confirmed this [with] the frozen fruit which, if put into cold water, the freezing leaves it, and it glows, and its taste gets better.

When the limb becomes dull-coloured, the way of its treatment is to make a deep incision and put it into hot water until the blood ascends so that nothing clots from the blood at the apertures of the cut and it restrains itself. Then coat [it] with Armenian bole soaked in vinegar and rose water, and [leave it to] harden for a day and a night. Then remove it and go back to coating it. Tar is useful simply and solely. If it goes past the blackness and greenness, and the organ gets more putrid, hurry to something that eliminates the putrid parts so that the healthy [part] next to it does not decay by boiling the outer parts of cabbage and beet, then make a medley of it with clarified butter, and put it on the organ until it causes the parts that became putrid to fall off. Warm bandages made from the leaf of marshmallow plant, mallow, and gooseberry powdered and mixed with violet oil two or three times a day makes the putrid part fall off. When it falls, it is treated with the treatment of the ulcers.

الفصل السادس في حفظ اللون

المسافر قد يعرض له في سفره تغيّر لون وجهه ويديه ورجليه، وذلك إمّا لحرّ مجفّف أو برد مكثّف، والاغتسال بالمياه القابضة أيضا يغيّر اللون.

فمن أولع بحفظ لونه فليطل وجهه بالأشياء اللزجة والتي فيها غروية، كلعاب بزر قطونا وبزر البقلة الحمقاء والكثيراء والصمغ المحلولان | C261v في الماء، ومثل بياض البيض وكعك السميد المنقوع في الماء، فإنّ هذه تحفظ اللون.

وأمّا إذا حصل للوجه أو اليدين أو الرجلين تشقّق من برد أو ريح أو شمس فيطلي بالقيروطي، وصفته: صندلان وورد، من كلّ واحد أربعة دراهم، اكليل الملك خمسة دراهم، زعفران درهمان، كافور نصف درهم، شمع عشر دراهم، دهن ورد إن كان في الشتاء فنصف رطل، وإن كان في الصيف فأربع أواق، ويخلط الجميع جيّدا، فإن لم يكن فبالأدهان والشحوم.

2 لحرّ] T: ابالحر 3 القابضة] C: العابضه 4 فليطل] M: فليطلى 6 تحفظ] T:— 7 وأمّا] T:— | تشقّق] T: تقشف 8 اكليل الملك] C: اكليل المكل 9 درهمان] M: درهمين | عشر] MT: عشرة | ورد] M: قرد

Sixth chapter on preserving the complexion

During his travel, change in the colour of his face, hands, and legs might befall the traveller, either because of drying hotness or thickening cold, and washing [oneself] with astringent waters changes the colour as well.

He who craves to preserve his complexion is to coat his face with sticky thinks and in which there is a glutionus agent, as the mucilage of psyllium seeds, purslane seeds, tragacanth, and gum, dissolved in water, and like the white of the egg and pastry of semolina soaked in water, for this preserves the complexion.

If the face, hands, or legs got fissures from the cold, wind, or the sun, he should coat it with the *qayrūṭī*, its recipe is: two [kinds of] sandalwood and rose, four *dirhams* from each, five *dirhams* of melilot, two *dirhams* of saffron, half a *dirham* of camphor, ten *dirhams* of wax, and half a *raṭl* of rose oil in the winter, four *ūqiyas*[15] in the summer, all of these mixed well. If this is not [possible], then [he is to coat it] with oils and solid fats.

15 One *ūqiya* is equal to 37,5 grams. (See the *Glossary, 1 Weights and Measures.*).

الفصل السابع | T105^{r} في أمور المياه

اختلاف المياه يوقع المسافر في أمراض أكثر | M5^{v} من اختلاف الأغذية، لأنّ احتياج الطبيعة إليه أكثر والصبر عنه أقلّ من الصبر عن الغذاء. وإذا كان كذلك، وجب أن أذكر في هذا الفصل بعض أحكام المياه لمسيس الحاجة إليه.

فأقول الماء لا يغذو ولكنّ يرقّق الغذاء. وأفضل المياه مياه العيون الجارية على الأراضي الطينية المنحدرة من مواضع عالية الغمرة المكشوفة، التي بعد منبعها وخفّ وزنها، ويكون مجراها نحو المشرق الصيفي أو الشمال. وماء المطر فاضل لطيف القوام، لا سيّما الذي من سحاب راعد، إلّا أنّه يعفّن سريعا، فإذا أُغلي بعد عن التعفّن. ومياه الأبار والقنى رديئة، وكذا المتوجّه إلى المغرب والجنوب، لا سيّما عند هبوب الجنوبية. والراكدة ثقيلة على المعدة. والأجمية، وهي ما بين الأشجار الكثيرة الملتفة، تولّد البلغم. والمارّ على المعادن رديء، إلّا الحديدي، | C262^{r} فإنّه يقوّي الأحشاء. والنوشادري يطلق. والشبّي يحبس. والماء المالح يسهل أوّلا ثمّ يعقل. والماء الحارّ يفسد الهضم ويؤدّي المواظبة عليه إلى حمّى الدقّ. والمسخّن إن كان فاترا أورث الغثيان أو أسخن منه غسل المعدة على الريق، وشديد السخونة تحلّل القولنج. والجمد والثلج يضرّان بالعصب، لكنّ الأولي أن يبرد بهما من خارج، لأنّ تبريده بهما من داخل يوجب مخالطة أجزائهما بالماء، ولا شكّ أنّ تلك الأجزاء ثقيلة كالراكد. وبالجملة، فالماء البارد المعتدل المقدار أوفق لمياه للأصحّاء.

وأمّا ما يدفع ضرر اختلاف المياه وتقلّل نكايتها فالتصعيد أو التقطير، لأنّ اختلاف المياه إنّما يكون لسبب ما يخالطها من الأجزاء الغريبة. وأمّا الماء فهو بسيط في نفسه، وحينئذ كلّما يزيد ذلك المخالط فهو يصلح الماء. وذلك المخالط أكثر ما يكون من أجزاء أرضية، لأنّ ما يكون من الهواء والنار يتحلّل ويفارق الماء للطافته. والتصعيد والتقطير يفعل ذلك. والمياه الكثيفة أيضا يصلحها

---

1 في ... المياه] C: — C^{1}: في أمور المياه صح 2 اختلاف المياه] T: — | يوقع] T: توقع 3 أقلّ] M: اكل 5 يغذو] C: نعدو M: يغدو | ولكنّ] T: اولكن | يرقّق] C: ىدرو T: يبذرق 6 وخفّ] M: خفت 7 المشرق] M: الشرق | الشمال] M: الشمالي | القوام] M: القواح 8 يعفّن] M: يغص T: يعص 9 والراكدة] M: والركدة 10 والمارّ] C: المار 11 والشبّي يحبس] M: والسمى محلس | يسهل] M: سهل | يفسد] T: يغسل 12 الغثيان] M: العان 15 كالراكد] C^{2}: ك 16 وتقلّل] CT: يقلل | إنّما] MT: اما ان 17 لسبب] MT: سبب | الأجزاء] T: + من الاجزا | الغريبة] M: الارض العدسه

Seventh chapter on the matters of the waters

The difference in waters makes the traveller sick more often than does the difference of food because the constitution needs it more, and the endurance of its lack is less than the endurance of the lack of food. Since this is the case, it is obligatory for me to mention in this chapter some of the principles of waters, should they be needed.

I say that the water does not nourish but refines nourishment. The best of the waters are waters of the springs running on clayey lands descending from elevated places, [being] abundant and uncovered, which are far from their source and lightweight, and their course is toward the summer sunrise or north. Rainwater is of excellent and delicate consistency, especially which is from plentiful clouds, except that it becomes putrid fast, and in that case, it is boiled afterwards against the putrefaction. Waters of the water pits and canals are bad, and likewise [the waters] facing toward the west and south, especially with southern winds. Tranquil [waters] are burdensome to the stomach. Swampy [waters], which are between thick and intertwined forests, produce phlegm. [Waters] passing over minerals are bad, except iron[-rich water], for it strengthens the bowels. Ammonic [water] loosens, aluminous [water] obstructs, and salty water firstly relieves [the bowels], then confines [them]. Hot water corrupts the digestion, and persistence in this leads to hectic fever and heated fever. If it is tepid, it causes nausea, or the water of the stomach heats up because of it on an empty stomach, and the strong heat dissolves colic. Ice and snow harm the nerves, but the first [thing to do is to] cool off with them from the outside, for cooling because of them from the inside makes the blending of their parts with water necessary, and without doubt these parts are heavy like the tranquil [water]. Altogether, the moderately cold water is the most appropriate of the waters for the healthy.

What repels the harms of the difference of waters and lessens their harm is vaporisation or distillation, for the difference of waters is because of what is mixed into them from the foreign parts. As for the water, it is plain in itself, and then whenever the mixing degrades it, it [= vaporisation or destillation] restores the water. This mixing, which is mostly due to earthy pieces, for what is due to the air or fire dissolves and leaves the water because of its fineness. Vaporisation and distillation do this. Boiling also restores dense waters, for the reason of the water's density is either the increase of the quality of cold or the mixing of tiny earthy pieces. These pieces are not able to dissolve the continuity of the water, and it all ceases with cooking, for cooking breaks

الطبخ، لأنّ سبب كثافة الماء إمّا اشتداد كيفية البرد أو مخالطة أجزاء أرضية صغار. لا تقوى تلك الأجزاء على أن تفرّق اتّصال الماء، وكلّ يزول بالطبخ، لأنّ الطبخ يكسر سورة البرد لامحالة ويخلخل أجزاء الماء خلخلة يسهل بها انفصال تلك الأجزاء.

T105v C262v والماء المالح يشرب ممزوجا بالخلّ والسكنجبين يلقى | فيه الخرنوب وحبّ الآس. فإن شرب | الماء المالح يسهل أوّلا، ثمّ يعقل وأدمانه يحرق الدم ويسحن البدن ويجفّفه. فشربه بالخلّ يكسر الحرارة الحاصلة منه والسكنجبين بارد يطفئ الصفراء ويسكن الدم ويلطفه إن لم يكن مفرط الحلاوة. والخرنوب فيه قوّة قابضة، فيها حلاوة تمنع من إسهاله، ويكسر ملوحته بحلاوتها. وحبّ الآس بارد يابس يمنع من استطلاق البطن.

والشيّ يشرب معه كلّما يلين الطبيعة، كلعاب بزر قطونا ونحوه. والنوشادري يشرب معه القوابض.

M6r والمياه الراكد في البطائح | والآجام، إذا كانت متعفّنة لم يستعمل عليها الأغذية الحارّة، لأنّها ترقّقها وتسرع في نفوذها إلى الأعضاء، وهي رديئة في نفسها. فتكون أقبل للعفونة، لكنّ يجب أن يستعمل عليها القوابض من الفواكه الباردة والبقول، مثل السفرجل والتفّاح القابض والريباس ونحو ذلك، فإنّها تحفظها عن العفونة وتتنافي الضرر الذي يحصل للمعدة من الاسترخاء يقبضها وعفوصتها وبردها.

C263r وينبغي للمسافر أن يستصحب من ماء بلده ليمزجه بكلّ ما ورد عليه إن أمكن، وإلّا فيمزجه بالماء الذي يليه، ثمّ يأخذ من الماء الذي يليه ويمزجه بالذي يليه، يفعل هكذا حتّى يبلغ مقصده. فيحمل معه من طين بلده ويخلطه بكلّ ما ورد عليه وتخضخضه ويتركه حتّى يصفو، ثمّ يشرب منه، لأنّ مياه بلد الإنسان قد ألفها وطبعه أقبل لها، لأنّه نشأ عليها ورطوبة بدنه أشبه بها. وينبغي | أن يشرب من وراء شيء يحجب ما يتولّد من الماء، كالدود والعلق ونحوه. وأن يستصحب من الربوب الحامضة ليمزجه بالمياه المختلفة، كربّ الحصرم والرمّان المزّ ونحوه.

---

1 إمّا] M: له ما | كيفية] C: كثفه | البرد] C: البرد⟦اه؟ـا⟧ 3 ويخلخل] M: يحلل | أجزاء] C: ا⟦بـ⟧ـجزا 9 كلّما ... معه] T: — 12 أقبل] C: اقتل 13 عليها] C: + ⟦...⟧ 16 بكلّ] C: كل M: من كل | ورد] M: يارد 18 بكلّ ما] M: بكلما 19 وطبعه] M: طبعه

the severity of the cold by all means, and shakes the parts of the water with a shake that facilitates the separation of those [earthy] parts.

Salty water [is to be] drank mixed with vinegar and oxymel[16] in which carob and myrtle seeds are thrown, for drinking salty water first causes diarrhea, then retention and its excess burns the blood, and warms and dries the body. Drinking it with vinegar in it breaks the heat occurring from it, and the oxymel is cold and it extinguishes yellow bile and calms and soothes the blood if it is not excessively sweet. The carob in it is a costive force, there is sweetness in it, protecting against its [= salty water] purging, and breaks its saltiness with its sweetness. The myrtle seed is cold and dry, protecting against the bowel movement.

With alumic [water] drink whatever makes the constitution tender, like mucilage of psyllium seeds and similar things, and with ammonic [water] drink costive [things].

Stagnant waters in the beds of *wādī*s and swamps, if they are putrid, warm food will not be of use against them, for it makes them [= stagnant waters] fine and hastens their passing through to the organs, and it is malicious alone. It is more lethal for the putridity, but the costives made of cold fruits and herbs must be used against it, like quince, sour apple, ribes, and the like, as these protect them [= organs] against the putridity and counteract the harms which befall the stomach because of the loosening occurring in it, its acridity, and its coldness.

The traveller should take with him water from his country to mix it with everything that comes to him, if possible. If not, then to mix it with the water which follows it [= which he drinks next], then to take from the water which follows it and mix it with the one which follows it, and to do like this until he reaches his goal. [He should] take with himself clay from his country, and mix it into everything that comes to him, shake it, and leave it until it becomes clear, then drink from it, for one gets used to his country's waters, and his temper is closer to those [waters], for it forms due to it and the moistness of hist body resembles those [waters]. He should drink through something that filters what originates from the water, like the worm, leech, and similar things. [He should] bring with himself sour robs to mix them into the different waters, like the rob of sour grape, sour pomegranate, and the like.

16 Oxymel is a syrup made from vinegar and sugar. Ibn al-Amshāṭī provides its recipe as well as the recipe of honey oxymel and discusses their various qualities and uses: see recipes SY1–2 and the short exposition before them.

الفصل الثامن في أحوال المسافر في البحر

الراكب في البحر يتخيّل أنّ دماغه وبدنه يدوران، وأنّ الأشياء تدور عليه، فلا يملك أن يثبت. وسبب ذلك أنّ الأخلاط الرقيقة تهيج عند حركة السفينة وتحرّك حركة غير طبيعية وتقابلها الروح بحركة طبيعية مضادّة لتلك الحركة وتتدافعان، فيحصل حركة دورية وقد يعرض له قيء وغثيان، إمّا لانصباب بعض الأخلاط إلى المعدة أو لتحرّك الخلط المستكنّ فيها وحينئذ لا يقطع القيء، إلّا إذا أفرط وخيف منه.

فمن أراد أن لا يعرض له قيء فليتناول من الفواكه القابضة، مثل السفرجل والرمّان المزّ والتفّاح المزّ، أو شراب الحصرم أو شراب الرمّان المزّ المنعنعين أو شراب التفّاح المزّ أو التمر | T106r
الهندي، هذه مفردة أو مجموعة، فإنّها تشتدّ المعدة وتقويها، وتمنع أيضا من انصباب الفضول إليها. ويشرب أيضا من بزر الكرفس، لأنّه يسكّن الغثيان بخاصّية فيه كما قيل، ولا يمنع أن يكون يقوّيه الحارّة اليابسة، إذ هي مذرّة مفتّحة تدفع الخلط إلى جهة أخرى أو محلّله، وكذلك الافسنتين. وأن يغتدي بالحموضات المقوّية لفم المعدة والمانعة من ارتفاع البخار إلى الرأس، مثل العدس بالحصرم والخلّ ونحوه. وأن يشمّ الصندل | والطين الارمني منقوعين في الماء الورد والخلّ. وأن يمسح أنفه C263v
من داخل بالاسفيذاج، فإنّه يمنع من الغثيان والقيء بخاصّية فيه.

والله تعالى أعلم، والبادي إلى الصواب، ومنه المبدأ، والله المعاد، وصلّى الله على سيّدنا محمّد وآله وصحبه وسلّم.

1 في ... البحر] C:— C^1: في أحوال المسا[.] فى البحر ح 2 يملك] MT: + نفسه 4 وتتدافعان] C: يتدافعا M: تتدافعان 7 قيء] T:— 8 أو] MT: و 8–9 التمر الهندي] MT: التمر هندي 9 تشتدّ] MT: تشد 10 يقوّيه] C: نعوية M: نقويه T: يقوته 11 تدفع] C: مدفع | وكذلك] T: وكذا 13 الصندل] C:— C^1: الصندل | الماء الورد] CM: الماورد 15 تعالى] M:— 15–16 والبادي ... وسلّم] MT:—

Eighth chapter on the circumstances of the traveller on the sea

Who travels on sea imagines that his brain and body are becoming dizzy and that the things are turning around him; therefore, he is not able to stand firm. The reason for this is that the fine humours are stirred up from the movement of the ship, and they move unnaturally, and the spirit opposes this with a natural movement contrary to this movement and opposes it. A circular movement occurs and results in vomiting and nausea. Either for the flowing of some of the humours to the stomach or the moving of the humours bundled in it, the vomiting does not stop, except when it becomes excessive and one has to be afraid of it.

Who wants to avoid vomiting is to eat costive fruits, for example, quince, sour pomegranate, sour apple, or minted sour grape syrup, or minted sour pomegranate syrup, or sour apple syrup, or tamarind, alone or together, for these strengthen the stomach and strengthen it and they also prevent the flowing of excrements towards it. He is to drink from [juice of] celery seeds as well, for it calms nausea because of a characteristic in it, as it is said, and it does not restrain the character of the dry warmth, since it is scattering and appetising, warding off the humour to another region or dissolves it, and absinthe as well. He is to feed with sour things that strengthen the cardia and prevent the rising of the vapours to the head, for example, lentils with sour grapes and vinegar and the like. He is to smell sandalwood and Armenian bole soaked in rose water and vinegar, and to wipe his nose from the inside with white lead, for it prevents nausea and vomiting because of a characteristic in it.

God Almighty knows best, the Revealer of the right way, the beginning is from Him and God is [where we] return. May the blessings of God be upon our lord Muḥammad, his family, and his companions, and [may He] grant them salvation.

وأمّا الخاتمة ففيما يحسن للمسافر نقلة وفيها فصلان

الفصل الأوّل فيما ينبغي أن يصحبه معه من الأدوية المفردة

وهي إمّا حارّة، كالفلفل والدار فلفل | والدار صيني والزنجبيل والهال والجوزبوا والحلتيت M6ᵛ والعاقر قرحا والرازيانج والآنيسون والكراويا وعرق السوس والبرشياوسان وهي كزبرة البئر وبزر المرو وبزر الرشاد وبزر الكرفس والبصل والثوم والقطران والزيت والشيرج ودهن البنفسج والسنا والمصطكاء والشبثّ والبابونج وإكليل الملك والسداب والجندبيدستر والسقمونيا والتربد والغاريقون والنانخواه والعنّاب والسبستان ولسان الثور والخيار شنبر والعسل النحل والزبيب والتين والخرنوب والفستق والصبر والمقل الأزرق. وإمّا باردة، مثل بزر قطرنا وبزر الخطمي وبزر الخبّازي وبزر الحماض وبزر الخسّ وبزر البقلة الحمقاء وبزر القثّاء وبزر الريحان وبزر القرع وبزر البطيخ العبدي وعيدان الخطمي | وبزر الملوخية وبزر الهندباء وبزر الكشوث وزهر البنفسج C264ʳ والإجّاص والقراصيا والأميرباريس وحبّ السفرجل والتمر الهندي والهليلج الكابلي والأصفر والأسود والهندي والبليلج والأملج وحبّ الآس والأفيون والخلّ.

1 ففيما] M: فيما | وفيها] C:— C²: وفيها 2 معه] MT: + المسافر 3 والجوزبوا] M: الخرنوب
4 وعرق] CT: عود M: وهى | والبرشياوسان] C: البرساوشان T: البرشاوشان 7 شنبر] MT: الشنبر
8 قطرنا] M: التعونا T: القطونا 10 العبدي] M: العندي | الملوخية] C: الملرضيا MT: الملوخيا | وزهر البنفسج] CMT:— C¹: وزهر البنفسج 11 الهندي] M: هندي 12 والهندي] C: الهندي | والبليلج] M: الهليلج | والأملج] T:—

Epilogue, on what is advisable for the traveller to carry, in two chapters
First chapter on what he should bring with him from the simple medicaments

These are either hot, like pepper, long pepper, cinnamon, ginger, true cardamom, fragrant nutmeg, assafetida, pellitory, fennel, anise, caraway, liquorice, *barshiyāwushān* which is the maidenhair, marjoram seeds, garden cress seeds, celery seeds, onion, garlic, tar, olive oil, sesame oil, violet oil, senna, mastic, dill, chamomile, melilot, rue, castoreum, scammony, turpeth, agaric, ajowan, jujube, manjack, borage, purging cassia, honey, date, raisin, fig, carob, pistachio, aloe, and bdellium; or cold, like psyllium seeds, marshmallow seeds, mallow seeds, bladder dock seeds, lettuce seeds, purslane seeds, Armenian cucumber seeds, basil seeds, pumpkin seeds, watermelon seeds, tall marshmallow tree, Egyptian spinach seeds, endive seeds, flax dodder seeds, flower of violet, pear/plum, cherry, barberry, quince seeds, tamarind, chebulic myrobalan, yellow myrobalan, black myrobalan, Indian myrobalan, beleric myrobalan, amla, myrtle seeds, opium, and vinegar.

الفصل الثاني فيما يصحبه معه من الأشربة والربوب والمعاجين والحبوب والشيافات والأقراص والسفوفات والأكحال وشيافات العين والأدهان والمراهم والذرورات والسنون

[الأشربة]

أمّا الأشربة فالمفرد منها الذي هو في غاية البساطة الماء | T106v القراح، هو أنفع شرابا المحمومين للطافته وسرعة نفوذه وخفّته على الطبع، لأنّ جميع الأشربة سواه فيها غدائية تحتاج أن يعمل فيها الطبيعة، فيثقل ورودها عليها عند شدّة اشتغالها لمقاومة المرض، فلا ينتفع بها كانتفاعها بالماء. وقد يحتاج الماء في نعض الأحوال إلى ما ينفذه إلى أقاصي البدن ويبلغه غاية التبريد، كالخلّ، وإلى ما يزيد في ترطيبه ويوصله إلى متون الأعضاء، كالسكّر، أو إليهما جميعا ويسمّى سكنجبينا.

[SY1] والسكنجبين السادج شراب جامع النفع في الحمّيات الحارّة لتسكين الحرارة ومنعه العفونة وتنقيصه الخلط وتفتيحه السدد. ويختلف بنسبة إجرائه بعضها إلى بعض بنسبة اختلاف الخلّ والسكّر، وبحسب حرارة الحمّى ومادّتها، واحتمال طبيعة الشارب له. فالمتّخذ من خلّ صادق الحموضة وسكّر شديد البياض مثليه الرفيق جدّا | C264v عند الطبخ. وعند الشرب يصلح في الحمّيات التي في غاية الحدّة والحرارة لمن يحتمل الحموضة ولا يكرهها. والمتّخذ من الخلّ الثقيف الخمري والسكّر الأحمر ثلاثة أمثاله الغليظ مداما للحمّيات المركّبة من الصفراء والبلغم. وقد يقلّل الخلّ من ذلك أيضا إلى نسبة الخمس فما دونها. وينبغي أن يغسل السكّر أوّلا غسلة خفيفة، ثمّ يلقى في القدر ويصبّ عليه الخلّ ويوضع على الجمر البادية حتّى يذوب السكّر، ثمّ يصبّ عليه | M7r الماء مثليه أو أقلّ أو أكثر بحسب الحاجة ويغلي ويؤخذ رغوته ويدفع.

[SY2] والسكنجبين العسلي لا يصلح للحمّيات الحارّة ويصلح للمركّبة منها والتي مادّتها باردة. ونسبة الخلّ إلى العسل على حسب الأخلاط في غلظها ولزوجتها وشدّة عفونتها، فإنّ الخلّ مبرّد والعسل مسخّن ملطّف.

---

1 يصحبه] MT: + المسافر 4 البساطة] M: السباطة | هو] M: فهو | شرابا] MT: شراب | المحمومين] C: المعحمومّين 6 ورودها] M: ودرها | لمقاومة] T: بمقاومة 7 ويبلغه] C²: صح 9 ومنعه] M: ومنع 10 وتنقيصه] M: ونقطعه T: تقطيعه | الخلط] M: الحلا T: الخلا | بنسبة] M: نسبة 12 وعند] M: اعتمد | وعند] C: ⟦و⟧عند 14 الغليظ] CT: الغليظ | مداما] MT: قوي من 15 غسلة خفيفة] M: غسلا خفيفا 17 ويدفع] M: تدفع

Second chapter on what he [is to] bring with himself from the syrups, robs, electuaries, pills, suppositories, pastilles, medicinal powders, collyriums, eye remedies, oils, liniments, powders, and dentifrices

[Syrups]

Regarding syrups, the simple from them is what is plain as clear water. It is the most useful as a syrup for those with fever for its fineness, the fastness of its effect, and its lightness on the natural disposition, for all syrups except this have nutritive substances in them, which require the constitution to process them. Its arrival to it [= constitution] is burdensome upon its intense engagement for the sake of fighting illness. It does not utilise it as it utilises water. Water in some cases needs something to lead it to the most remote places of the body and get it to the purpose of cooling, like vinegar, and [it needs something] that increases its moistening and gets it to the main part of the organs, like sugar, or [it needs] both of them, and [that] is called oxymel.

[SY1] Pure oxymel is a syrup with extensive usefulness regarding hot fevers, because of its alleviation of the heat, its prevention of putridity, its reducing of blending, and its opening of obstructions. One [oxymel] varies from another according to the difference of the vinegar and sugar, and according to the fever's heat and its base and the endurance of the drinker's constitution of it. The one made from genuinely sour vinegar and twice as much truly white and tender sugar by cooking, when drank, is useful against fevers which are extremely vehement and hot for [those] who can stand sourness and do not hate it. The thick one made from very acidic golden brown vinegar and thrice as much red sugar [is taken] as wine for fevers consisting of yellow bile and phlegm. Sometimes the [quantity of] vinegar is reduced from this to the rate of one fifth and below. The sugar should be washed first gently, then put into the kettle. Vinegar is poured upon it. [The kettle] is put onto plain embers until the sugar dissolves. Then twice as much water, or less, or more, according to the need, is poured to it. It [should be] boiled, and its foam [should be] removed.

[SY2] Honey oxymel is not useful for hot fevers, but for those which are composed of it and for those with a cold component. The ratio of the vinegar to the honey depends on the humours in its [= fever] thickness, viscidity, and the strongness of its putridity, for the vinegar is cooling, and the honey is warming and soothing.

[SY3] وأيضا يصحب معه من شراب الرمّان المنعنع، فإنّه لتسكين القيء الصفراوي والغثيان. وصفته: تؤخذ الرمّان المزّ وتخلط معه من السكّر، وهو على النار ما لا يبطل مزوزته بالكلّية، ويصبّ عليه ماء النعناع مقدار ما لا يحدث فيه مرارة، ويلقى فيه عند الطبخ من قشر الفستق البرّاني مقدار قليل ومن ورق الأترجّ أو قشره مقدار ما تطهّر رائحته فيه، ويطبخ حتّى يصير له قوام الأشربة، ويرفع، ويترك قشر الفستق فيه، ويمصّها العليل.

[SY4] وأيضا شراب الحصرم. وصنعته: كالرمّان.

[SY5–8] وشراب الورد والبنفسج والنيلوفر ولسان الثور. | وقانون اتّخاذها أن يطبخ بالماء حتّى C265r يأخذ الماء قوّتها وطعمها ولونها، ثمّ يصفّي ذلك الماء ويلقى عليه من السكّر أو يصبّ على السكّر منه ما يعذبه قليلا وقوّته بعد | باقية، ويقوم بنار ليّنة حتّى لا يفور، فإن فار مسح عن القدر بعد سكونه T107r بخرقة مبلولة حتّى لا يحترق ويختلط به في الفورة الثانية، فيغسله، ويؤخذ له قوام الأشربة، ويرفع.

[SY9] وشراب الصندل لحرارة القلب. يؤخذ من الصندل المقاصيري ويبرد منه ثلاثون درهما بالمبرد، وينقع في نصف رطل خلّ يوما وليلة، ويطبخ من الغد في ثلاثة أرطال ماء حتّى يرجع إلى رطل ويصفّي، ويضاف إليه نصف رطل من ماء الرمّان المزّ ونصف رطل من ماء التمر الهندي وثلاثة أرطال سكّر الطبرزد، ويقوم على النار، وينزل حتّى يبرد، ثمّ يلقى عليه طباشير وصندل مسحوق درهمان، وكافور نصف درهم، وزعفران درهمان، ثمّ يرفع.

[الربوب]

وأمّا ما يحتاج إليه من الربوب

[R1–6] فربّ التفّاح المزّ والسفرجل والحصرم والرمّان والليمون والأميرباريس، وكلّ واحد منها مفردا أقوى في بابه، لكنّها إذا ركبت مع السكّر صارت ألطف. وقانون صنعتها أن يعتصر مياه الفواكه ويوضع في قدر برام على نار ليّنة حتّى يبقى النصف أو الثلث، وإن شئت أضفت إليه من السكّر الطبرزد قدر الحاجة.

---

2 تؤخذ] T: + ماء | ما] M:— 3 النعناع] MT: النعنع | مقدار ما] M: مقداره 4 مقدار] C:— C¹: مقدار صح | ما] C: ما⟦.⟧ | تطهّر] MT: يظهر 6 وأيضا] T:— 9 عن] M: على | القدر] M: العدد 10 فيغسله] C: فيغسِله MT: فيغسده 11 الصندل] M: العسد | لحرارة] C: الحرارة M: للحرارة 12 ويطبخ] M: يطبخ | ماء] M:— 13 ماء] T:— | الهندي] MT: هندي 15 وزعفران] C: زعفران | درهمان] M:— 19 أن] M:— | يعتصر] C²: صح

[SY3] He [is to] bring with himself pomegranate syrup flavoured with mint as well, for it alleviates bilious vomiting and nausea. Its recipe is: sour pomegranate is taken, sugar is mixed into it, and it is put onto the fire which does not suppress its sourish sweetness at all. Juice of mint is poured onto it in a quantity that does not cause sourness. At cooking, a small amount of the outer shell of pistachio is put into it, and leaves or peel of citron in an amount that cleans its odour. It is cooked until its consistency is that of the juices. Then it is stored, and the pistachio shell is left in it. The ill person sips it.

[SY4] [He is to bring with himself] sour grape syrup as well. It is made like the pomegranate [syrup].

[SY5–8] Rose syrup, violet syrup, water lily syrup, and borage syrup. The rule of the making of these is to cook [them] in water until the water takes their potency, taste, and colour, then strain that water, and throw sugar into it or pour from it into sugar, which sweetens it a bit while its potency remains. It is put onto a low fire so that it does not boil. If it boils, it is wiped off the kettle after it settles with a wet cloth so that it does not burn, and it is mixed with it in the second boiling. Then it is cleaned, and its consistency is that of the syrups. Then it is stored.

[SY9] Sandalwood syrup for the warmness of the heart. It is made from *Maqāsīrī* sandalwood. Thirty *dirhams* of it are filed with a rasp, and it is soaked in half a *raṭl* of vinegar for a day and a night. The following day, it is boiled in three *raṭls* of water until it boils down to one *raṭl* and it is purified. Half a *raṭl* of sour pomegranate juice and tamarind juice, and three *raṭls* of solid white sugar are added to it, and it is put onto the fire. [Then] it is left until it cools down. Then two *dirhams* of both chalk and powdered sandalwood, half a *dirham* of camphor, and two *dirhams* of saffron are added to it; then it is stored.

[Robs]

As for what he needs from the robs:

[R1–6] [These are] rob of sour apple, quince, sour grapes, pomegranate, lemon, and barberry. All are stronger as a single medicament in their category, but if they are prepared with sugar, they become finer. The rule of making these is to squeeze out the juices of the fruits and put it in an soapstone cooking pot on feeble fire until half or third [of the juice] remains. If you want, mix into it as much solid white sugar as needed.

[المعاجين]

وأمّا المعاجين التي تشتدّ الحاجة إلى حملها فخمسة.

[E1] الأوّل معجون الأطريفل. ولفظة الأطريفل معرّبة من اللغة الهندية. تقع على الهليلج | C265v الكابلي والبليلج والأملج، ثلاثتها مقوّية للأعضاء العصبية دابغة لآلات الغذاء، جمّعت وركّبت لمشاركتها في المنفعة ومعونة بعضها بعضا، وجعلت متساوية الوزن لتساوي قوّاها ومنافعها. وقد يضاف إليها الهليلج الأصفر والأسود بمثل أوزان الأدوية لقربها منها في المنفعة والمزاج والتقوية، فتصير أكمل وأقوى فعلا. ولتّت بعد سحقها بالسمن أو دهن اللوز لكسر شدّة يبوستها، لأنّ | M7v اليبوسة ضارّة للقوّة الهاضمة إذا جاوزت حدّ التقوية لآلات الغذاء. وكذلك إدمان الأطريفل يورث الهذال. والسمن أولى الأدهان بلتّها لموافقته لمزاج الإنسان، هذا إن استعمل في الوقت. فأمّا إذ أريد ادّخاره فدهن اللوز أولى، لأنّ السمن يتغيّر رائحته سريعا. ثمّ تجمع الأدوية كلها بالعسل، لأنّ العسل فيه خواصّ وأفعال شريفة وحفظ لما يخلط به من الأشياء عن التغيّر والفساد، وتبرّكا به لما ورد في الكتاب والسنة من مدحه، مع إنّه لذيذ في الذوق حبيب للطبع. ومن خواصّه بعد التغذية واللذاذة وإزالة كراهة الأدوية وبشاعتها الجلا | T107v للغضلات الغليظة وتنقيتها. ومن خواصّه أيضا أنّه يمتزج بأجزاء ما تركب معه ويستخرج قوّاها ويخلط بعضها ببعض ويخمرها حتّى يحصل لها مزاج ويكسّبها قوي لم يكن حاصلة قبل ذلك، ويصدر عنها خواصّ وأفعال شريفة ليست في الأدوية المفردة. فلذلك اختير لجمعها وعجنها العسل. والعسل نيئا أحرّ وأحدّ | C266r وأقرب للدوائية، ومطبوخا منزوع الرغوة أكثر حدّة. وينبغي أن يجعل العسل ضعف للأدوية حيث يراد تمام فعل الأدوية وكمالها. وقد يجعل ثلاثة أضعافها يصير أحرّ وألطف وأقلّ بشاعة. ثمّ يرفع.

[E2] الثاني معجون الخيار شنبر للقولنج الحارّ والعلل الصفراوية والبلغمية من الأحشاء. يوخذ من البنفسج الإصفهاني والتربد من كلّ واحد أربعون درهما، ومن الملح الهندي سبعة دراهم ونصف، ومن بزر الرازيانج والآنيسون والمصطكاء من كلّ واحد خمسة دراهم، ومن ربّ

---

3 تقع] C: يقع 6 بمثل] M: مثل 7 فتصير] C: فيصير 8 لآلات] M: آلات 9 أولى] C: أَوْلى | الأدهان] C: للادهان 10 إذ] T: اذا | تجمع] M: بجتمع 11 لأنّ] T: فان | وأفعال] M: افعال | التغيّر] MT: التعفن 12 الكتاب] M: + العزيز | حبيب] C: حبب 13 الجلا ... وتنقيتها] MT: الجلا ونضج الفضلات 14 يمتزج] C[1]: يمترج | تركب] T: يركب 15 ويصدر] MT: فيصدر 16 فلذلك] T: ولذلك 17 يجعل] M[2]: ص | للأدوية] M: الادوية 18 يصير] MT: ليصير 20 والتربد] M: + والمصطكى | درهما] C: — 21 والمصطكاء] M: —

[Electuaries]
As for the electuaries which are highly needed to be carried, these are five.

[E1] The first is the triphala (*iṭrīfal*) electuary. The word *iṭrīfal* is Arabized from the Indian language. It consists of chebulic myrobalan, beleric myrobalan, and amla. These three are strengthening for the nervy organs and softening for the digestive organs, combined and prepared together for their collaboration in beneficial use and their aiding of the other. Their weight is the same for the equity of their taste and benefit. Yellow and black myrobalan is added to them, the same weight as the medicaments, for their similarity in benefit, disposition, and strengthening. Thus, it becomes more complete and strong in effect. It is kneaded after it is crushed with clarified butter or almond oil to break the strongness of its dryness, for the dryness is harmful to the digestive power if it exceeds the verge of strengthening the digestive organs. Likewise, the excess of triphala causes skinniness. Clarified butter is better than oils for kneading them for its accordance with the temperament of man, that is if it is used right away. If its preservation is wanted, almond oil is better, for clarified butter changes its smell quickly. Then all of the medicament is combined in honey, for in honey there are eminent characteristics and effects, and it preserves what is mixed into it from the things from changing and spoiling, and they are blessed in it for what is said in the Quran and Sunna on its praising, besides that it has a tasty flavour and it is pleasant for the natural disposition. Its characteristics thereupon are nourishment, tastiness, elimination of the disgust of medicaments and their evident ugliness due to the thick residues and cleaning them. Its characteristics are also that it mixes with the parts which are prepared with it and extracts their power, it mixes them and ferments them until it becomes a mixture, lets them attain a power that was not attained before, and eminent characteristics and effects originate from them which were not [present] in the simple medicaments. For this, honey is preferred for their [= medicaments] mixing and kneading. Raw honey is the warmest, sharpest, and closest to medicative [purposes]. Cooked [honey with its] foam removed is its greatest sharpness. The honey should be made double [the amount] of the medicament when the whole and complete effect of the remedy is wanted. If it is made thrice as much, it becomes more warm, mild, and less ugly. Then it is stored.

[E2] The second is the electuary of purging cassia against warm colic and yellow bilious and phlegmatic illnesses of the intestines. It is prepared from Isfahanian violet and turpeth, 40 *dirhams* of each, seven and a half *dirhams* of Indian salt, fennel seeds, anise seeds, and mastic, five *dirhams* of each,

السوس أربعة عشر درهما، ومن السقمونيا خمسة عشر درهما، ومن فلوس الخيار شنبر مائة درهم، يوزن هذا الأدوية منخولة، ويجمع مع لبّ الخيار شنبر مائة درهم فانيذ ومائة درهم عسل، ويجمع الأدوية بها، والشربة من خمسة دراهم إلى عشرة.

[E3] الثالث ترياق الأربع نافع من سموم الحيوانات القاتلة بلدغها، لا سيّما العقرب، ومن العلل البلغمية. وصفته: جنطيانا رومي وحبّ الغار ومرّ مكي وزراوند طويل من كلّ واحد جزء، ويدقّ الأدوية، ويعجن بعسل منزوع الرغوة، والشربة مثقال.

[E4] الرابع معجون النانخواه لتفتيت الحصاة وتنقية آلات البول. يدقّ النانخواه ناعما، وتعجن بعسل منزوع الرغوة، ويرفع، والشربة مثقال.

[E5] الخامس معجون لنضج السعال البلغمي. يؤخذ بزر الكتّان، يقلي قليا خفيفا | C266v لتنقّص رطوبته الفضلية ويكتسب غروية وسخونة أزيد، ثمّ يدقّ، ويعجن بعسل منزوع الرغوة.

[الحبوب المسهلة]

وأمّا ما يحتاج إليه من الحبوب المسهلة

[PP1] لحب لتنقية البدن من الأخلاط المختلفة. تربد مثقال، هليلج أصفر نصف درهم، افتيمون دانق ونصف، غاريقون نصف درهم، شحم حنظل دانق، زنجبيل دانق، مصطكى دانق، مقل أزرق دانقان، كثيراء طسوج | M8r ورد أحمر دانق، تدقّ الأدوية، وينقع الكثيراء ويعجن به الأدوية، ويحبّب، وهو شربة واحدة.

[PP2] وحبّ يسهل السوداء والبلغم. تربد مثقال، أيارج فيقرا درهم، أصطوخودوس دانقان، غاريقون نصف درهم، | T108r سقمونيا دانق ونصف، زنجبيل وورد أحمر من كلّ دانق، مقل أزرق دانقان، يدقّ الأدوية، وينقع المقل في الماء ويعجن به الأدوية، ويحبّب.

---

2 هذا الأدوية] T: هذه | مع ... فانيذ] M:— | لبّ ... شنبر] T: ⟦ ⟧ | ومائة] M: ماله 4 الحيوانات] C: الحيونات 5 رومي] C: رومس C²: ٢ | من] M:— 6 ويدقّ] M: ندق T: تدق 7 وتنقية] M: نفعيه | يدقّ] M: تدق 8 ويرفع] M: + وبـــسل T: + وتستعمل 10 الفضلية] M: لتمص | ويكتسب] M: وتكسر 14–15 مصطكى ... دانق] C:— C¹: + صح 15 الأدوية] T: + الادوية | وينقع] M: تنقع 17 تربد] MT: تريد | أصطوخودوس] MT: اسطوخودس 18 من كلّ] MT:— 19 يدقّ] T: تدق | وينقع] M: تنقع

14 *dirhams* of liquorice rob, 15 *dirhams* of scammony, and 100 *dirhams* of the scales of purging cassia. These drugs are weighed after they have been sieved. 100 *dirhams* of purging cassia kernels are mixed with pulled taffy and 100 *dirhams* of honey, and the drugs are mixed into this. The dose is from five to ten *dirhams*.

[E3] The third is quadruple theriac, [which is] useful against the poisons of animals killing with their stings, especially the scorpion, and against phlegmatic illnesses. Its recipe is: Byzantine gentian, bay kernels, Meccan myrrh, long aristolochia, one part of each. The medicament is pulverised and kneaded with honey, the foam of which was removed. The dose is one *mithqāl*.

[E4] The fourth is the electuary of ajowan, for the dismemberment of the calculus and purification of the urinary organs. The ajowan is pulverised finely and kneaded with honey, the foam of which was removed. It is stored. The dose is one *mithqāl*.

[E5] The fifth is an electuary for the ripeness of phlegmatic cough. It is made of flaxseed slightly roasted to decrease its excess moistness and let it obtain greater viscosity and warmth. Then it is pulverised and kneaded with honey, the foam of which has been removed.

[Purgative pills]
As for what he needs from the purgative pills:

[PP1] A pill for the purification of the body from the different humours. One *mithqāl* of turpeth, half a *dirham* of yellow myrobalan, one and a half *dāniq* of dodder, half a *dirham* of agaric, one *dāniq* of colocynth pulp, one *dāniq* of ginger, one *dāniq* of mastic, two *dāniq*s of bdellium, one *ṭassūj* of tragacanth, one *dāniq* of red rose. The medicament is pulverised, the tragacanth is soaked, and the medicament is kneaded with it, and it is made into a pill. It is one dose.

[PP2] A pill that purges black bile and phlegm. One *mithqāl* of turpeth, one *dirham* of hiera picra, two *dāniq*s of lavender, half a *dirham* of agaric, one and a half *dāniq* of scammony, one *dāniq* of both ginger and red rose, two *dāniq*s of bdellium. The medicaments are pulverised, the bdellium is soaked in water, and the medicaments are kneaded with it. It is made into a pill.

[PP3] وحبّ يطيّب النكهة، يؤخذ في الفم غدوة وعشية ويبلع ماؤه. مسك وقرنفل وقرفة وجوزبوا وسعد وسنبل وقشر الأترجّ بالسوية، يدقّ، ويجمع بربّ المشمش، ويتّخذ حبّاً كالحمّص.

[PP4] وحبّ الملوك لمن يعاف المسهل ويتعيّاه. تربد درهم، غاريقون ثلثي درهم، [هليلج] أصفر دانق ونصف، هليلج أسود دانق ونصف، افتيمون نصف درهم، مصطكاء ربع درهم، بادرنبوية سدس درهم، سقمونيا انطاكي سدس درهم، زعفران سدس درهم، طباشير سدس درهم، ورد أحمر سدس درهم، تدقّ الأدوية، ويعجن بجلاب.

[الأشياف]

وأمّا ما يحتاج إلى حمله من الأشياف

فإن كانت ليبس البطن | والقولنج وتنقية الأمعاء وما يليها، فينبغي أن يكون مستطيله في طول C267r الأصبع أو أزيد ليقع في المعاء المستقيم ويصل أثرها إلى المعاء قولون. وإمّا إذا اتّخذت لوجع الورك والنسا فتجعل مدودة ليطول مقامها في موضع قريب من العلّة. أمّا الليّنة منها المستعملة في الحمّيات، فأقواها:

[SU1] أشياف البنفسج. وصفته: بنفسج وسكّر أحمر ورجبين، وهو ماء اللبن المنعقد، من كلّ واحد خمسة دراهم، سقمونيا وتربد وبورق من كلّ واحد ثلاثة دراهم، ملح هندي درهمان، تجمع الأدوية، ويعمل شيافا.

[SU2] وأمّا الشيافات الحارّة المحتاج إليها في القولنج البارد وتسخين الظهر وإسهال البلغم، فأشرفها الصابون الذي من الزيت إذا خرط منه شيافة وأحمل بها، أو جمعت مع الفانيذ أو العسل على النار ويذرّ عليها الملح المسحوق والبورق والتربد والزنجبيل وشحم الحنظل والسقمونيا ونحوها من الأدوية المسهلة، أو المحلّلة للرياح، مثل الشونيز والكمّون والجندبيدستر، أو يجمع هذه مع الصموغ الحارّة، كالجاوشير والسكبينج.

---

1 غدوة] M: عديره | مسك] M: سكر   2 وسعد] C^2: صح | وقشر] M: قشر | بربّ] M: شرب 5 سقمونيا] C:— | زعفران سدس] M: راعون قليدس   5–6 سدس درهم] C: ~~سدس درهم~~ 8 الأشياف] M: الشيافات   9 مستطيله] C: مپستطيله M: مسطتيلة   10 المستقيم] M: المستقيمة | المعاء قولون] C: قولون المعا | الورك] C: الور⟦ق⟧   11 الليّنة] M: الكيفية   13 أشياف] M: شنيان | ماء] M: + بقه T: مابه   14 خمسة ... واحد] M:—   15 شيافا] C: اشيافا M: شيافات   16 الحارّة] M^2: صح   17 وأحمل بها] MT:—   19 أو] M: و

[PP3] A pill that makes the smell of the breath pleasant [and it is] put into the mouth in the morning and the evening and its liquid is swallowed. Musk, clove, cinnamon, fragrant nutmeg, cyperus, spikenard, and citron peel in an equal amount are pulverised and mixed with apricot rob and taken as pills [sized] like the chickpea.

[PP4] The pill of kings for he who loathes suffering from diarrhoea and it makes him ill. One *dirham* of turpeth, two thirds *dirham* of agaric, one and a half *dāniq* yellow [myrobalan], one and a half *dāniq* of black myrobalan, half a *dirham* of wormwood, quarter *dirham* of mastic, sixth *dirham* of lemon balm, sixth *dirham* of Antiochian scammony, sixth *dirham* of saffron, sixth *dirham* of chalk, sixth *dirham* of red rose. The medicament is pulverised and kneaded with julep.

[Suppositories]
As for what he needs to carry from the suppositories:

If it is for the dryness of the stomach, colic, purification of the bowels, and what follows them, it should be prolongated to the length of a finger or more to get to the rectum and for its effect of getting to the colon. If it is taken for the pain of the hip and sciatica, it is to be extended so that its place reaches a position close to the illness. The gentle of these are used against the fevers, and the strongest of them is:

[SU1] Suppository of the violet. Its recipe is: violet, red sugar, whey, which is the liquid of the curded milk, five *dirhams* of each, scammony, turpeth, borax, three *dirhams* of each, and two *dirhams* of Indian salt. The medicaments are mixed and made into a suppository.

[SU2] As for the warm suppositories, which are needed for cold colic, warming of the back, and purging black bile. The most eminent of these is the soap which was made from olive oil if a suppository is cut off from it and it is born; or it is combined with pulled taffy or honey on fire, and sprinkled with powdered salt, borax, turpeth, ginger, colocynth pulp, scammony, and purging remedies similar to these; or [with] flatulence dissolvants like nigella, cumin, castoreum, or these mixed with warming melted [herbage] like opopanax[17] and sagapenum.[18]

---

17 Yellow, more opaque gum resin of *Opopanax chironium* mainly used in perfumery today; or the plant itself. Dietrich, *Dioscurides triumphans*, II/398–399 (no. III/47); Löw, *Aramaeische Pflanzennamen*, 190–191 (no. 145).

18 Yellow, translucent gum resin of a species of *Ferula* (*Ferula scowitziana* DC. and var.) with a smell similar to assafetida; or the plant itself. Dietrich, *Dioscurides triumphans*, II/432–433 (no. III/76); Löw, *Aramaeische Pflanzennamen*, 190–191 (no. 145); Dietrich, *Ṣamgh*.

[الأقراص]

وأمّا ما تشتدّ الحاجة إليه من الأقراص فثلاثة.

[PA1] الأوّل قرص الكافور للحمّيات الحارّة والخفقان مع الحرارة. طباشير وورد وصندل أبيض وبزر الخيارين وبزر الهندباء | C267v والخسّ والبقلة الحمقاء أجزاء سوية، تجمع مسحوقة، ويخلط بكلّ مثقال من الجميع من شعيرة إلى نصف قيراط من الكافور بمقدار الحاجة، ويعجن بماء التفّاح، ويقرّص أقراصا رقاقا، ويجفّف في الظلّ، والشربة | T108v منه مثقال.

[PA2] الثاني قرص العود للقيء والهيضة مع البرودة. كندر ثلاثة دراهم، ورد ستة دراهم، عود قرنفل مسك سنبل طين الأكل طباشير من كلّ واحد درهم، مصطكاء ثلاثة دراهم، سويق حبّ | M8v الرمّان درهمان، يدقّ الأدوية، ويجمع، ويقرّص.

[PA3] الثالث قرص الورد لتقوية المعدة. ورد أحمر عشرة دراهم، ربّ سوس درهمان، سنبل طيّب درهم، مصطكاء درهم، تدقّ الأدوية، وتقرّص أقراصا رقاقا.

[السفوفات]

وأمّا ما يضطرّ إليه من السفوفات فثلاثة.

[MP1] الأوّل سفوف المقلياثا للسحج والحرارة والمغص. برر قطونا وبزر المرو وبزر الخشخاش الأبيض وبزر الحماض وبزر الفرنخ وحبّ الآس والصمغ العربي والطين الارمني أجزاء سوية، يقلي البزور سوى بزر الحماض، لأنّه ليس من البزور اللعابية، فتقلي لتصير لعابتها غروية، ويجفّ الرطوبة، وتدقّ الأدوية ما سوى البزر قطوتا، لحدّة ما في باطنه، وسوى بزر المرو، لأنّ المقصود منه ظاهره ولعابه الغليظ، ويستّف بمعونة ربّ السفرجل أو ربّ الآس إذا كان هناك سعال.

---

5 شعيرة] CM: سعيره | قيراط] M: مثقال T: ~~مثقال~~ قيراط | بمقدار] M: بقدر 7–8 دراهم ... عود] M: — 8 قرنفل] M: وقرنفل | طين] M: — 11 طيّب] T: الطيب | تدقّ] C: يدق | وتقرّص] C: ويقرص 14 المقلياثا] M: المقليات | والمغص] M: والعصر 15 الفرنخ] CT: القرنخ M: الفرمح | العربي] M: المغربي | سوية] CMT: سوا 16 يقلي] M: ىنقلى | بزر] C: برب | ويجفّ] M: ىخف 17 وتدقّ] C: يدق | ما ... باطنه] MT: — | وسوى] MT: سوى | بزر] C: البزر

[Pastilles]
As for what is strongly needed from the pastilles, those are three.

[PA1] The first is the camphor pastille for warm fevers and heartbeat with warmness. Chalk, rose, white sandalwood, seeds of both types of cucumber [?], endive seeds, lettuce, purslane in equal parts. They are put together grounded, and into each *mithqāl* of the mixture up to half a *qīrāṭ* of barley and camphor according to the need is mixed. It is kneaded with apple juice and made into small pastilles and dried in the shade. The dose of it is one *mithqāl*.

[PA2] The second is the aloeswood pastille for vomiting and summer cholera with coldness. Three *dirhams* of frankincense, six *dirhams* of rose, aloeswood, clove, musk, spikenard, *Naysābūr* clay, and chalk, one *dirham* of each, three *dirhams* of mastic, two *dirhams* of pomegranate seed stems. The medicaments are pulverised, mixed, and made into pastilles.

[PA3] The third is the rose pastille for strengthening the stomach. Ten *dirhams* of red rose, two *dirhams* of liquorice rob, one *dirham* of sweet-scented spikenard, one *dirham* of mastic. The medicaments are pulverised and made into small pastilles.

[Medicinal powders]
As to what he needs from the medicinal powders, those are three.

[MP1] The first is the *muqliyāthā* [= roasted] powder[19] for abrasion, warmness, and gripes. Psyllium seeds, marjoram seeds, white poppy seeds, bladder dock seeds, seeds of purslane,[20] myrtle seeds, gum arabic, and Armenian bole, in equal parts. The seeds are roasted except the bladder dock, for that is not from the mucous seeds. They are roasted so that their mucousity becomes viscous and the wetness dries up. The medicaments are pulverised except for the psyllium seeds for the vehemence of what is inside it, and except the marjoram seeds, for its outside and thick mucus is wanted from it. It is arranged with the help of quince rob or myrtle rob, if there is a cough.

19 See Fellmann, *Das Aqrābāḏīn al-Qalānisī*, 263. I would like to thank one of my anonymous reviewers for this reference.

20 Maybe it stands for *qirfa* with a *tā' marbūṭa* instead of a *ḥā'* (which would mean a kind of cinnamon; however, *dār ṣīnī* is used through the text for cinnamon; it is also worth noting that seeds of cinnamon (tree) are not listed in any of the other recipes). While the diacritical marks in manuscripts C and T are quite clear, another possibility could be *farfakh* (being a synonym of *baqla ḥamqā'*, purslane; the latter is used through the text, therefore using another name for the same ingredient would not make sense, just like with *dār ṣīnī* and *qirfa*; however, seeds of purslane seem more plausible than seeds of cinnamon).

C268r [MP2] | الثاني سفوف البزور لحرقة البول. وصفته: لبّ بطّيخ مقشّر ثلاثون درهما، لبّ الخيار المقشّر والقرع وبزر البقلة الحمقاء والخشخاش من كلّ واحد عشرة دراهم، نشا وكثيراء وربّ السوس من كلّ واحد ثلاثة دراهم، بزر البنج درهمان، سكّر مثل الكلّ، يستفّ منه ثلاثة دراهم غدوة ومثله عشية بشراب البنفسج أو شراب الجلاب.

[MP3] الثالث سفوف ينفع من السلس بلا حرقة ولا عطش. لحاء لبّ بلّوط خمسون درهما، كندر ثلاثون درهما، كزبرة يابسة وطين ارمني وصمغ عربي من كلّ واحد عشرة دراهم، والشربة منه ثلاثة دراهم غدوة وعشية مثله.

[الأكحال والشيافات للعين]

وأمّا ما تمسّ الحاجة إليه من الأكحال والشيافات للعين

[C1] فشياف أحمر ينفع من بقايا الرمد وغلظ الأجفان والحرب الخفيف. وصفته: شادنج مغسول خمسة دراهم، نحاس محرق ثلاثة دراهم، بسّذ ولؤلؤ وكهرباء واسرنج من كلّ واحد درهمين، صمغ عربي وكثيراء من كلّ واحد خمسة دراهم، دم الأخوين وزعفران من كلّ واحد نصف درهم، يدقّ وينخل، ويعجن بماء الورد والحصرم.

[C2] وبرود وينفع من حرارة العين والسلاق والدمعة. وصنعته: يؤخذ التوتيا. فتسحّق ناعما، وتربّى بماء الحصرم الذي قد اعتصر منه، وجعل في الشمس أيّاما، ثمّ يصفي وتربّى به، ثمّ يترك ليجفّف، ويسحق ناعما، | ويكتحل به. C268v

T109r [C3] وأمّا ما يحفظ صحّة العين وينشف الدمعة | والقروح فالإثمد، وهو المعروف بالكحل الأسود وأيضا كحل الزعفران، ينفع من الظلمة والحكّة. وصنعته: زعفران وسنبل الطيّب من كلّ واحد درهمان، دار فلفل درهم فلفل أبيض دانق ونصف، نوشادر نصف درهم، عفص ثلاثة درهم، كافور نصف دانق، يدقّ وينخل بخرقة حرير، ثمّ ينعم، ويكتحل به.

---

1 لبّ] C: — C^2: + | لبّ] C: — C^2: + T: بزر   2–3 وربّ السوس] M: رب سوس T: ورب سوس
3 واحد] C: — | دراهم] T: —   5 لحاء لبّ] C: تحالب M: عالب T: غالب   6–7 كزبرة … دراهم]
M: —   9 ما] C: — C^2: +   10 والحرب] M: والربو   11 مغسول] C: مغپسول | بسّذ ولؤلؤ] C: بپسدولولو
M: حرسدولولو   12 واحد] C: —   13 والحصرم] C^2: صح   14 التوتيا] M: المرتيا   15 وتربّى] C: تعربى
C^1: وتربي صح   16 ليجفّف] M: ويخف   18 الأسود] M: الازود | الطيّب] M: طيب   20 ويكتحل]
C: ويكون يكتحل

[MP2] The second is the powder of seeds for burning urine. Its recipe is: thirty *dirhams* of peeled watermelon kernel, peeled cucumber kernel, pumpkin, purslane seeds, and poppy, ten *dirhams* of each, cornstarch, tragacanth, and liquorice rob, three *dirhams* of each, two *dirhams* of henbane seeds, and sugar like these together. Three *dirhams* of it are swallowed in the morning and the same in the evening with violet syrup or julep syrup.

[MP3] The third is a powder useful against incontinence of urine without burning and without sneezing. Fifty *dirhams* of acorn peels,[21] thirty *dirhams* of frankincense, dry coriander, Armenian bole, and gum arabic, ten *dirhams* of each. The dosage from this is three *dirhams* in the morning and evening likewise.

[Collyriums and eye remedies]

As for what is necessary from the collyriums and remedies for the eye:

[C1] A red eye remedy useful against the residues of eye inflammation, the coarseness of the eyelids, and slight scabies. Its recipe is: five *dirhams* of washed hematite, three *dirhams* of burnt copper, coral, pearl, amber, and red lead, two *dirhams* of each, gum arabic and tragacanth, five *dirhams* of each, dragon's blood and saffron, half a *dirham* of each. It is pulverised, sieved out, and kneaded with rose water or sour grape juice.

[C2] A collyrium useful against the warmness of the eye, the roughness of the eyelids, and epiphora. Its preparation is: zinc oxide is taken, it is pulverised finely, and cooked [like a jam] with sour grape juice which was squeezed from it, and put under the sun for some days. Then it is cleared and cooked [like a jam]. Then it is left to dry and it is pulverised. The eyelids are coloured with it.

[C3] As to what preserves the health of the eye and cures epiphora and ulcers. It is antimony, known as black kohl and also the saffron kohl, which is useful for darkness and itching. Its recipe is: saffron and sweet-scented spikenard, two *dirhams* of each, one *dirham* of long pepper, one and a half *dāniq*s of white pepper, half a *dirham* of ammonia, three *dirhams* of gallnuts, half a *dāniq* of camphor. It is pulverised and sieved with a silk cloth. Then it becomes fine, and the eyelids are [to be] coloured with it.

21 I would like to thank one of my anonymous reviewers for the reading *liḥā'*.

[الأدهان]

وأمّا ما يحتاج إليه من حمل الأدهان

[O1–13] فدهن البنفسج والورد والخشخاش والخسّ والقرع ودهن السوس والياسمين ودهن البلسان والخروع والبابونج والخيار والآس والسفرجل. وأمّا كيفية عملها فقد تركب الأدهان مع الأدوية بواسطة الماء والنار. إمّا بأن تطبخ الأدوية التي تريد تسمية ذلك الدهن بها من بنفسج وورد وغيره في الماء حتّى يأخذ الماء قوّاها، | ثمّ يصفي ذلك الماء، ويمزج بأيّ دهن أردت من زيت M9r وغيره، ثمّ يغلي حتّى يذهب الماء ويبقى قوّة ذلك الدواء في الدهن. فإن كان الدواء الذي طبخ في الماء وردا فهذا دهن ورد أو كان بنفسجا فهو دهن بنفسج إلى غير ذلك. إمّا بأن تلقى الادوية وهي عفصة طرية في الدهن ويشمّس حتّى يكتسب الدهن قوّاها، وقد تركب الأدهان مع قوى الأدوية بواسطة الهواء، بأن تجمع الرياحين الرطبة | واللبوب الدهنة في خرائط صفيقة ويستوثق C269r من رأسها، ثمّ يترك حتّى يذيّل، ثمّ تبدل ويتّخذ غيرها عفصة طرية ويكرّر ذلك حتّى يأخذ اللبوب قوى الأدوية ورائحتها، ثمّ تعتصر اللبوب عند الحاجة وتؤخذ دهنها. وهذا ضعيف جدّا بالقياس إلى الصنفين المتقدّمين. وقد استأثروا هذا الطريق في الأدهان الباردة الرطبة، مثل البنفسج واللينوفر، احترازا عن استيلاء حرارة النار أو الشمس عليها وأفنا رطوبتها التي هي المطلوب منها، وحذارا أن تزنخ سريعا وتصير حارّة.

[المراهم والذرورات]

وأمّا ما تدعوا الضرورة إليه من المراهم والذرورات

[L1] فمرهم لإنبات اللحم والإلحام. يؤخذ أوقية مرداسنج مسحوق، مثل الكحل، ويصبّ عليه ثلاثة أواق زيت، ويطبخ ويحرس حتّى ينحلّ، ثمّ يؤخذ كندر وأنزروت ودم الأخوين وقنّا وزفت يابس من كلّ واحد درهمان، فتلقى عليه مسحوقة، ويطبخ حتّى يغلو، ويرفع اخر.

4 والخيار] C: الحنا M: الحيار 5 بأن] M: ان | تطبخ] CM: يطبخ | بها] MT: — 6 قوّاها] C: فواها 7 الماء] M: الا | ويبقى] M: وينعى | كان] M: — T: + ذلك 8 وردا] T: ورد | فهذا] M: فهو | تلقى] C: يلقى 9 ويشمّس] C: ويشمش | قوّاها] C: فواها 10 الأدوية] C: الادهان ويه | صفيقة] M: صفته 11 عفصة] C: غصه M: عصة | ويكرّر] M: وبكسر 12 تعتصر] C: تعصر 13 واللينوفر] M: والنيْلُوفر T: النيلوفر 14 وأفنا] M: واضار | رطوبتها] M: طوتها | وحذارا] C: حذور⟦ا⟧ M: وحدرا T: وحذرا 15 سريعا] C: بسريعا | وتصير] M: وقصير 19 ثلاثة] T: ثلاث | ويحرس] M: ويحرل T: يحرك 20 ويرفع] C: — C¹: + صح T: —

[Oils]

As to what he needs to carry from the oils:

[O1–13] Oil of violet, rose, poppy, lettuce, and pumpkin, oil of iris and jasmine, and oil of lemon balm, castor bean, chamomile, cucumber,[22] myrtle, and quince. The manner of their preparation: the oils are prepared with the medicaments by means of water and fire. Either by cooking the medicaments which are needed according to the naming of these oils from violet, rose, and the others in water until the water takes their power, then that water is cleaned, and it is mixed into whichever oil you want from olive oil and the others, then it is boiled until the water evaporates and the power of that remedy remains in the oil. If the remedy which was cooked in the water was rose, then it is rose oil, if it was violet, it is violet oil, and so on. Or [these are prepared by] throwing the medicament which is sour and fresh into the oil, and it is laid out to the sun until the oil acquires their power. The oils take the power of the remedies by means of the air, in that the aromatic plants collect the moistness and the pulps [collect] the odour in thick receptacles, and it bonds to their extremities. Then it is left to continue [like this]. Then it is replaced and another [part] form thick pieces. This is repeated until the pulps collect the powers and odours of the medicaments. Then the pulps are squeezed out when needed, and their oil is used. This is really weak in comparison with the previously mentioned kinds. This method is appropriate for cold and moist oils, like the violet and water lily, as a precaution against the continued heat of the fire or sun on them destroying their moistness, which is required of them, being aware of it turning rancid quickly and becoming hot.

[Liniments and powders]

As for what is necessary from the liniments and powders:

[L1] A liniment for the growth of flesh and tissue growth. It is prepared from one *ūqiya* of litharge pulverised like kohl, three *ūqiya*s of olive oil is poured into it, it is boiled and watched over until it dissolves. Then frankincense, anzerot, dragon's blood, galbanum, and dry pitch is taken, two *dirhams* of each. These are thrown into it [after being] pulverised, and it is cooked until it boils, then it is stored.

22 In MS C, it is [oil of] henna.

[L2] وهو مرهم الباسليقون ينبت اللحم ويصلّح المواضع العصبية والجرّاحات التي لا حرارة فيها. وصنعته: زفت وراتينج وشمع من كلّ واحد عشرون مثقالا، قنّا أربعة دراهم، يجمع بزيت، ويذاب به بقدر الحاجة، | ويرفع. T109v

وأمّا الذرورات

[PO1] فذرور ملحّم. | كندر وأنزروت مرّ مكّي ودم الأخوين أجزاء سوية، وهو المعروف بالأربعة الأدوية. C269v

[PO2] وذرور مجفّف. مرداسنج وورق السوسن وقشور البليلج وعفص جزء ومن كلّ واحد، قشر الرمّان نصف جزء، ويدقّ ناعما، ويرفع.

[ما يقطع الدم]

وأمّا ما يقطع الدم

[H1–2] فالزاج القبرصي أو الشب المحرق.

[السنونات]

وأمّا ما يحتاج إليه من السنونات

[D1] فسنون يجلو الأسنان. زبد البحر محرق ورماد الصدف ورماد أصل القصب الفارسي وزراوند مدحرج أجزاء سوية.

[D2] وسنون يشتدّ اللثّة والأسنان. قرن أيّل محرق ملح أندراني محرق هليلج أصفر ورد من كلّ واحد جزء، وجلنار نصف جزء، ،

---

1 والجرّاحات] C²: ح | حرارة] M: مرارة 2 أربعة] M: اربع 3 به] M: — 5 وأنزروت] C: انزروت 6 الأدوية] M: ادوية 7 وورق السوسن] T: وورق ~~السوسن~~ السوسن 8 نصف] M: مصفى 11 القبرصي] M: القبرجو 16 قرن أيّل] M: قمدايل

[L2] This is the basilicon liniment. It grows the flesh, restores the nerved places, and the wounds which do not have warmness in them. Its preparation is: pitch, resin, and wax, twenty *mithqāls* of each, and four *dirhams* of galbanum are put together in olive oil and dissolved in it according to the need, and is stored.

As for the powders:

[PO1] A soldering powder. Frankincense, anzerot, Meccan myrrh, and dragon's blood in equal parts. It is known as the four medicaments.

[PO2] A drying powder. Litharge, iris leaves, beleric myrobalan peels, and gallnut, one part of each, and half part of pomegranate peel is pulverised finely and stored.

[Against bleeding]

As for what stops bleeding:

[H1–2] Cyprian vitriol or burnt alum.

[Dentifrices]

As for what he needs from the dentifrices:

[D1] A dentifrice which clears the teeth. Burnt sea foam, seashell ashes, Persian sugarcane trunk ashes, and smearwort in equal parts.

[D2] A dentifrice which strengthens the gums and the teeth. Burnt antler of red deer, burnt *Andarānī* salt, yellow myrobalan, and rose, one part of each, and half a part of pomegranate flowers.

، وهذا ما اردنا عمله قد كمل ، نسأل الله تعالى أن يجعله من صالح العمل ،
، منقذا من الأوصاب والعلل ، مبرئا من كلّ أمر حلل ،
، والحمد لله ربّ العالمين وصلّى الله على سيّدنا ،
، محمّد وآله وصحبه وسلّم ،
غفر الله لكاتبه ولصاحبه
ولمصنّفه ولمن
قرأ لهم ودعا
بالمغفرة
ولجميع
المسلمين
أجمعين.

1–11 وهذا ... أجمعين] M: ، هَذا اخر مَا اردنا عمَله ، تم الكتاب ، بعون | الملك الوهاب ، والله اعلم بالصّواب ، واليه المرجع والماب ، | ، على يد اقل عباد الله واحوجهم الى عفوه وغفرانه ، | ، محمد بن على بن محمد بن عمر القلتى الازهرى عفى الله ذنوبه ،| ، وستر عيوبه وعفى عنه وسامحه ، | ، ولمانِحه ولجميع المسامين ، | ، في سادس عسر ، | ، ربع الاول ، | سنه | ، ٩٧٦ ، T: وهذا آخر | ما اردناه والله سحانه وتعالى اعلم | تمه الفقر أبو الصلاح محمد | الحنفى | ى ١٧ جمادى الاولى | من شهور سه ١٠٨٣ بمصر

This is what we wanted to carry out, and it is completed. We
ask God Almighty to make it a useful accomplishment,
a saviour from illnesses and maladies, a recoverer of all things.
Praise be to God, Lord of the worlds, and may
the blessings and peace of God be upon our lord
Muḥammad, his family, and his companions.
May God give forgiveness for its writer, its possessor,
its compiler, and for who
read to them, and pray
for forgiveness
and for all the Muslims
completely.

Commentary

Ibn al-Amshāṭī's travel regimen entitled *al-Isfār ʿan ḥikam al-asfār* encompasses several aspects worth of analyses. In this Commentary, I focus on three such features.

In Chapter *1 Preface: A Literary Analysis* I examine the preface of the work separately due to the contrast between the genre of literary prefaces and the rest of the work (a technical, medical text), which warrants distinct aspects and criteria.

In Chapter *2 Introduction and Chapters 1–8: The Isfār as a Travel Regimen* I take under scrutiny the medical content of the treatise following the structure of the treatise itself, leaning on the results of the discussion of travel regimens in the Introductory part of the present book.

In Chapter *3 Epilogue: Simple and Compound Medicaments for Travellers* I employ both simple statistical and comparative methods to offer a preliminary evaluation of the most unique feature of Ibn al-Amshāṭī's travel regimen.

1 Preface: A Literary Analysis

A systematic analysis of the whole text would not do much to further an evaluation of its literary qualities, due to the fact that it is mostly a technical text. The literary aspect, however, is of particular importance since the author dedicated the work not only to a simple *kātib*, 'scribe', but to the *kātib al-sirr*, 'head of the chancery'. A necessary qualification for fulfilling this post, besides many other things, was eloquence and mastery of the ornate prose style (*inshāʾ*) of the chancery. Therefore, one would expect the author to strive to showcase his literary prowess to his patron or to not embarrass himself at the very least. As opposed to that of the whole text, a thorough scrutiny of the preface would provide a perfect testing-ground to appraise the author's belletristic capabilities for the following reasons.

The *muqaddima* (plural *muqaddimāt*, 'introduction, preface, foreword, exordium'), the preface to prose works emerging in the 3rd/9th centuries, is an independent literary form from the 4th/10th century onwards.[1] It consists of three distinct parts (initial commendations, a middle part, and closing praises), and its construction relies on the use of standardised patterns, expressions,

1 Freimark, *Muḳaddima*, 495; Freimark, *Das Vorwort*, 161–162.

 DOI:10.1163/9789004708204_004

and topoi. Nevertheless, it provides the author with an opportunity to present these elements with his unique twists integrated into the formulae and topoi. This way, the *muqaddima* can incorporate the specific functions desired by the author and allows him to showcase his literary skills as well. As a result of this, it proves to be a rewarding ground for a survey, as Freimark demonstrated.[2] Another point to make is what Bauer notes in his article on Mamluk literature: one of "the major fields of activity of the Mamluk *adīb*" is the *inshāʾ*, which includes "drawing up of [...] related texts (such as prefaces to books) in elaborated and rhymed prose".[3] The fact that literary anthologies include examples of *sajʿ* and *inshāʾ* besides poetry[4] indicates that such texts were considered a part of literature and therefore had literary qualities.

Returning to the treatise *al-Isfār ʿan ḥikam al-asfār*, Ibn al-Amshāṭī conforms to the language of medical works throughout the whole work. Still, he has the opportunity to abandon this style and participate in a kind of "literary communication" in the *muqaddima*.[5]

In this analysis, I will first examine the content following its tripartite structure, focusing on its functions and topoi besides its literary quality, taking note of some possible Quranic allusions found in the preface, relying on the works of Freimark for the most part and thus using the terms 'function' and 'topoi' in a 'Freimarkian' sense. Then I will analyse the *sajʿ*, 'rhymed prose' of the preface.

However, looking at the structure of the work, we must notice that there is another, 'second' *muqaddima* or introduction following the one analysed here. Therefore, to avoid any further confusion, I will use the term 'preface' when talking about this 'first' one and reserve the terms *muqaddima* and 'introduction' for the other one, as that is the part which was explicitly named so by the author.

1.1 *Content*

The initia, as a rule, begins with the obligatory doxological formulae. In this case, these are a *basmala*, immediately followed by a *ṣalwala* for Muḥammad. The following parts are in *sajʿ*. The initia continues with a *ḥamdala*, where Ibn al-Amshāṭī begins implementing the rhetorical concept of *ḥusn al-ibtidāʾ* or

2 Freimark, *Das Vorwort*.

3 Bauer, *Mamluk literature*, 119, 125.

4 For examples, see Bauer, *Mamluk literature*, 125–126.

5 While this part of Bauer's article regarding the "adabization of the ulama" focuses on poetry, some of his observations definitely hold for the *sajʿ* of a preface, since it also possessed literary qualities, as shown above. Bauer, *Mamluk literature*, 108–111.

barāʿat al-istihlāl, 'skilful opening',[6] meaning that in the following parts of the initia he alludes to the main theme of the work. He praises God who commanded men to travel, then elaborates the allusion by invoking the concepts of religiosity, pilgrimage, *ʿumra*,[7] and of course, medicine. All these images are conjured in connection to the praising of God, as they are expressed in relative clauses connected to the phrase *al-ḥamd lillāh alladhī*, 'praise be to God who'. The initia concludes with a *ṣalwala* for Muḥammad (who is now the curer of harms, *al-shāfī min al-maḍārr*), his family, and his companions.

The middle part starts with the *baʿdiyya*, the epistolary and textual formula separating the doxologies from the preface proper.[8] In this case, its exact form is *wa-baʿdu*. Instead of immediately jumping to more 'practical' functions of the preface proper, Ibn al-Amshāṭī starts with building up the scene with the use of powerful religious concepts so as to provide a compelling setting for the introduction of the patron. These blend into the initia quite smoothly as the invoked images unfold, to wit the inner preparation for religious travel, crucial elements of the pilgrimage, trust in God's forgiveness, the abolishment of sins, the Hereafter, and the end of times. It is as if the reader himself is part of this preparation in a heightened religious state. This elevated background provides the stage for the patron to appear as none other than the *imām*, the 'leader' of people (*ahl al-amṣār*, 'cities' folk'). Here, there might be a wordplay, as the singular form of *amṣār* is *miṣr*, which also stands for Egypt (albeit with different declension and without a plural form). First, the patron's various qualities are praised (generosity, knowledge, magnificence, and splendour). Then, after some honorific adjectives, Ibn al-Amshāṭī gives the patron's name and office, using the most exalted designation possible for the latter.[9] Then, Ibn al-Amshāṭī asks God to keep his patron safe from harm and in the best circumstances. While this form of addressing the patron is more formal than personal, the setting created for his introduction, the level of laudation, and the following blessing fulfils the function of *captatio benevolentiae*.[10] It is interesting to note that the completion of this function takes up approximately half of the preface proper.

In the middle part of the preface proper, a new train of thought begins, in which we can detect various functions. The first of these is the specification

6 Bonebakker, *Ibtidāʾ*, 1006.

7 The "lesser pilgrimage" to Mecca. The *ʿumra* can be performed at any time of the year and consists of fewer rituals compared to the *ḥajj*; however, it is also possible to perform it alongside the *ḥajj* in specific ways. For a detailed analysis of the *ʿumra*, see Chaumont, *ʿUmra*.

8 Gacek, *The Arabic manuscript tradition*, 14.

9 For more details on this, see the Introduction, sub-chapter 3.2 *Dating the Work*.

10 Freimark, *Das Vorwort*, 58–60.

of the reason for compilation. Ibn al-Amshāṭī states that the most important of the great principles is the preservation of health and offering useful things for those travelling in desolate places, alone and without medicaments. These latter specifications are expressed through parallelism. We find two phrases for both conditions ('without a companion, a servant, without medicaments, or remedies') and all four words are negated the same way in the Arabic original. The preface continues; to quote the author: 'I decided to compile a book for His Highness, His Excellency, in which I show the way for this, following the best methods.' This testimony makes it clear that Ibn al-Amshāṭī keeps away from the most popular topos for justification of writing his book, namely, being asked to do so (whether it is a real or fictitious request).[11] It is his own decision to compile this work, in all probability wishing to live up to the great principles mentioned at the beginning of this section by providing a useful compilation for those in need of it. To some extent, this can be connected to the topos that it is meritorious to write a book and share knowledge.[12]

The reason for writing is followed by the purpose of the work. Quoting Ibn al-Amshāṭī once more, his book is 'being a substitute for carrying those books on the crossroads of travels and [being] a collection of all which split from it, by means of summarising.' This clearly corresponds to the popular topos of composing a book that makes the previous ones on the topic superfluous.[13] His reason to do so, as can be seen, is not the unsatisfying quality of the works he aims to replace with his book; rather, it is a practical issue. This premise might serve Ibn al-Amshāṭī to maintain his modesty. His humility is further emphasised by the fact that he does not mention his name throughout the preface;[14] his person only appears due to the use of verbs in the first-person singular on three occasions. The method of compilation (summarising) can be linked to the topos of shortness;[15] instead of all the excessive works on the topic, this one will be concise. Besides the functions and topoi, this part contains literary features as well. The terms 'books' and 'travels' are homonyms in the Arabic original (*asfār*),[16] and the terms 'crossroads' and 'split' are derived from the same roots (*f-r-q*). Another element of this section is the repeated use of singular indefinite nominals in the accusative.

---

11 Freimark, *Das Vorwort*, 36–40.

12 Freimark, *Das Vorwort*, 48.

13 Freimark, *Das Vorwort*, 48–49.

14 Freimark, *Das Vorwort*, 54–56.

15 Freimark, *Das Vorwort*, 50.

16 On the *s.f.r* root and its meanings related to 'travel' and 'book', see Rosenthal, *On the Semitic root s/š-p-r*.

After this section, the author states that this is why he named his book *al-Isfār ʿan ḥikam al-asfār*, translated as *The unveiling of the wisdoms of the books*. The original title fits the common tendency of witty intitulations for two reasons. Firstly, both *isfār* and *asfār* go back to the same root (*s-f-r*). Secondly, *asfār* is a homonym, and while the title 'The unveiling of the wisdoms of the journeys' would also make sense, I favour rendering *asfār* as books for the following reasons. While according to Arabic scholars, the phrase would primarily refer not to ordinary books but rather those of the Scriptures or those on religious sciences, the term's additional meaning is a book that reveals truths.[17] Moreover, such volumes are depicted as "large, heavy books of religious knowledge" carried by donkeys on journeys.[18] While Ibn al-Amshāṭī certainly does not refer to religious books when using *asfār*, he surely utilises the additional layers of meaning related to books. To quote Ibn al-Amshāṭī: 'I decided to compile a book for His Higness, His Excellency in which I show the way for this, following the best methods. Containing secrets, praise be to God, came the books (*kutub*) of this great discipline [medicine]. Being a substitute for carrying those books (*al-asfār*) on the crossroads of travels (*al-asfār*) and being a collection of all which split from it, by means of summarising, I named it *al-Isfār ʿan ḥikam al-asfār*.' As it is carrying of the books which contain the knowledge needed on journeys that Ibn al-Amshāṭī wants to spare his patron, in my opinion it is clearly the wisdoms (*ḥikam*) of these knowledge-bearing books (*asfār*) on medicine that he wishes to uncover in his treatise.

In the third part of the preface, the author praises God and asks Him to grant him a favourable reception and completeness for his work and deem it an undertaking worthy of redemption from Hell.

The preface ends with a table of contents, enumerating the book's chapters and their titles.

Lastly, before moving on to the *sajʿ* of the preface, I would like to take note of some words which likely allude to terms found in the Quran, due to the role of such allusions in prefaces.[19] Therefore, a short list of these words follows, arranged according to the lines of the preface and giving the *sūra* and *āya* in which the terms appear in the Quran. While the list presented below is likely not exhaustive, it nevertheless shows Ibn al-Amshāṭī's attention to detail.

Line 10, *abrār*: 3:193, 3:198, 76:5, 82:13, 83:18, 83:22: those having piety and devotion to God, future dwellers of Paradise.[20]

---

17 See Rosenthal, *On the Semitic root s/š-p-r*, 8, 9.

18 See Rosenthal, *On the Semitic root s/š-p-r*, 9, 18.

19 See Freimark, *Das Vorwort*, 63–65.

20 Kinberg, *Piety*.

Line 15, *mashāʿir* in its singular form, *mashʿar*: 2:198: a place or places where a religious ritual or rituals of the pilgrimage take place.[21]

Line 17, *al-Ghaffār*: 20:82, 38:66, 39:5, 40:42, 71:10: one of the names and attributes of God, the all-forgiving, much forgiving,[22] rendered here as repeatedly forgiving.

Line 18, *yamḥū*: 13:39: the verb *mahā*, 'to erase' occurs three times in the Quran. In 13:39, its form is the same as in line 18 of the preface ("God erases or confirms whatever He wills").[23]

Line 18, *awzār*: 16:25: the plural form occurs in another *sūra* as well (47:4) but in 16:25 the term 'burdens' is mentioned along with the Day of Judgment. There are other examples for this association with the singular form of the term.[24]

Line 19, (*rafʿ*) *al-darajāt*: 6:83, 40:15, 58:11: the levels of Paradise, degrees or rankings by which people are raised in this world and in the afterlife by God's decision.[25]

Line 19, *Dār al-Qarār*: 40:39: this exact term for Paradise, 'the abode of permanence', appears in the Quran only once.[26]

Line 22, *aqṭār*: 33:14, 55:33: the term 'regions' appears only in this plural form in the Quran.

Line 23, *hammār* in the active participle form of stem VII, *munhamir*: 54:11: this root occurs only once in the Quran when telling the story of the people of Noah ("so We opened the gates of the sky with torrential water").[27]

Line 43, *asfār* with the meaning of 'books': 62:5: while *asfār* as 'journeys' appears on numerous occasions, it means 'books' only in one instance, in 62:5 ("those who have been charged with obedience to the Torah, but have failed to carry it out, are like asses carrying books").[28]

Line 50, *najāt* [*min al-nār*]: 40:41: 'deliverance' or 'salvation', which appears in this exact form only once in the Quran ("why do I call you to salvation when you call me to the Fire").[29]

---

21 Hawting, *Pilgrimage*, esp. 96; Rubin, *Sacred precincts*.

22 Peterson, *Forgiveness*; Böwering, *God and his attributes*, 321.

23 Badawi—Abdel Haleem, م/ح/و *m–ḥ–w*.

24 Gaffney, *Load or burden*.

25 Afsaruddin, *Garden*, 284; Hermansen, *Talent*.

26 Asrafuddin, *Garden*, 283.

27 Badawi—Abdel Haleem, ه/م/ر *h–m–r*.

28 Badawi—Abdel Haleem, س/ف/ر *s–f–r*; Rosenthal, *On the Semitic root s/š-p-r*, 9.

29 Badawi—Abdel Haleem, ن/ج/و *n–j–w*; Borrmans, *Salvation*; Renard, *Deliverance*.

1.2 *Form*

Regarding *sajʿ*, 'rhymed prose', its medieval analyses in Abū Hilāl al-ʿAskarī's (d. ca. 400/1010) *Kitāb al-ṣināʿatayn*, Ḍiyāʾ al-Dīn Ibn al-Athīr's (d. 637/1239) *al-Mathal al-sāʾir*, and al-Qalqashandī's (d. 821/1418) *Ṣubḥ al-aʿshā* are frequently consulted. During the following analysis, I relied on encyclopaedia entries[30] and modern analyses[31] as well. I adopted the term rhymeme: "The rhymeme is a particular group of sounds which repeats at the end of every line throughout the entire poem. [...] The rhymeme includes the *rawiyy* and all successive sounds if any exist; under certain conditions, preceding sounds are also included, even if they do not form a continuous sequence with the *rawiyy*."[32] Since this term is also used in the case of *sajʿ*, it allows a clear description of elements of the rhyme other than the concurring consonant or rhyme letter, which ends the rhythmic units. As the last words of the rhythmic units were pronounced in their pausal form,[33] I observed this rule throughout the following analysis. In this part of the book, I deviate from transliteration in favour of transcription. I separate the preface into numbered lines according to the rhythmic units. First I divide the numbered rhythmic units into words (*alfāẓ*)[34] and syllables, and then I list the rhymemes of the units and the morphological patterns of the last words of the units. This is followed by an analysis of the use of rhymemes and patterns in the rhythmic units, the length of the rhythmic units, and some additional aspects of the *sajʿ*.

1.2.1 Rhythmic Units of the Preface

1. (الحمد / لله / الذي) / أمر / بالأسفار
al/ḥam/du/lil/lā/hil/la/dhī/ʾa/ma/ra/bil/as/fār
⏑ - ⏑ - - - ⏑ - ⏑ ⏑ ⏑ - ⏑ -

2. للتفكّر / والاعتبار
lil/ta/fak/ku/ri/wal/iʿ/ti/bār
- ⏑ - ⏑ ⏑ - ⏑ ⏑ -

30 Ben Abdesselem, *Sadj*; Borg, *Sajʿ*.
31 Frolov, *Classical Arabic verse*; Drory, *Models and contacts*; Orfali, *The art of the muqaddima*.
32 Drory, *Models and contacts*, 64.
33 See Stewart, *Sajʿ in the Qurʾān*, 109–110.
34 Here, I attempted to follow the method of Ibn al-Athīr (Ibn al-Athīr, *al-Mathal al-sāʾir*, 1/255–257). As he only gives a few examples of groups of rhythmic units and their word counts without any further explanation, mistakes on my part are probable. According to Stewart, Hayim Sheynin's system in his study of the *maqāmāt* is "virtually identical" to Ibn al-Athīr's system (Stewart, *Sajʿ in the Qurʾān*, 114); however, I could not access Sheynin's analysis for further explanation and examples of this method.

3. وأداء / فرائض / الحجّ / والاعتمار
wa/ʾa/dā/ʾi/fa/rā/ʾi/ḍil/ḥaj/ji/wal/iʿ/ti/mār
⏑ ⏑ - ⏑ ⏑ ⏑ - ⏑ - - - ⏑ - ⏑ ⏑ ⏑ -

4. وجعل / في الطبّ / من / الأسرار
wa/ja/ʿa/la/fiṭ/ṭib/bi/mi/nal/as/rār
⏑ ⏑ ⏑ ⏑ - - - ⏑ ⏑ - ⏑ -

5. ما / يحفظ / الصحّة / ويبرئ / من / الأضرار
mā/yaḥ/fa/ẓuṣ/ṣiḥ/ḥa/ta/wa/yub/ri/ʾu/mi/nal/ʾaḍ/rār
- - ⏑ - - - ⏑ ⏑ ⏑ - ⏑ ⏑ ⏑ ⏑ - - -

6. (وصلّى / الله / على / سيّدنا / محمّد / عبده / ورسوله) / الشافي / من / المضارّ
wa/ṣal/lā/al/lā/hu/ʿa/lā/say/yid/nā/mu/ḥam/ma/din/ʿab/di/hi/wa/ra/
sū/li/hish/shā/fī/ mi/nal/ma/ḍārr
⏑ - - ⏑ - ⏑ ⏑ - - - - - ⏑ - ⏑ - - ⏑ ⏑ ⏑ ⏑ ⏑ - ⏑ - - - - ⏑ - ⏑ -

7. وعلى / آله / وأصحابه / الأخيار
wa/ʿa/lā/ā/li/hi/wa/aṣ/ḥā/bi/hil/ʾakh/yār
⏑ ⏑ - - ⏑ ⏑ ⏑ ⏑ - ⏑ - - -

8. ما / طرد / الليل / النهار
mā/ṭa/ra/dal/lay/lan/na/hār
- ⏑ ⏑ - - - ⏑ -

9. وأضاء / فجر / وأنار
wa/ʾa/ḍā/ʾa/faj/run/wa/ʾa/nār
⏑ ⏑ - ⏑ - - ⏑ ⏑ -

10. (وبعد / فلمّا) / عزم / على / سير / الأبرار
wa/baʿ/du/fa/lam/mā/ʿa/za/ma/ʿa/lā/si/ya/ril/ab/rār
⏑ - ⏑ ⏑ - - ⏑ ⏑ ⏑ ⏑ - ⏑ ⏑ ⏑ - ⏑ -

11. واحتزم / لزيارة / البيت / المختار
waḥ/ta/za/ma/li/zi/yā/ra/til/bay/til/mukh/tār
- ⏑ ⏑ ⏑ ⏑ ⏑ - ⏑ - - - - -

12. من / كلّ / جبّار
min/kul/li/jab/bār
- - ⏑ - -

13. ولزم / العجّ / بالانتقار
wa/la/zi/mal/ʿaj/ja/bi/lin/ti/qār
⏑ ⏑ ⏑ - - ⏑ ⏑ - ⏑ -

14. والثجّ / والاعتذار
wal/thaj/ji/wal/iʿ/ti/dhār
- - ⏑ - ⏑ ⏑ -

15. وجوار / تلك / المشاعر / الكبار
wa/ji/wā/ri/til/kal/ma/shā/ʿi/ril/ki/bār
⏑ ⏑ - ⏑ - - ⏑ - ⏑ - ⏑ -

16. بالذلّ / والانكسار
bidh/dhal/li/wa/lin/ki/sār
- - ⏑ ⏑ - ⏑ -

17. رجاء / كرم / الغفّار
ra/jā/ʾu/ka/ra/mil/ghaf/fār
⏑ - ⏑ ⏑ ⏑ - - -

18. يمحو / الذنوب / والأوزار
yam/ḥūdh/dhu/nū/ba/wal/ʾaw/zār
- - ⏑ - ⏑ - - -

19. ورفع / الدرجات / في / دار / القرار
wa/ra/fa/ʿad/da/ra/jā/ti/fī/dā/ril/qa/rār
⏑ ⏑ ⏑ - ⏑ ⏑ - ⏑ - - - ⏑ -

20. خلاصة / الأعصار
khu/lā/ṣa/tal/ʾaʿ/ṣār
⏑ - ⏑ - - -

21. وإمام / أهل / الأمصار
wa/ʾi/mā/mu/ʾah/lil/am/ṣār
⏑ ⏑ - ⏑ - - ⏑ -

22. عين / أعيان / ساكني / الأقطار
ʿay/nu/ʾaʿ/yā/ni/sā/ki/nīl/ʾaq/ṭār
- ⏑ - - ⏑ - ⏑ - - -

23. من / إذا / ذكر / جوده / استغنى / عن / السحاب / الهمّار
man/ʾi/dhā/dhu/ki/ra/jū/du/hus/tagh/nā/ʿa/nis/si/ḥā/bil/ham/mār
- ◡ - ◡ ◡ ◡ - ◡ - - - ◡ - ◡ - - - -

24. وإذا / تُأُمِّل / علمه / استصغر / في / جنبه / البحر / الزخّار
wa/ʾi/dhā/tu/ʾum/mi/la/ʿil/mu/hus/taṣ/gha/ra/fī/jan/bi/hil/baḥ/ruz/
zakh/khār
◡ ◡ - ◡ - ◡ ◡ - ◡ - - ◡ ◡ - - ◡ - - - - -

25. وإذا / تحدّث / عن / المجد / والسودة / علم / أنّه / القطب / الذي / عليه / المدار
wa/ʾi/dhā/tu/ḥud/di/tha/ʿa/nal/maj/di/was/saw/da/ti/ʿu/li/ma/ʾan/na/
hul/quṭ/bul/la/dhī/ ʿa/lay/hil/ma/dār
◡ ◡ - ◡ - ◡ ◡ ◡ - - ◡ - - ◡ ◡ ◡ ◡ ◡ - ◡ - - - ◡ - ◡ - - - ◡ -

26. (المقرّ الأشرف الكريم العالي الأمامي العالمي العلّامي الكمالي ابو المعالي محمّد الجهني البارزي الشافعي ناظر دواوين الإنشاء الشريفة) / بالديار / المصرية
al/mu/qir/rul/ash/ra/ful/ka/rī/mul/ʿā/līl/ʾa/mā/mīl/ʿā/la/mīl/ʿal/lā/mīl/
ka/mā/lī/ʾa/būl/ma/ʿā/lī/mu/ḥam/ma/dun/al/ju/ha/nīl/bā/ri/zīsh/shā/
fi/ʿī/nā/ẓi/ru/da/wā/wī/nil/ʾin/shā/ʾish/sha/rī/fa/ti/bid/di/yā/ril/miṣ/
riy/ya
◡ ◡ - - ◡ ◡ - ◡ - - - - ◡ - - - ◡ - - - - ◡ - - ◡ - ◡ - - - ◡ - ◡ ◡ ◡ - - ◡ - - - - - ◡ ◡ ◡ - -
- - - - ◡ - ◡ ◡ - ◡ - - - - - ◡

27. وسائر / الممالك / الإسلامية
wa/sā/ʾi/ril/ma/mā/li/kil/ʾis/lā/miy/ya
◡ - ◡ - ◡ - ◡ - - - - ◡

28. رجّعه / الله / بعد / بلوغ / الأوطار
raj/ja/ʿa/hul/lā/hu/baʿ/da/bu/lū/ghil/ʾaw/ṭār
- ◡ ◡ - - - ◡ - ◡ ◡ - - - -

29. سالما / من / الآفات / والأخطار
sā/li/man/mi/nal/ā/fā/ti/wal/akh/ṭār
- ◡ - ◡ - - - - ◡ - ◡ -

30. على / أجمل / الأوصاف / وأجلّ / الأخطار
ʿa/lā/ʾaj/ma/lil/ʾaw/ṣā/fi/wa/ʾa/jal/lil/ʾakh/ṭār
◡ - - ◡ - - ◡ ◡ ◡ ◡ - - - -

31. وكان / من / القواعد / الكبار
wa/kā/na/mi/nal/qa/wā/ʿi/dil/ki/bār
⏑ - ⏑ ⏑ - ⏑ - ⏑ - ⏑ -

32. جلب / المصالح / ودرء / المفاسد / والمضارّ
jal/bul/ma/ṣā/li/ḥi/wa/dar/ʾul/ma/fā/si/di/wal/ma/dārr
- - ⏑ - ⏑ ⏑ ⏑ - - ⏑ - ⏑ ⏑ ⏑ - ⏑ -

33. وكان / من / أهمها / حفظ / الصحّة / والأخيار
wa/kā/na/min/ʾa/ham/mi/hā/ḥif/ẓuṣ/ṣiḥ/ḥa/ti/wal/ʾakh/yār
⏑ - ⏑ - ⏑ - ⏑ - - - - - ⏑ ⏑ - - -

34. والنذور / بما / لعّله / ينفع / لذي / البراري / والقفار
wan/nu/dhū/ru/bi/mā/la/ʿal/la/hu/yan/fa/ʿu/li/dhīl/ba/rā/rī/wal/qi/fār
- ⏑ - ⏑ ⏑ - ⏑ - ⏑ ⏑ - ⏑ ⏑ ⏑ ⏑ - ⏑ - - - - ⏑ -

35. (حيث) / لا / صاحب / ولا / جار
ḥay/thu/lā/ṣā/ḥi/ba/wa/lā/jār
- ⏑ - - - ⏑ ⏑ ⏑ - -

36. ولا / عقاقير / ولا / عقّار
wa/lā/ʿa/qā/qī/ra/wa/lā/ʿaq/qār
⏑ - ⏑ - - - ⏑ ⏑ - - -

37. (رأيت / أن / أجمع) / لحضرته / الشما
ra/ʾay/tu/ʾan/ʾaj/ma/ʿa/li/ḥaḍ/ra/ti/hish/sha/mā
⏑ - ⏑ - - - ⏑ ⏑ ⏑ - ⏑ ⏑ ⏑ - ⏑ -

38. وحومته / العليا
wa/ḥaw/ma/ti/hil/ʿul/yā
⏑ - ⏑ ⏑ - - -

39. (كتابا) / أرشد / فيه / إلى / ذلك
ki/tā/ban/ʾur/shi/du/fī/hi/ʾi/lā/dhā/lik
⏑ - - - - ⏑ - ⏑ ⏑ ⏑ - - -

40. سالكا / فيه / أجمل / المسالك
sā/li/kan/fī/hi/ʾaj/ma/lal/ma/sā/lik
- ⏑ - - ⏑ - ⏑ - ⏑ - -

41. فجاء / بحمد / الله / حاويا / لأسرار
fa/jā/ʾa/bi/ḥam/dil/lā/hi/ḥā/wi/yan/li/as/rār
⏑ - ⏑ ⏑ - - - ⏑ - ⏑ - ⏑ ⏑ -

42. كتب / هذا / الفنّ / الكبار
ku/tu/bi/hā/dhāl/fan/nil/ki/bār
⏑ ⏑ ⏑ - - - - ⏑ -

43. مغنيا / عن / حمل / تلك / الأسفار
mugh/ni/yan/ʿan/ḥa/ma/li/til/kal/ʾas/fār
- ⏑ - - - ⏑ ⏑ ⏑ - - - -

44. في / مفارق / الأسفار
fī/ma/fā/ri/qil/ʾas/fār
- ⏑ - ⏑ - - -

45. جامعا / لانتشار / ما / تفرّق / منها / على / سبيل / الاختصار
jā/mi/ʿan/lin/ti/shā/ri/mā/ta/far/ra/qa/min/hā/ʿa/lā/sa/bī/li/likh/ti/ṣār
- ⏑ - - - ⏑ - ⏑ - - - ⏑ ⏑ - - ⏑ - ⏑ - - ⏑ -

46. فلذلك / سمّيته / الإسفار / عن / حكَم / الأسفار
fa/li/dhā/li/ka/sam/may/tu/hul/ʾis/fā/ra/ʿan/ḥi/ka/mil/ʾas/fār
⏑ ⏑ - ⏑ ⏑ - - - ⏑ - - - - ⏑ - ⏑ ⏑ - - -

47. والله / تعالى / المسؤول / وهو / الكريم / الغفّار
wal/lā/hu/ta/ʿā/lāl/mas/ʾū/lu/wa/hu/wal/ka/rī/mul/ghaf/fār
- - ⏑ ⏑ - - - - - ⏑ ⏑ - ⏑ - - - -

48. (إن) / يتحفه / بالقبول / فلا / يبتغي / له / عثار
ʾin/yut/ḥi/fu/hu/bil/qu/bū/li/fa/lā/yub/ta/ghī/la/hu/ʿi/thār
- - ⏑ ⏑ ⏑ - ⏑ - ⏑ - - - ⏑ - ⏑ ⏑ ⏑ ⏑ -

49. ويسعفه / بالكمال / فلا / يحتاج / إلى / اعتذار
wa/yus/ʿi/fu/hu/bil/ka/mā/li/fa/lā/yuḥ/tā/ju/ʾi/lāʿ/ti/dhār
⏑ - ⏑ ⏑ ⏑ - ⏑ - ⏑ - - - - ⏑ ⏑ - ⏑ -

50. ويجعله / سببا / للنجاة / من / النار
wa/ja/ʿa/la/hu/sa/ba/ban/lin/na/jā/ti/mi/nan/nār
⏑ ⏑ ⏑ ⏑ ⏑ ⏑ ⏑ - - - ⏑ - ⏑ ⏑ - -

51. والفوز / بمرافعة / الأبرار
wal/faw/zi/bi/mu/rā/fa/ʿa/til/ʾab/rār
- - ⏑ ⏑ ⏑ - ⏑ ⏑ - - -

1.2.2 Rhymemes:

- ār: 43 times; ārr: 2 times (lines 6, 32)
- iyya: 2 times (lines 26, 27)
- ālik: 2 times (lines 39, 40)
- ā: 2 times (lines 37, 38)

1.2.3 Patterns:

- afʿāl [A]: 18 times (lines 1, 4, 5, 7, 10, 18, 20, 21, 22, 28, 29, 30, 33, 41, 43, 44, 46, 51)
- faʿʿāl [B]: 6 times (lines 12, 17, 23, 24, 36, 47)
- iftiʿāl [C]: 6 times (lines 2, 3, 13, 14, 45, 49)
- fiʿāl [D]: 5 times (lines 15, 31, 34, 42, 48)
- faʿāl [E]: 3 times (lines 8, 9, 19)
- mafāʿil [F]: 3 times (lines 6, 32, 40)
- faʿal [G]: 2 times (line 35, 50)
- feminine *nisba* ending: 2 times (lines 26, 27)
- fuʿlā: 1 time (line 38)
- infiʿāl [H]: 1 time (line 16)
- mafʿal [I]: 1 time (line 25)
- muftaʿal [J]: 1 time (line 11)

The two lines unaccounted for above are lines 37 and 39. *Shamā* in line 37 is 'politeness' or 'refinement' used to elevate, praise, or exalt one's rank. Line 39 ends with the demonstrative pronoun *dhālika*.

1.2.4 The Use of Rhymemes and Patterns

In the previous section on the contents and topoi of the preface, I used a tripartite division. However, breaking up the preface into more sections facilitates some observations regarding the patterns employed at the ends of lines and the changes of the rhymeme. Lines 1–5 [section 1] are dependents of the *ḥamdala*, while lines 6–9 [section 2] are dependents of the *salwala*. Lines 10–30 [section 3] are connected to the patron; 10–20 [3a] serve as the introduction to the patron's appearance, 21–25 [3b] are the patron's praise, 26–27 [3c] are the naming of the patron, while 28–30 [3d] are asking God's favours for the patron. Lines 31–36 [section 4] are the transition to the topic and matters of the treatise. Lines 37–46 [section 5] are connected to the treatise; 37–40 [5a] state the aim of writing the treatise, 41–45 [5b] describe the methods of compilation, and 46 [5c] is the naming of the treatise. Lines 47–51 [section 6] plead to God for favourable intervention regarding the treatise's merits.

The low number of different rhymemes present in the preface is striking. Except for three pairs of rhyme members (2–2–2), all other rhyme members (45) end with the rhymeme *ār/ārr*. In *sajʿ*, the rhymeme can change even after a few rhyme members; despite this, Ibn al-Amshāṭī chose to stick to one rhymeme for the majority (~88%) of his preface. When analyses of more 15th-century prefaces become available, they would provide data necessary for determining whether this is a general characteristic or tendency of the *sajʿ* formulated in this period or if this construction was a deliberate choice on the part of Ibn al-Amshāṭī. If the latter is true, it would mean that Ibn al-Amshāṭī created an opportunity to parade his talents, as adhering to one rhymeme while avoiding clumsy repetition of the same words (but not of patterns) becomes increasingly difficult and demanding the longer the rhymeme goes on.

Where changing of rhymemes occurs, it is obviously connected to the functions or content of the rhythmic units. The main rhymeme changes to the feminine *nisba* ending in section 3c, stating the name and title of the patron. The subsequent two deviations from the main rhymeme come nine lines later, in section 5a, expressing the aim of writing. Lines 37–38 have the rhymeme *ā*, the last words of these rhythmic units are both laudatory phrases of the patron, while lines 39–40 end with the rhymeme *ālik*. All three instances concur with clearly definable sections of the preface.

For the rest of the lines, analysing the combinations of the same rhymeme and various patterns does not provide such clear-cut results. The first and last rhyme members end with the most common pattern of the preface, *afʿāl*, framing the whole preface. The patterns in section 1 are ACCAA; after the opening and framing rhythmic unit, the patterns are in pairs. The pattern formula for section 2 is FAEE; the first two rhythmic units match each other only in their rhymemes but the second two share the same pattern as well. Section 3 is more problematic in this regard. The patterns of 3a are AJ(BCC)DHBA(E)A. The parentheses indicate rhythmic units omitted in the Cairo manuscript but included in the Mosul and Tarīm manuscripts. The first inclusion is more skilful, with a pair of rhythmic units sharing a pattern besides the rhymeme. The second inclusion separates a pair of rhythmic units that would form a couple based on their patterns; however, it observes the rhymeme and also contains a fitting Quranic allusion. The patterns in section 3b are AABBI, where it can be reasoned that the fifth pattern is a variation before the change of the rhymeme occurring in section 3c. Section 3d again shows a more orderly composition, as its patterns are AAA. Section 4 seems yet again to be irregular in this regard, as its pattern formula is DFADGB. In the last two rhythmic units, however, the parallel structure of the Arabic text (essentially both units are formed by the same type of negation used twice in both units) aptly makes up for not ending the section by employing the same pattern for the rhythmic units. Section 5a works through the two variant rhymemes discussed above. The formula of sections 5b and 5c is ADAAC/A, where the slash separates the subsections. The pair in 5b is where the homonym *asfār* occurs. As in the case of 3b, here too it can be theorised that the uncoupled pattern before 5c is yet again a variation before the content-wise quite important rhythmic member containing the title of the treatise. Section 6 is also mixed, as its pattern formula is BDCGA. Nothing much can be said about this section's patterns other than observing that the last rhythmic unit ends with the most prominent pattern of the preface as a kind of framing. In total, from the 45 rhythmic units with the rhymeme *ār/ārr*, there are six pairs and two trios that share the same pattern for their last words, which means 18 rhythmic units (40 %).

1.2.5 The Length of the Rhythmic Units

After looking at the length of the rhythmic units, it is apparent that the shorter type of *sajʿ* was preferred by Ibn al-Amshṭī when he composed the preface. The word count of the rhythmic units of the short *sajʿ* does not exceed ten words, according to Ibn al-Athīr.[35] This is true for the rhythmic units of Ibn al-Amshāṭī's preface, with the notable exception of line 26, which contains the name and title of the patron, and line 25 immediately before it. It can easily be argued, however, that the name and title are not part of the *sajʿ*, in which case the actual *sajʿ* would be *bi-d-diyāri / 'l-miṣriyya*, making line 26 a proper short rhythmic unit. Other than this, there are two somewhat lengthier (but still short) rhythmic units, namely line 6, which is the first line of section 2, and line 45, which is the one before the line containing the title of the treatise. Lines 23–25 also tend to be slightly longer, leading up to the line containing the name and title of the patron. Therefore, these elongated short lines are likely compiled so on purpose to call the listener's or reader's attention to a change of content or of an important part of the content. In the case of lines 23–25, it also serves as a transition and further escalation of the scene for the introduction of the patron.

While the unit of measurement in *sajʿ* is traditionally the single word, examining the syllables is more and more common.[36] In the case of this preface, however, the results of such an inquiry are not so impressive. It seems that Ibn

35 Ibn al-Athīr, *al-Mathal al-sāʾir*, 1/257–258; Ben Abdesselem, *Sadj*, 737.

36 On this, see Orfali, *The art of the muqaddima*, 195, esp. n. 77; Stewart, *Sajʿ in the Qurʾān*, 113–116.

al-Amshāṭī was not paying special attention to the balance or parallelism of the syllables in his rhythmic units. There are no obvious repeating patterns in the length of the syllables, other than those at the end of rhythmic units coupled due to their last words sharing the same morphological pattern. Yet again, in the light of other studies on prefaces of this period, it would be possible to decide whether this is a tendency and possibly a norm as well or rather a lack of additional refinement.

However, it is important to note that if we turn back to the 'original' measurement of word count, there are examples where the rhythmic units are balanced, especially if the introductory phrases, which are not a part of the *sajʿ* in Ibn al-Athīr's analysis, are not counted.[37] This way, already lines 1 and 2 are balanced: if the words *al-ḥamdu li-llāhi 'l-ladhī* are the introductory phrase, then *amara / bi-l-asfār* and *li-l-tafakkuri / wa-l-iʿtibār* are both two-two words as per Ibn al-Athīr's counting system. This way, lines 3 and 4 are also balanced: *wa-adā'i / farā'iḍi / 'l-ḥajji / wa-l-iʿtimār* and *wa-jaʿala / fiṭ-ṭibbi / min / al-asrār* both contain four words. Applying this method, many additional balanced couples of rhythmic units can be identified. The lack of frequent changing of the rhymeme and the lower ratio of rhythmic units sharing the same pattern for their last words makes the grouping of the rhythmic units difficult. Focusing only on the word count, the following consecutive lines are of the same length: 1–2 (2 words), 3–4 (4 words), 7–8 (4 words), 10–11 (4 words), 12–13 (3 words), 17–18 (3 words), 23–24 (8 words), 35–36 (4 words), 37–38 (2 words), 39–40 (4 words), and 46–49 (6 words). This gives a total of 24 lines, nearly half of the rhythmic units.

When looking at the sections, there is an interesting rhythm of wordcounts. The rhythmic units of section 1 grow longer towards the end of the section (2–2–4–4–5). The wordcount for the lines of section 2 is 3–4–4–3. While concurrence of morphological pattern would enable the rhythmic units to cross-reference one another ('XYXY'), I have not found a reference to such a phenomenon based on word count or length in Ibn al-Athīr's analysis of *sajʿ*. Section 3a shows a decreasing tendency, as the wordcount here is 4–4-(3–3–2)–4–2–3-3-(5)–2, where the parentheses indicate the lines given only in the Mosul and Tarīm manuscripts. Section 3b is something of an explosion (3–4–8–8–11) with the patron's praising, while section 3d returns to a more moderate wordcount (5–4–5). Section 4 shows a neat increase and a closure with a balanced couple (4–5–6–7–4–4). Section 5a is neatly balanced (2–2–4–4), but the rest of the section is more irregular (5–4–5–3–8–6). The beginning of section 6 is also

37 Ibn al-Athīr, *al-Mathal al-sā'ir*, 1/255–257; Stewart, *Sajʿ in the Qur'ān*, 113–118.

balanced, with decreasing length of the last units (6–6–6–5–3). To make sense of these numbers, it is important to note that balanced couples were deemed the best, second best is where the second unit is longer (although not excessively so) than the first, and if the second part of a couple is shorter than the first, it is considered faulty. The increasing trends present in sections 1, 3, 4, and 5 likely fall in the second category in general, while they contain perfectly matched couples as well. While the decreasing closure of sections 2 and 6 might be faulty based on the strict rules, I would argue that these 'deviations' are well used since section 2 ends the obligatory doxological section and section 6 closes the entirety of the preface.

1.2.6 Some Additional Aspects

As shown above, Ibn al-Amshāṭī managed in this preface to conform to Ibn al-Athīr's preference for the short type of *sajʿ*, albeit without paying attention to balancing the syllable-length of the rhythmic units. However, it seems that Ibn al-Amshāṭī avoided repetition. Looking at the rhythmic units and their contents, it is noticeable that reiteration of the same meaning with different words is not apparent anywhere in the preface, except for lines 37–38. Avoiding this kind of repetition, or "excess", is another "literary principle" of Ibn al-Athīr.[38]

Internal rhyming of the rhythmic units is relatively rare throughout the preface. There is one instance where it seems to be the result of conscious compilation, namely in line 45 (other than the internal rhyme in line 46 due to the title). The few resemblances to an internal rhyme are clearly partial and occasional, governed by the content of the rhythmic units instead of a stylistic choice.

Parallelism of syntactical structures is more expressed in the second half of the preface. It is employed within a rhythmic unit as well as between rhythmic units. Examples of the first would be lines 30, 32, 35–36. Examples of the latter are lines 35–36, 37–38, 48–49. The indefinite accusatives of lines 39, 40, 41, 43, and 45 also provide some sense of connectedness, even if these cannot be considered as proper parallelisms.

An additional matter to consider is the following. According to Ibn al-Athīr, *sajʿ* is more than balance and a concurring consonant of the last word of the units: the words should be nice, glowing, humming, and buzzing instead of being meagre and dull, and the form should follow the meaning instead of making the meaning a dependant of the form.[39] It is obvious when reading the preface as a whole that the content progresses and the functions and plot advance

38 Ibn al-Athīr, *al-Mathal al-sāʾir*, 1/214; Gully, *The culture of letter-writing*, 146.

39 Ibn al-Athīr, *al-Mathal al-sāʾir*, 1/212–213.

nicely and flawlessly. The near-monorhyme might offset the loose adherence to balance, especially since balance is applauded but not imperative. The preface meets the fundamental formal requirements of *sajʿ*, and the meaning or content obviously enjoys priority over adhering to a complicated form or strict observance of balance.

1.3 *Further Considerations*

The literary style of Mamluk *muqaddima*s is not frequently analysed. Due to the paucity of such works, we do not have a precise picture of what was common practice and considered aesthetically pleasing. Surely, comparing a 15th-century *muqaddima* of a scientific work to the standards of the *maqāmāt* of al-Hamadhānī (d. 398/1008) or al-Ḥarīrī (d. 516/1122) or other earlier examples of *sajʿ* is deceptive and pointless if we try to evaluate how Ibn al-Amshāṭī's *sajʿ* was looked at, as the functions and topoi of the preface are not representative of the whole picture. While this means that a decisive conclusion cannot be reached as of now, the above analysis perhaps suffices to show that such prefaces are indeed rewarding objects for study.

The study of the contents shows that the beginning of the preface already bears literary qualities, as the initia with the doxological formulae adheres to *ḥusn al-ibtidāʾ*, 'skilful opening'. In the middle part of the preface, Ibn al-Amshāṭī endeavours to describe a scene with powerful religious imagery that carries the reader to the more matter-of-fact functions of the preface. As demonstrated above, even through these more pragmatic functions, Ibn al-Amshāṭī takes care to embellish his text with the use of various literary devices.

The *sajʿ* of the preface has a distinct tendency to monorhyme, a feature prevalent in Quranic *sajʿ*.[40] Changing of the rhymeme concurs with parts of the preface having a distinct content and function. Grouping of rhythmic units by last words of the same pattern is only moderately present. Still, due to the near-monorhyme, this feature is apparent only upon closer inspection of the preface. In terms of syllables, identical syllable patterns and partial correspondences are not evident. Lengthwise, the *sajʿ* is short, as the rhythmic units do not exceed ten words, except for one unit. Although a syllable-analysis of the preface does not show much patterning, the wordcount-analysis unravels a nicely flowing rhythm in which the two parts not conforming to the standard aesthetics of the length of units and couples are obvious tools of closure.

Once similar analyses of prefaces, especially those of scientific works, become available, they will provide the context that is necessary to accurately

---

40 Stewart, *Sajʿ in the Qurʾān*, 109.

evaluate the literary qualities of this preface of Ibn al-Amshāṭī and identify which of the above characteristics are part of the trends and/or norms and which are reflections of his own literary style. One such element might be the use of some variant of *sālikan* [...] *al-masālik*, 'following the [...] methods' as one of the rhythmic units. This phrase seems to be either commonly employed in general or favoured by Ibn al-Amshāṭī, considering the fact that it can be found in the prefaces of all of his works in one version or another.[41]

2 Introduction and Chapters 1–8: The *Isfār* as a Travel Regimen

After the preface, the text that follows is a technical text belonging to the literature of the learned medical tradition. In order to evaluate the medical contents and arrangement of Ibn al-Amshāṭī's *Isfār* as a travel regimen, I compare it with other specimens of this corpus. Throughout this comparison, I follow the structure of the *Isfār*. My main focus is identifying the sources Ibn al-Amshāṭī uses, his methods of engaging with these sources, and the innovations of his regimen both regarding its contents and arrangement of material. Still, in some cases it can also prove useful to compare these sub-chapters with those in the Introduction on the relevant topics, for example regarding the *samūm* or the different waters to provide further context to Ibn al-Amshāṭī's text if needed.

For ease of referencing, I refer to Ibn al-Amshāṭī's travel regimen in its edited form and its translation present in this book in the footnotes of this chapter as "Ibn al-Amshāṭī, *al-Isfār*, [page number(s)]:[line number(s)]".

2.1 *'Introduction on the Need for Compiling This Book'*

In a short but theoretically dense introduction (*muqaddima*), Ibn al-Amshāṭī states that the sudden deviation from the usual circumstances of life can be the cause of dangerous diseases, and the exertion and fatigue of travelling strengthen this effect. He briefly explains the underlying reasons (the dissolved harmful humours cause swellings or diseases) and articulates his approach to

41 *Al-Kifāya*: *sālikan awḍaḥ al-masālik*, 'following the clearest methods', MS Istanbul, Feyzullah Efendi 848, f. 1^{v}:8–14. *Al-Munjaz*: *sālikan fīhi ajmal al-masālik*, 'following in it the best methods', MS Istanbul, Feyzullah Efendi 1319, f. 2^{v}:14–24. *Ta'sīs al-ṣiḥḥa*: *sālikan fīhi ajmal al-masālik*, 'following in it the best methods', MS Princeton, Garrett 570H, ff. 1^{v}:7–2^{r}:11, MS Paris, BnF Arabe 3025 ff. 2^{v}:9–3^{v}:7. *Ta'sīs al-itqān wa-al-matāna*: *sākikan fīhi bi-luṭf Allāh ajmal al-masālik*, 'following in it, by the grace of God, the best methods', MS Mashhad, Āstān-e Qods-e Rażavī 6339, f. 1^{v}:4–11; MS Istanbul, Süleymaniye Kütüphanesi, Shahīd 'Alī 2006, f. 1^{v}:5—f. 2^{r}:2. *Al-Qawl al-sadīd*: *sālikan fīhi bi-'awn Allāh ajmal al-masālik*, 'following in it, with the help of God, the best methods', Ibn al-Amshāṭī, *al-Qawl al-sadīd*, 32.

the topic; the traveller should know what is useful and what is harmful to avoid illnesses. In other words, he advocates prophylaxis or prevention.

Ibn al-Amshāṭī discloses the general dangers of travelling in his introduction. The main danger is quite simply the abrupt and sudden deviation from one's regular regimen, leading to dangerous diseases (*amrāḍ khaṭira*). Two necessary occurrences of travelling, exertion (*taʿab*) and fatigue (*naṣab*) warm the body and dissolve harmful humours, facilitating their transfer from place to place, thereby furthering the emergence of diseases besides possibly causing swellings (*waram*). Additionally, these harmful humours can mix with and corrupt good humours resulting in burdensome diseases (*amrāḍ ṣaʿba*). According to Ibn al-Amshāṭī, this is the reason the traveller should be aware of what is harmful or useful for him so that via treating oneself avoidance of such diseases is possible.

It is interesting to note that Ibn Sīnā expresses himself as *fa-yajibu an yaḥraṣa ʿalā mudāwāt amr nafsihi li-allā tuṣībahu amrāḍ kathīra*,[42] 'it is necessary to strive for treating his own matter so that he is not affected by many diseases', in comparison to Ibn al-Amshāṭī's *wajaba* (*ʿalā al-musāfir an yaʿrifa mā yaḍurruhu wa-yanfaʿuhu li-*)*yaḥraṣa ʿalā mudāwāt nafsihi li-an lā yuṣībahu shayʾ min dhālika*,[43] 'it is necessary (for the traveller to know what harms him and what benefits him to) strive for treating himself so that none of these [diseases] affects him'. Even though the points made in both texts before the quoted sections are identical (leaving the usual habits, fatigue), the wording of these parts is different altogether. In addition, while Ibn Sīnā mostly lists these and then moves on to giving general advice, Ibn al-Amshāṭī offers more detailed explanation and sticks to providing a short but nevertheless theoretical reasoning for the need for his treatise and the genre of travel regimens in a broader sense, due to the universality of his argument. Therefore, it is a possibility that Ibn al-Amshāṭī was inspired by this part of Ibn Sīnā's travel regimen, especially since similar parts are not found in other guides; however, it is important to stress that if this is the case, Ibn al-Amshāṭī's introduction is elaborated in a way that it is very much his own product and not just a heavily reworked copied material.

2.2 *'First Chapter on What Is Necessary for the Traveller to Do'*

This chapter is titled simply as 'the first chapter' in the main text but a more descriptive title appears at the end of the preface where Ibn al-Amshāṭī lists

42 Ibn Sīnā, *al-Qānūn*, 1/321.
43 Ibn al-Amshāṭī, *al-Isfār*, 120:6–7.

his chapters. This chapter is dedicated to preparatory measures with the three essential components thereof (purification, getting accustomed to certain things, and exercise), and to prevention of hunger, and prevention of thirst. The analysis of this chapter therefore follows this tripartite structure of preparation, hunger, and thirst.

Ibn al-Amshāṭī does not detail why purifying the harmful humours from the traveller's body is necessary, nor does he say whether it should be done via purgation or bloodletting, as the rest of the physicians do apart from Ibn Sīnā who remains silent on this issue. Despite this, Ibn al-Amshāṭī offers something unique: ten principles to observe in regard to purging (*istifrāgh*). These are having harmful humours, adequate strength, a warm and moist temperament, adequate symptoms, not being too thin or fat, too young or old, the weather not being too hot or cold, the country one is in not being too hot or cold, being accustomed to purging, and one's profession. The second unique element in this chapter by Ibn al-Amshāṭī is five additional things to consider for venesection, namely the pulse, strength, state of the muscles, age of the person, and the redness of his complexion. Such rules or propositions are not mentioned in any of the previous travel regimens as a set of conditions or factors to consider. Therefore, antecedents of these principles are to be uncovered from outside the genre of travel regimens. This fact also means that inclusion of these rules is Ibn al-Amshāṭī's original addition to the issue of pre-travel purification.

The ten principles of purging can be found in Ibn Sīnā's *Qānūn*.[44] Ibn Sīnā first enumerates these principles, then he explains their meaning. In comparison, Ibn al-Amshāṭī's approach is to give short clarifications immediately after stating each one of these principles. In addition to this, while both explanations convey the same meaning, they are structured and worded in a noticeably different way. After general remarks on purging, Ibn Sīnā moves on to discuss the various methods of purging, including venesection. Despite the detailed discussion he dedicates to venesection, there is no parallel there for Ibn al-Amshāṭī's five issues to consider in regard to venesection. Properly identifying the source of these ideas in general and a particular Arabic text Ibn al-Amshāṭī might have relied on would require further scrutiny, especially since the issues of purging and particularly venesection is a much-discussed topic already in the Greek medical tradition[45] and a comprehensive analysis of

44 Ibn Sīnā, *al-Qānūn*, 1/334.

45 See for example Peter Brain's study and translation of three Galenic texts on venesection: Brain, *Galen on bloodletting*. Galen's principles regarding venesection are discussed in Brain, *Galen on bloodletting*, 122–134 (Chapter 7, *Galen's practice of venesection*), esp. 131–132.

various methods of purging (and purging in general) in the Arabic medical tradition is still a *desideratum*.[46]

After purification, Ibn al-Amshāṭī discusses exercise and getting accustomed to new habits and circumstances as part of preparing for a journey. He recommends exercising more in general, besides walking or riding more and more each day depending on the mode of travel during the journey. These recommendations conform to the usual instructions previous physicians recommended. On closer inspection, however, it becomes obvious that Ibn al-Amshāṭī must have relied on al-Majūsī's text, as al-Majūsī writes: *wa-man lam yakun lahu ʿādat al-mashy fa-l-yaruḍ nafsahu bi-al-mashy qabla dhālika wa-yuʿawwiduhā dhālika qalīlan qalīlan wa-yazīdu fī miqdārihi fī kull yawm ʿalā tadrīj ḥattā yuʾallifuhu wa-yahūnu ʿalayhi*,[47] 'and who is not accustomed to walking is to exercise himself with walking before that and get used to it bit by bit and increase its quantity gradually each day until he is accustomed to it and it becomes no trouble for him'. Compared to this, Ibn al-Amshāṭī's text has only the following minor differences: it begins as [*fa-in kāna mimman yurīdu al-safar māshiyan*] *wa-lam yakun lahu ʿāda bi-al-mashy fa-l-yartāḍa*, using the stem VIII verb of the r-w-ḍ roots[48] instead of al-Majūsī's stem I form, then it has *ḥattā taʾallafa*, using the stem V form of the ʾ-l-f roots instead of al-Majūsī's stem II form, and ends with the slight variant *wa-yahūnu ʿalā al-ṭabīʿa ḥamluhu*, 'and its bearing becomes easy for the constitution'. The changes at the beginning and end of this section are to fit the quote into the flow of Ibn al-Amshāṭī's text, while the two occasions where the stem of the verbs changed might even originate in the manuscript copy Ibn al-Amshāṭī had access to, since the meaning remains the same and the difference between the written Arabic variants of the words can be minuscule depending on the script of a manuscript in both cases.

From the circumstances and conditions of travel, Ibn al-Amshāṭī names sleeplessness, hunger, and thirst to which the traveller should gradually get accustomed to if these are expected to happen during his journey.

---

46 Ambjörn gives a brief summary of issues related to purgative drugs and lists related works from the contemporaries of Qusṭā ibn Lūqā: Qusṭā ibn Lūqā, *Qusṭā ibn Lūqā on purgative drugs and purgation*, i–iii and Qusṭā ibn Lūqā, *Qusṭā ibn Lūqā on the preparation of purgative drugs*, 125–129.

47 Al-Majūsī, *Kāmil al-ṣināʿa*, II/81.

48 As noted in the critical apparatus of the Arabic text, this form (*fa-l-yartāḍa*, Ibn al-Amshāṭī, *al-Isfār*, 122:12–13) is a conjecture. The stem VIII form of the verb appears in line 16 on the same page, while for the verb in line 14 M and T have the same stem I form as in al-Majūsī's text but in C it is clear that two letters were scraped off the paper from the middle of the word.

In the second part of the first chapter, Ibn al-Amshāṭī discusses hunger. In this part, it becomes obvious that Ibn al-Amshāṭī relied on Ibn Sīnā's travel regimen, as Ibn Sīnā writes: *al-aṭʿima al-muttakhidha min al-akbād al-mashwīya wa-naḥwahā, wa-rubbamā uttukhidha minhā kubab maʿa lazūjāt wa-shuḥūm mudhāba qawīya wa-lawz wa-duhn lawz wa-al-shuḥūm mithla al-baqar, fa-idhā tanāwala minhā wāḥida ṣabara ʿalā al-jūʿ zamānan lahu qadr*,[49] 'food made from roasted livers and similar things, and perhaps kebabs made from them with viscid things and melted greasy solid fats and almonds and almond oil and solid fats like [that of] the cattle, and if [somebody] eats from these one [piece] he endures hunger for an amount of time'. Ibn al-Amshāṭī starts with *fa-al-aṭʿima al-muttakhidha min al-akbād al-mashwīya*[50] to fit the quoted section into his paragraph, then amends Ibn Sīnā's text by inserting an explanation that livers are digested slowly and once digested, they are nutritionally abundant and approvable and do not descend fast. Then, Ibn al-Amshāṭī returns to his source: *wa-idhā uttukhidha minhā kubab maʿa lazūjāt wa-shuḥūm qawīya ka-shuḥūm al-baqar al-mudhāba wa-lawz wa-duhnihi fa-idhā tanāwala minhā wāḥida ṣabara ʿalā al-jūʿ zamānan ṭawīlan*.[51] As can be seen, the only changes Ibn al-Amshāṭī makes are to include the example of melted cattle fat in a more concise and logical way and switching 'for an amount of time' [lit.: for a time which has an amount or scope] to 'for a long time'. While Ibn Sīnā ends his list here, Ibn al-Amshāṭī yet again offers an explanation for his reader: he advises this food because oil and fat added to livers increase the slowness of digestion, since fats generate phlegm which blots the stomach. The continuation of this explanation is also Ibn al-Amshāṭī's own: he states that those with carnal appetite are to eat fatty foods such as oils, solid fats, and fatty tails of sheep for this reason. Following this second amendment, Ibn al-Amshāṭī returns once more to his source text and includes with some modifications the practice of drinking a *raṭl*[52] of violet oil mixed with wax to not feel hungry for ten days. To illustrate the slight changes, Ibn Sīnā writes: *wa-qīla: law anna insānan shariba qadr raṭl min duhn al-banafsaj, wa-qad adhāba fīhi shay'an min al-shamʿ ḥattā ṣāra qīrūṭiyyan lam yashtahi al-ṭaʿām ʿashara ayyām*.[53] Meanwhile, Ibn al-Amshāṭī's text is as follows: *wa-qīla annahu man shariba raṭlan min duhn al-banafsaj idh baththa fīhi qalīl min al-shamʿ ḥattā ṣāra qayrūṭiyyan* (*bi-fatḥ al-qāf wa-iskān al-taḥtiyya wa-ḍamm al-rā' al-muhmala thumma wāw wa-ṭā' muhmala*) *lam*

49 Ibn Sīnā, *al-Qānūn*, 1/321.
50 Ibn al-Amshāṭī, *al-Isfār*, 122:18.
51 Ibn al-Amshāṭī, *al-Isfār*, 122:19–20.
52 One *raṭl* equals to approximately 450 g. Hinz, *Islamische Masse*, 28–29.
53 Ibn Sīnā, *al-Qānūn*, 1/321.

yashtahī [sic] *al-ṭaʿām ʿashara ayyām*.[54] The most striking difference is a unique feature of Ibn al-Amshāṭī's regimen, namely the inclusion of the description of pronunciation of foreign words.

In the third part of the first chapter, Ibn al-Amshāṭī discusses what prevents thirst. He divides his advice into two sections, the first is what the traveller should consume and the second is what the traveller is to avoid consuming. He recommends consuming foodstuffs with moist and cooling properties and gives specific examples as well as materials to cook with, amongst them *dūgh*, 'buttermilk', where the pronunciation and explanation of a foreign word appears again. In case of extremely hot weather, Ibn al-Amshāṭī advises drinking certain drinks and either sucking on quince seeds or taking a thirst-quenching pastille, for which he includes the recipe, in addition to naming two substitutes for the pill, a lead coin or a dirham. This part is clearly based on al-Majūsī's regimen with some alterations, omissions, and amendments. As these sections are somewhat lengthier, they are presented parallel to each other. The differences are highlighted in bold. The words Ibn al-Amshāṭī omitted from al-Majūsī's text are in red, the words added by Ibn al-Amshāṭī are in green.

al-Majūsī[55]		**Ibn al-Amshāṭī**[56]
(*wa-*)***yastaʿmilu*** *al-aghdhiya al-mubarrida ka-sawīq al-shaʿīr wa-sawīq al-burr bi-al-māʾ al-bārid wa-al-sukkar wa-al-khass wa-al-baqla al-ḥamqāʾ wa-al-biṭṭīkh wa-bizr al-baqla wa-al-qarʿ wa-al-māsh* ***wa-mā yajrī hādhā al-majrā***	[1]	(*fa-yanbaghī an*) ***yatanāwala*** *al-aghdiya al-raṭba al-mubarrida ka-sawīq al-shaʿīr bi-al-māʾ al-bārid wa-sukkar wa-baqlat al-ḥamqāʾ bi-al-khall wa-al-biṭṭīkh al-hindī wa-al-qarʿ wa-al-māsh* ***wa-mā shākala dhālika***
wa-mā ***ʿumila*** *bi-al-khall wa-al-ḥiṣrim wa-al-dūgh*	[2]	*wa-ka-dhālika mā* ***uttukhidha*** *bi-al-ḥiṣrim wa-al-khall wa-al-dūgh lafẓ fārisī bi-ḍamm al-muhmala wa-ākharuhu muʿjama wa-huwa al-laban al-makhīḍ*
wa-lā yastakthiru min al-ghidhāʾ fa-in kathurathu taʿaṭṭasha	[3]	–

54 Ibn al-Amshāṭī, *al-Isfār*, 124:2–4.
55 Al-Majūsī, *Kāmil al-ṣināʿa*, II/82.
56 Ibn al-Amshāṭī, *al-Isfār*, 124:6–14.

(*cont.*)

al-Majūsī		Ibn al-Amshāṭī
wa-in kāna al-ḥarr shadīdan aw khāfa min al-ʿaṭash fa-l-yashrab qabla masīrihi luʿāb al-bizr qaṭūnā wa-ʿuṣārat bizr al-baqla maʿa shayʾ min māʾ al-rummān wa-duhn al-lawz wa-duhn ḥabb al-qarʿ	[4]	*wa-in kāna al-ḥarr shadīdan fa-l-yashrab qabla masīrihi luʿāb bizr qaṭūnā wa-bizr al-baqla al-ḥamqāʾ maʿa shayʾ min māʾ al-rummān al-muzz wa-duhn ḥabb al-qarʿ*
wa-l-yamsuk fī ***fīhi*** *shayʾan min ḥabb al-safarjal wa-min al-ḥabb al-musakkin li-l-ʿaṭash wa-hādhihi ṣifatuhu yuʾkhidhu lubb ḥabb al-qarʿ wa-lubb al-qiththāʾ wa-lubb al-khiyār wa-bizr al-baqla min kull wāḥid khamsat darāhim nashā wa-kuthayrāʾ wa-ṭabāshīr min kull wāḥid wazn dirhamayn yudiqqu al-jamīʿ nāʿiman wa-yuʿjinu bi-luʿāb al-bizr qaṭūnā wa-yuʿmilu ḥabban kibāran mufarṭaḥan wa-yumsku fī al-fam*	[5]	*wa-yamsuk fī* ***al-fam*** *min ḥabb al-safarjal aw min al-ḥabb al-musakkin li-l-ʿaṭash wa-hādhihi ṣifatuhu lubb ḥabb al-qarʿ wa-lubb ḥabb al-qiththāʿ wa-bizr al-baqlat al-ḥamqāʾ min kull wāḥid khamsat darāhim nashā wa-kuthayrāʾ wa-ṭabāshīr min kull wāḥid dirhamayn yudikku al-jamīʿ nāʿiman wa-yuʿjinu bi-luʿāb bizr qaṭūnā wa-yuʿmilu ḥabban kibāran mufarṭaḥan wa-yumsaku fī al-fam*
fa-in lam ***yaḥḍur*** *fa-l-yamsuk fī fīhi qiṭʿat* ***raṣāṣ*** *aw dirhaman aṭlasan fa-inna dhālika mimmā yaskunu al-ʿaṭash wa-yuqallilu al-ḥāja ilā shrub al-māʾ*	[6]	*wa-in lam* ***yūjad*** *fa-l-yamsuk fī fīhi qiṭʿat* ***usrubb*** *aw dirhaman aṭlasan fa-inna dhālika yaskunu al-ʿaṭash wa-yuqallilu al-ḥāja ilā shrub al-māʾ*

The second section of the third part of Ibn al-Amshāṭī's first chapter lists the foodstuffs forbidden for the traveller to eat: foods that make one thirsty, such as salty or fresh fish, salted food, seasoned cheese, cooked fava beans, as well as acrid and sweet foods. Ibn al-Amshāṭī likely relied on al-Majūsī's text for this section as well, omitting only dairy products (*albān*) from al-Majūsī's list and slightly rearranging the rest of the mentioned foodstuffs. This is followed by the advice to drink water with vinegar if water is scarce, as even a small quantity of the mixture quenches thirst. Here, Ibn al-Amshāṭī returned to Ibn Sīnā, indicated by the identical wording: *wa-idhā shariba al-māʾ bi-al-khall kāna al-qalīl minhu kāfiyan fī taskīn al-ʿaṭash ḥaythu lā yūjadu māʾ kathīr.*[57]

57 Ibn Sīnā, *al-Qānūn*, 1/322; Ibn al-Amshāṭī, *al-Isfār*, 124:16–17.

Two main characteristics of this chapter can be pointed out as a summary. The first is that the chapter gradually moves from the discussion of more theoretic concepts and issues towards providing rather practical and particular advice. The second is that Ibn al-Amshāṭī relied on the travel regimens of al-Majūsī and Ibn Sīnā heavily; Ibn al-Amshāṭī compiled his text by way of copying his sources with minor alterations to adapt the source materials to his needs and amended the material when he deemed it lacking. It must be stressed, however, that these addenda seem to be Ibn al-Amshāṭī's own products and add clarity, theoretical backing, and explanation to the compiled text, besides his original inclusion of the material on purification, not witnessed in any of the earlier travel regimens scrutinised in this book.

2.3 *'Second Chapter on Travelling in Hot Weather'*

In this chapter, Ibn al-Amshāṭī presents a concise theoretical discussion of what happens in the body when travelling in hot weather. Some general advice is followed by Ibn al-Amshāṭī's recommendations for those who have a dry temperament with short explanations added throughout the section. While in the first chapter pinpointing the exact passages Ibn al-Amshāṭī incorporated into his treatise was straightforward, this seems hardly possible for this chapter. The one source which is identifiable is al-Majūsī's regimen, as some of its unique points recur; however, in this case, there are no substantial quotes at all, nor is the structure of the source material observed.

Ibn al-Amshāṭī begins by stating: *al-safar fī al-ḥarr muḍirr yuḥdithu amrāḍan radīʾa*,[58] 'travelling in the hot [weather] is harmful, [it] brings forth malicious diseases', compared to al-Majūsī who writes after some other things *fa-innahu rubbamā aḥdatha al-sayr fī al-shams wa-al-ḥarr amrāḍan radīʾa*,[59] 'travelling in the sun and the hot [weather] likely brings forth malicious diseases'. Al-Majūsī proceeds to give headache, hectic fever (*ḥummā al-diqq*), and dryness and withering of the body as examples, then writes that these occur *lā siyyamā li-aṣḥāb al-amzija al-ḥārra al-yābisa wa-al-abdān al-qaḍīfa*,[60] 'especially in those of hot and dry temperaments and thin bodies'. Ibn al-Amshāṭī does not list specific diseases. Instead, he gives an explanation: travelling in hot weather weakens the strength, as hotness dissolves the moist fluids, thereby weakening the innate heat. To counter this, the constitution demands drinking water to moisten, cool, and strengthen the dissolved fluids. In Ibn al-Amshāṭī's opinion, this more frequent drinking causes many diseases, as well as thirst

58 Ibn al-Amshāṭī, *al-Isfār*, 126:2.
59 Al-Majūsī, *Kāmil al-ṣināʿa*, II/81.
60 Al-Majūsī, *Kāmil al-ṣināʿa*, II/81.

if there is no water to drink. Additionally, the sun can harm the brain, causing headache and fever due to its drying effect, *lā siyyamā fī al-mizāj al-ḥārr al-yābis wa-al-abdān al-qaḍīfa*,[61] 'especially in [those with] the hot and dry temperament and [those with] thin bodies'. As can be seen, while it is a possibility that the beginning and end of this theoretical section is indeed based on al-Majūsī's regimen, the explanation provided by Ibn al-Amshāṭī instead of some examples of such diseases is clearly Ibn al-Amshāṭī's own, even more so considering the fact that a similar line of argumentation is not present in any of the other regimens from where he might have borrowed the idea.

In the following part, Ibn al-Amshāṭī advises those not accustomed to moving in hot weather to not journey during the daytime. If they must do so, they are to cover their head, face, and chest with a turban, hood, or kerchiefs so that the heat of the sun is mitigated and inhaling of the hot air is lessened. While al-Majūsī also continues with this point after finishing the previous train of thought with an additional element, the two texts are so different that it is safe to say Ibn al-Amshāṭī relied on his source only for the general idea instead of simply copying it. Nevertheless, this reliance is easy to pinpoint as it is only al-Majūsī (and Ḥājjī Bāshā, who obviously copied al-Majūsī) who is concerned with the issue of inhaling hot air.

The last part of this chapter contains specific recommendations for those with dry temperaments. Ibn al-Amshāṭi advises to consume barley *sawīq*[62] and fruit syrups or fruit juices before the travel. While these are also generally suggested by other physicians, Ibn al-Amshāṭī goes further by explaining why barley *sawīq* is particularly useful. Firstly, those with a dry temperament have excess bile. Secondly, the dissolution [of moisture and fluids] is increased in such persons, due to the innate heat dissolving from the inside and the external heat dissolving from the outside, in addition to the movement necessary for travelling furthering this warming effect besides weakening of the strength. Barley *sawīq* is not only cold and moistening but also a repellent of yellow bile. Such an explanation is not found in the other travel regimens. Additionally, Ibn al-Amshāṭī instructs to wait after consuming the recommended foodstuffs to let them settle in the stomach instead of shaking them up to the cardia and ruining their digestion by movement. The last of the recommendations is to

61 Ibn al-Amshāṭī, *al-Isfār*, 126:7–8.

62 *Sawīq* is a meal of toasted and crushed seeds which can be prepared into a gruel by mixing it with water, sugar, or fats. It is most commonly made from barley or wheat but other seeds or fruits can also be added to it. For additional information and some recipes, see Nasrallah, *Treasure trove*, 475–476, 221–222, 231, 232; Ibn Sayyār al-Warrāq, *Annals*, 126–127.

use oil of rose and violet with cold water and vinegar on the temples hourly, as these cold and moist materials help prevent headache.

The evidence indicates that in compiling this chapter, Ibn al-Amshāṭī relied on his own discretion for the most part on what to include and omit and how to structure the material. It is interesting to note that besides his unique explanatory addenda Ibn al-Amshāṭī chose to omit listing prohibited foodstuffs, the use of mucous materials besides clothing to cover oneself, and the proper way of resting when travelling in the heat.

2.4 *'Third Chapter on What Pertains to This Concerning Burning Winds'*

This chapter discusses the *samūm* in two sections. The first one focuses on preventive measures, while the second one is dedicated to treating the afflictions caused by the *samūm*. It is al-Rāzī, Ibn Sīnā, and Ḥājjī Bāshā who include the *samūm* in their regimens. They treat the topic in a similar manner, giving advice on prevention and then treatment.

Ibn al-Amshāṭī advises those who travel in the *samūm*, 'a very hot and burning wind making the body dry and chapped'[63] to cover the face and nose and endure scarce inhaling and breathing, as it could lead to serious diseases or even death. He recommends eating onion soaked in *dūgh*, 'buttermilk'. He explains that the two materials work well together because the *dūgh* strengthens the onion if it was already a stronger one. The last of Ibn al-Amshāṭī's preventive advice is to inhale rose oil or pumpkin seed oil, since both are cold and moistening, thereby countering the warming and drying properties of the *samūm* and keeping the brain safe. He also notes that putting these on the head with some vinegar is beneficial against *sirsām* and melancholia. Ibn al-Amshāṭī's advice agrees with that of the other physicians. Nevertheless, it is not possible to identify a direct source for his material. We find short explanations which are lacking in the other texts besides omission of certain issues included in those texts (advised or prohibited foodstuffs and beverages, coating the chest with mucous materials, regularly rinsing the mouth with water, detailed instructions for the *dūgh*-soaked onion), in addition to the lack of identifiable quotes or even heavily reworked sections from the other physicians' works. Based on the omitted issues with the inclusion of the two oils and enduring the state of difficult breathing due to the covered face and nose, Ibn Sīnā's section on the *samūm* is the closest to Ibn al-Amshāṭī's text. However, for this first part, Ibn Sīnā was at most an inspiring guideline for Ibn al-Amshāṭī when compiling his own text, since it is so decidedly different from the source material.

---

63 Ibn al-Amshāṭī, *al-Isfār*, 129:2–3.

For the part on treatment, however, Ibn al-Amshāṭī relied more heavily on Ibn Sīnā. First, Ibn al-Amshāṭī instructs the afflicted traveller to pour cold water on his limbs, wash his face, eat foodstuff prepared from cold herbs, and put cold oils and saps on his head. Ibn al-Amshāṭī does not list rose oil and willow oil (*khilāf*)[64] but adds many examples of cold herbs. Otherwise, he follows Ibn Sīnā's text. Ibn al-Amshāṭī recommends abstaining from intercourse, however, he includes this point at a later part of his regimen. He omits only one statement of Ibn Sīnā, namely that salty fish is beneficial once the afflicted person's constitution settles, but the fact that milk is the best if such a person does not have a fever is repeated together with recommending *dūgh* for those having a fever which is not putrid. Ibn al-Amshāṭī forbids drinking plenty of water and provides a detailed explanation for this: a bigger quantity of water cannot be stopped by any organ from reaching the heart, abound in heat, and thus the cold water can extinguish the innate heat. If the water is only a draught, the stomach retains it first and thus when it gets to the heart, the heart becomes content and the innate heat is not harmed. In comparison, Ibn Sīnā only warns that drinking a lot of cold water leads to immediate death. Therefore, both Ibn Sīnā and Ibn al-Amshāṭī recommend drinking gulp after gulp, as well as to begin drinking rose oil and water mixed together before drinking pure cold water. Then, it is advisable to rest in a cold place, wash the legs with cold water, and eat food that is easily digestible. Ibn al-Amshāṭī follows his source in this part while amending it with examples. Due to the length of these sections, they are presented parallel to each other in order to better illustrate the similarities, omissions, and addenda. The differences are highlighted in bold. The words Ibn al-Amshāṭī omitted from Ibn Sīnā's text are in red, the words added by Ibn al-Amshāṭī are in green.

Ibn Sīnā[65]		**Ibn al-Amshāṭī**[66]
*wa-**idhā ḍarabahu** al-samūm sukiba ʿalā aṭrāfihi māʾ bārid aw ghusila bihi wajhuhu wa-**yujʿalu** ghidhāʾuhu min al-buqūl al-bārida, wa-yaḍaʿu ʿalā raʾsihi al-adhān al-bārida mithla duhn al-ward*	[1]	*wa-**man aṣābahu** shayʾ min al-samūm sukiba ʿalā aṭrāfihi māʾ bārid aw ghusila wajhuhu wa-**juʿila** ghidhāʾuhu min al-buqūl al-bārida ka-al-isfānākh wa-baqlat al-ḥamqāʾ wa-al-qarʿ wa-*

64 Dietrich, *Dioscurides triumphans*, II/163–165.
65 Ibn Sīnā, *al-Qānūn*, I/322–323.
66 Ibn al-Amshāṭī, *al-Isfār*, 128:9–20.

(*cont.*)

Ibn Sīnā		Ibn al-Amshāṭī
wa-al-ʿuṣārāt al-bārida mitla ʿuṣārat ḥayy al-ʿālam, wa-duhn al-khilāf		*al-khass wa-mā shākala dhālika wa-yaḍaʿu ʿalā raʾsihi al-adhān al-bārida wa-al-ʿuṣārāt al-bārida mithla ʿuṣārat ḥayy al-ʿālam wa-naḥwahu*
*thumma yaghtasilu, wa-l-**yaḥdhar** al-jimāʿ*	[2]	moved to [5]
wa-al-samak al-māliḥ yanfaʿuhu idhā sakana mā bihi	[3]	–
*wa-al-sharāb al-mamzūj ayḍan yanfaʿuhu, wa-al-laban min ajwad al-**ghidhāʾ** lahu in lam yakun bihi ḥummā, fa-in kāna bihi ḥummā laysat min al-ḥummayāt al-**ʿafina** bal al-yawmiyya **istaʿmala** al-dūgh al-ḥāmiḍ*	[4]	*wa-al-laban min ajwad al-**aghdhiya** lahu in lam yakun bihi ḥummā fa-in kāna bihi ḥummā laysat min al-ḥummayāt al-**ʿafīna** fa-l-**yastaʿmil** al-dūgh*
	[5]	*wa-l-**yajtanib** al-jimāʿ*
*wa-idhā ʿaṭasha ʿalā al-nawm tajazzā bi-al-maḍmaḍa wa-**lam yashrab** rayyah* [*sic*] *fa-innahu ḥīnaʾidhan yamūtu ʿalā al-makān*	[6]	*wa-**yajib an lā yashrabu** rayya min al-māʾ* […; explanation]
*bal yajibu an **yatajazzā bi**-al-maḍmaḍa wa-in lam **yajid** buddan min **an yashraba, yashrabu** jurʿa baʿda **jurʿa***	[7]	*bal **yaktafī** al-maḍmaḍa wa-in lam **yakun** budd min **al-shurb shariba** jurʿa baʿda **ukhrā***
*fa-idhā sakana mā bihi wa-sakana al-hāʾij min ʿaṭashihi shariba, **wa-in badaʾa awwalan qabla shurbihi fa-shariba** duhn ward wa-māʾ mamzūjayn, thumma **shariba** al-māʾ, kāna aṣwab*	[8]	*fa-idhā sakana mā bihi min ʿaṭash shariba **wa-yanbaghī an yabtadī bi-shurb** duhn ward wa-māʾ mamzūjayn thumma **yashrabu** al-mā*

(*cont.*)

Ibn Sīnā		Ibn al-Amshāṭī
wa-bi-al-jumla fa-in maḍrūb al-ḥarr yajibu an yajʿala majlisahu ***mawḍiʿan*** *bāridan wa-yaghtasila* ***rijlahu*** *bi-al-māʿ al-bārid, wa-in kāna ʿaṭashān shariba al-bārid qalīlan qalīlan wa-yaghtadiya bi-shay sarīʿ al-inhiḍām*	[9]	*wa-yajʿala majlisahu* ***munkhafiḍan*** *bāridan wa-yaghtasila* ***rijlayhi*** *bi-al-māʾ al-bārid wa-yaghtadiya bi-ghidhāʾ sarīʿ al-inhiḍām mithla aṭrāf al-jidāʾ wa-al-qarʿ al-maʿmūl bi-māʾ al-ḥiṣrim wa-al-khall wa-naḥwa dhālika*

These observations suggest that the main source for this chapter was Ibn Sīnā's section on the *samūm*. In the first half of the chapter, Ibn al-Amshāṭī follow his source only in general. In the second half, he observes it more closely with some modifications and rearrangement, and even though he omits a few words, he expounds it greatly by providing explanations and additional examples. In the end, he changes and augments it to the degree that justifies concluding with confidence that he adds extra value to the source material.

2.5 *'Fourth Chapter on the Matter of Travelling in Winter'*

This chapter can be separated into three parts, as Ibn al-Amshāṭī first discusses the general dangers of cold, then moves on to preventive measures, and finally to treatment of those afflicted by the cold.

In the first part, Ibn al-Amshāṭī explains why travelling during wintertime or in cold places is dangerous: the cold quenches the innate heat, causing spasms (*kuzāz*), convulsion (*tashannuj*), and freezing of the body. Another possibility is *būlīmūs* or the hunger of the cattle, when the organs are in need of nutrition even when the stomach is full, likely due to the corrupted cold temperament afflicting the cardia, according to Ibn al-Amshāṭī. Additional dangers are the limbs falling off, especially when one is riding, or weakening of the vision due to looking at the ice and snow. The only physicians who included a list of typical diseases are al-Rāzī and Ibn Sīnā. From these two, only the latter includes *būlīmūs* and on the grounds of some expressions it is even more likely that Ibn al-Amshāṭī took inspiration from Ibn Sīnā here. The changes Ibn al-Amshāṭī made, however, are so profound that comparing the two texts side by side would be pointless. Besides omitting a brief descriptive section and some reasons of possible death, Ibn al-Amshāṭī includes the explanations mentioned above which cannot be found in any of the other travel regimens. Additionally, he includes the limbs and eyes at the end of his list with which he presents a more rounded picture about the dangers of travelling in cold at the beginning of his chapter.

In the second part, Ibn al-Amshāṭī presents general advice for those travelling in the cold. He begins with stating that the traveller's journey should be during daytime and his rest during nighttime. Al-Majūsī's *fa-yanbaghī li-ṣāḥib dhālika an yakūna masīruhu bi-al-nahār wa-rāḥatuhu bi-al-layl*[67] is obviously recognisable in Ibn al-Amshāṭī's *fa-yanbaghī li-l-musāfir fīhi an yakūna masīruhu bi-al-nahār wa-rāḥatuhu bi-al-layl*.[68] However, Ibn al-Amshāṭī briefly explains that the reason for this is that during the daytime, the traveller benefits from the heat of the sun but during the night, the cold becomes more severe, and thus it is recommended to rest and seek shelter during the night. After this, Ibn al-Amshāṭī recommends anointing oneself with oil of Egyptian willow, lily, olives, bay laurel, or similar oils to prevent the cold reaching the organs inside the body. This comes from al-Majūsī's guide, although from a bit later section of his text. Ibn al-Amshāṭī finishes this thought with that this is due to the oils clogging the pores. With this notion, Ibn al-Amshāṭī goes back to Ibn Sīnā's regimen, where we find the same idea, followed by the advice to protect the nose and mouth from the cold air getting into them,[69] which is the next one in the list of Ibn al-Amshāṭī's advice. Ibn al-Amshāṭī adds that this is especially important when it is windy, then mentions the importance of the protection of the limbs which he discusses later—Ibn Sīnā does the same regarding the limbs. As the last topic of the second part, Ibn al-Amshāṭī moves on to discussing how to warm oneself when resting. He advises the traveller not to proceed to warming himself straightaway but to protect himself from sudden exposure to warmth after exposure to cold, since this would exhaust and weaken the body and the strength. This effect is present also when one warms oneself in a hurry, going close to a fire and then leaving it, therefore Ibn al-Amshāṭī does not recommend this. It is best to warm oneself gradually. This idea in general is mentioned by Ibn Sīnā in a much briefer way;[70] while Ibn Sīnā's sentences might be the inspiration for this discussion by Ibn al-Amshāṭī, due to the level of elaboration, it is definitively not an expanded copy of Ibn Sīnā.

In the last, third part, Ibn al-Amshāṭī presents the general regimen of those weakened by the cold. This includes oils to use, proper places for a campsite, warming oneself, as well as what and when to eat. The first instruction for the

67 Al-Majūsī, *Kāmil al-ṣināʿa*, II/82.
68 Ibn al-Amshāṭī, *al-Isfār*, 130:9–10.
69 Ibn Sīnā, *al-Qānūn*, I/324.
70 Ibn Sīnā, *al-Qānūn*, I/323.

traveller is to warm himself and use warm oils such as oil of iris, lily, castor, chamomile, and similar oils. From the warming oils in general, al-Majūsī names oil of Egyptian willow, lily, and bay laurel; Ibn al-Quff lists oil of violet, lily, and chamomile; Ibn al-Khaṭīb names iris oil; and al-Ṭabarī and Ibn Sīnā refrain from giving examples. In this case, the most probable scenario is that Ibn al-Amshāṭī gives examples of warming oils based on his own knowledge instead of borrowing a list from another physician. After this topic, Ibn al-Amshāṭī moves on to the issue of the proper resting place. He recommends choosing a warm place sheltered from the wind and away from the passage of streams, and to place the riding animals close to the tent to utilise their warmth. In addition to this, Ibn al-Amshāṭī instructs the traveller to take all his garments off if possible, or at least those most afflicted by the cold and put something else on. While al-Rāzī, al-Majūsī, Ibn al-Khaṭīb, and Ḥājjī Bāshā all give instructions for travellers afflicted by the cold, their passages differ greatly from Ibn al-Amshāṭī's discussion of this topic, as they focus for the most part on massage, bathing, warming oils, sleeping under blankets, and consuming warming foodstuffs. The only similarity is al-Rāzī's recommendation to choose a warm, leeward resting place; this is, however, only a similarity and does not indicate a closer relationship between the passages. An interesting feature to point out is the inclusion of placement of riding animals by Ibn al-Amshāṭī, since this instruction only appears in the regimens meant for armies. The rest of Ibn al-Amshāṭī's advice pertains to foodstuffs and nutrition. The foodstuffs in this case should be warm and richly seasoned with warming herbs, such as garlic, nutmeg, mustard seeds, assafetida, onion, pepper, cinnamon, long pepper, and ginger, not listed in a similar way by the rest of the physicians. As for nutrition, Ibn al-Amshāṭī states that the traveller should not travel on an empty stomach. Therefore, he should eat the recommended foodstuffs and wait for it to descend to the bottom of the stomach properly. In general, this last section seems to be geared more towards a traveller afflicted by the cold who decides to rest on the road, while bathing and massage often recommended by the other physicians would presuppose access to certain facilities (although al-Rāzī advises massage even if a bathhouse and its services are not available).

In summary, Ibn al-Amshāṭī's chapter on travelling in winter is inspired by al-Majūsī's and Ibn Sīnā's relevant passages. This is most noticeable in the first half of the chapter, where we can occasionally find the same expressions, not just similar ideas. As we progress towards the end of the chapter, Ibn al-Amshāṭī moves away from his sources, as there are no parallels to find in the other regimens. Additionally, there are examples of Ibn al-Amshāṭī's tendency to include concise theoretical explanations in this chapter as well as in the previous ones.

2.6 *'Fifth Chapter on the Guarding of the Limbs and Their Treatment'*

In this chapter, Ibn al-Amshāṭī discusses various methods of protecting the limbs and the eyesight, then dedicates approximately two-thirds of the chapter to the treatment of the limbs according to the severeness of their affliction.

Ibn Sīnā[71]		Ibn al-Amshāṭī[72]
yajibu an yadlukahā al-musāfir awwalan ḥattā taskhunu	[1]	*yajibu an yadluka al-musāfir fī al-bard* ***aṭrāfahu*** *ḥattā taskhunu*
thumma yaṭliyahā bi-duhn ***ḥārr*** *min al-adhān al-ʿaṭira mithla duhn al-sawsan wa-duhn al-bān wa-al-maysawsan luṭūkh jayyid lahum*	[2]	*thumma yaṭliyahā bi-al-adhān* ***al-ḥārra*** *al-ʿaṭira mithla duhn al-bān wa-al-sawsan*
fa-in lam yaḥḍur *fa-al-zayt, wa-khuṣūṣan idhā* ***juʿila fīhi*** *al-fulful wa-al-ʿāqir qarḥā, aw al-farbiyūn wa-al-ḥiltīt aw al-jundibādistar*	[3]	***wa-illā*** *fa-bi-al-zayt wa-khuṣūṣan idhā* ***khuliṭa maʿahu*** *al-ʿāqir qarhā wa-al-fulful wa-al-ḥiltīt*
–	[4]	*aw duhn al-yāsamīn ayḍan*
wa-min al-aḍmida al-ḥāfiẓa li-l-aṭrāf an yajʿala ʿalayhā qinna wa-thawm	[5]	*wa-al-thawm yalṭakhu bihi al-aṭrāf*
fa-innahu amān wa-lā ka-al-qaṭrān	[6]	*wa-al-qaṭrān nāfiʿ jiddan*
–	[7]	*wa-kull dhālika mimmā yamnaʿu taṭarruq al-fasād ilayhā*

As for prevention, Ibn al-Amshāṭī advises massaging the limbs until they warm up, then coating them with warm, aromatic oils, such as oil of Egyptian willow or iris, or if these are not available, then olive oil, especially if it was mixed with pellitory, pepper, and assafetida. Jasmine oil is another alternative, as well

71 Ibn Sīnā, *al-Qānūn*, 1/324.
72 Ibn al-Amshāṭī, *al-Isfār*, 134:3–6.

as sprinkling the limbs with garlic. The usefulness of tar is stressed but Ibn al-Amshāṭī deems all the materials that he listed good for preventing decay of the limbs. Here, Ibn al-Amshāṭī obviously borrows from Ibn Sīnā; however, in the second half of this section, Ibn al-Amshāṭī omits the bandages mentioned by Ibn Sīnā and recommends garlic separately, in addition to stating that tar is useful, while Ibn Sīnā deems it unsafe. While Ḥājjī Bāshā writes that tar is the most effective of such materials as it protects the limbs from putrefaction, it is not likely that this is Ibn al-Amshāṭī's source. The similarities and differences of Ibn Sīnā's and Ibn al-Amshāṭī's passages are illustrated by the side by side comparison on the previous page. The differences are highlighted in bold. The words Ibn al-Amshāṭī omitted from Ibn Sīnā's text are in red, the words added by Ibn al-Amshāṭī are in green.

The next set of preventive measures Ibn al-Amshāṭī recommends is properly padding and covering the limbs. He advises putting the undercoat hair of goats with hare fur or something similar between the fingers, then wrapping the legs with *kāghad*, 'paper', putting on stockings, then shoes. Here, al-Majūsī seems to be the likely source, even if Ibn al-Amshāṭī added hare fur but omitted additional garments mentioned by al-Majūsī (fur boots and fur gloves). The relation of the two texts is shown below with the differences in bold and the addenda in green.

al-Majūsī[73]		**Ibn al-Amshāṭī**[74]
[...] (*bi-*)*an* ***yaḍaʿa*** *bayna* ***al-*** *aṣābiʿ shaʿr al-marʿaz*	[1]	(*wa-yanbaghī*) *an* ***yajʿala*** *bayna aṣābiʿ****ihi*** *shaʿr al-maʿz* ***al-marʿazī*** *wa-ʿalayhā wabr al-arnab aw ghayrahu*
wa- *yaluffa****hā*** *bi-al-kāghad*	[2]	***thumma*** *yaluffa* ***al-rijl*** *bi-al-kāghad* (*bi-al-muʿjama al-maftūḥa wa-al-dāl al-muhmala wa-huwa al-waraq fārisī muʿarrab*)
wa- *yalbasa ʿalayhā al-jawārib thumma al-khuff* [...]	[3]	***thumma*** *yalbasa ʿalayhā al-jawārib wa-hiya al-lafāʾif thumma al-khuff*

73 Al-Majūsī, *Kāmil al-ṣināʿa*, II/82–83.
74 Ibn al-Amshāṭī, *al-Isfār*, 134:6–8.

The last bit of information regarding prevention by Ibn al-Amshāṭī concerns protection of the eyes. Weakening of the vision due to looking at the sharp whiteness of the snow and ice can be prevented by hanging black, green, or dark blue rags in front of the eye and wearing a turban and garments of these colours, although black is the most effective of these colours. This part also relies heavily on al-Majūsī's text. In this case, virtually nothing pertaining to content is omitted or added, despite the changes Ibn al-Amshāṭī makes to al-Majūsī's text. These are illustrated below, with the differences in bold, the omissions in red, and the addenda in green. The comparison here does not mark the rearrangement of words, as those are obvious on a closer reading of the sections.

al-Majūsī[75]		**Ibn al-Amshāṭī**[76]
(wa-yanbaghī ayḍan) an yataḥarraza min an yanāla al-baṣar al-ḍaʿf ***bi-sabab*** *al-naẓar ilā al-thalj* ***fa-inna*** *dhālika* ***yafruqu*** *al-nūr al-bāṣir*	[1]	*(wa-)an yataḥarraza an yanāla al-baṣar daʿf* ***min*** *al-naẓar ilā al-thalj wa-al-jamad* ***li-anna*** *shiddat bayāḍihimā* ***yufarriqu*** *al-nūr al-bāsir*
wa-yuqallilahu bi-an ***yuʿalliqa*** *ʿalā al-ʿayn al-khiraq al-****sūd*** *wa-takūna al-ʿimāma sawdāʾ wa-in amkana an* ***takūna*** *thiyābuhu sawdāʾ kuḥliyya aw khuḍran fa-l-yafʿal dhālika*	[2]	*wa-yuqalliluhu wa-yamnaʿu min dhālika* ***taʿlīq*** *al-khiraq al-****sawdāʾ*** *ʿalā al-ʿayn wa-al-ʿimāma* ***al-****sawdāʾ aw* ***lubs*** *al-thiyāb al-sawdāʾ in amkana wa-kadhālika al-khuḍr wa-al-kuḥliyya yaqūmu maqām al-sūd*
fa-inna hādhihi al-alwān tajmaʿu al-nūr al-bāṣir wa-tamnaʿu ***min tafarruqihi*** *wa-al-lawn al-aswad aqwāhā fiʿlan fī dhālika*	[3]	*fa-inna hādhihi al-alwān tamnaʿu* ***an yufarriqa*** *al-nūr al-bāṣir wa-yajmaʿuhu wa-al-aswad aqwāhā*

After means of prevention, Ibn al-Amshāṭī moves on to treatment. Other than the above measures against less serious freezing, the physicians focus their discussion on the various stages of the affliction of the limbs, namely decay

75 Al-Majūsī, *Kāmil al-ṣināʿa*, II/83.
76 Ibn al-Amshāṭī, *al-Isfār*, 134:8–11.

without discolouration, green or black discolouration, and putrefaction. Before treatments, Ibn al-Amshāṭī includes the symptoms of decay caused by the cold and a short theoretical explanation on what happens inside the body. When moving on to treatments, Ibn al-Amshāṭī separates his advice in a different way than the previous physicians, discussing treatment of various external and internal ulcers, stiff but not discoloured limbs, and discoloured and already putrefying limbs.

According to Ibn al-Amshāṭī, the symptom of decay reaching the limbs due to the cold is that the traveller does not feel the pain and cold in the affected limbs. Either the cold suppresses the innate heat of the organ and restrains what would dissolve from it, or it harms the organ without reaching this suppressing effect. The first of these happens because the severe cold and the obstruction of the pores causes the heat, vapour, and blood to move to the inside of the organ. When these materials dwell in the inside of the organ, they burn it and putrefy, causing ulcers. Previous physicians discuss treatment of frozen limbs, discoloured limbs, and discoloured and putrefied limbs; however, they do not include a theoretical explanation of how and why the cold affects the limbs, neither do they mention ulcers as a possible affliction and therefore their treatment is likewise not included in their travel regimens. The only exception to this is Ibn Sīnā who writes that if the cold has afflicted the organ, suppressed the innate heat, and restrained what would dissolve from it, exposing the organ to putrefaction, it is to be treated in accordance with his instructions in his chapter on ulcers.[77] Therefore, his exposition is shorter and refers his reader to another part of his encyclopaedia. This means that this brief theoretical explanation as well as the treatment of various kinds of ulcers is another novelty of Ibn al-Amshāṭī's travel regimen; even if he utilises additional medical literature and his knowledge, his inclusion of these topics is unparalleled.

Ibn al-Amshāṭī advises the following treatments for ulcers. External, clean ulcers (*qarḥa naqīya*) are to be dried, while external, putrid ulcers ([*qarḥa*] *ʿafina*) are to be cured with warm, consuming remedies and cauterisation if the ulcer is not painful. For ulcers with nothing being consumed from their middles, it is sufficient to bind their edges together. However, if the skin perishes from an ulcer, it is treated with sealing medicaments such as gallnuts and pomegranate peel, and if the meat is perishing, then with medicaments facilitating tissue growth besides having drying properties, such as red anemones and basilicon liniment. After these types of external ulcers, Ibn al-Amshāṭī moves

77 Ibn Sīnā, *al-Qānūn*, 1/324.

on to internal ulcers (*qurūḥ bāṭina*). In case of internal ulcers, their draining medicaments should be prepared with additional drying agents such as honey and medicaments according to the specific place of the ulcer. For citatrisation, a sticky material similar to Lemnian earth is to be produced by gripping the ulcers. Internal ulcers should not be distressed further by using hot water. When looking for a source material of this section, Ibn Sīnā's more detailed discussion of the various kinds of ulcers and their treatments is an obvious choice for three reasons: Ibn Sīnā refers his reader to this part of his encyclopaedia, he is the only physician mentioning ulcers in his travel regimen, and it is evident that Ibn al-Amshāṭī relied on Ibn Sīnā's text when compiling. On closer inspection of Ibn Sīnā's chapter on ulcers,[78] there are short sections which are similarly worded, especially the one pertaining to internal ulcers. However, Ibn al-Amshāṭī's discussion is more simplified and streamlined, and for the other kinds of ulcers, he does not repeat and copy the medicaments recommended by Ibn Sīnā. It is a possibility that this section of Ibn Sīnā was a looser inspiration for Ibn al-Amshāṭī, similarly to the ten principles of purging discussed previously. However, just as in that case, here too it is impossible to assert with certainty that Ibn al-Amshāṭī used the *Qānūn*'s chapter on ulcers when compiling his text; the similarities might be a result of a profound knowledge of the *Qānūn* and meanwhile it is a plausible possibility that he mostly relied on his own medical knowledge and compiled this section without closely using a source text.

In the second affliction Ibn al-Amshāṭī discusses, when the cold harms the organ but does not suppress the innate heat and drives materials to the inside of the organ, the afflicted organ is either swollen or not. If the organ is not swollen, it is to be massaged and anointed with warm oils, such as olive oil. If the organ is swollen, it is to be put into water of rapeseed or water in which fig and cabbage, hot aromatic plants, dill and chamomile, or similar plats were boiled alone or together. This section seems to be a combination of al-Majūsī's and Ibn Sīnā's advice.[79] The former is the only one of the physicians who also mentions swelling as a symptom, and recommends chamomile, melilot, and dill to be boiled in the water used to treat the organ. Ibn Sīnā mentions snow water or fig, cabbage, basil, dill, chamomile, wormwood (*shīkh*), pennyroyal (*fūdanaj*), and a kind of mint (*nammām*) to be boiled in the water. Al-Majūsī includes anointing as a treatment for swollen limbs, and Ibn Sīnā continues with compresses, approaching a fire, slightly exercising the limbs, then massaging and anointing it. Ibn al-Amshāṭī omits all these and sticks to putting the organ into the aforementioned water. Then he moves on to describe

78 Ibn Sīnā, *al-Qānūn*, I/375–377.

79 Al-Majūsī, *Kāmil al-ṣināʿa*, II/83; Ibn Sīnā, *al-Qānūn*, I/324.

the treatment of the empiricists: immersing the organ in cold water, driving the pain away, comparing it to the frozen fruit put into cold water resulting in the freezing leaving the fruit. This section likely originates from Ibn Sīnā's account of the same treatment, as he is the only physician to include this in his travel regimen; while Ibn Sīnā says some people do this (*min al-nās*), Ibn al-Amshāṭī links the treatment to some of the empiricists (*baʿḍ al-mujarribīn*). To further illustrate the relationship of the two sections, they are presented side by side, with the differences in bold, the omissions in red, and the addenda in green.

Ibn Sīnā[80]		**Ibn al-Amshāṭī**[81]
(*wa-min al-nās man*) *yaghmisuhu* *fī māʾ bārid*	[1]	**(*wa-qāla baʿḍ al-mujarribīn innahu*) *ghamasa al-ʿuḍw*** *fī māʿ bārid*
*fa-**yajidu** li-dhālika manfaʿa ka-anna al-adhā yandafiʿu ʿanhu*	[2]	*fa-**wajada** li-dhālika manfaʿa wa-ka-anna al-adhā yandafiʿu ʿanhu*
***ka-mā yaʿriḍu li**-l-fākiha al-jāmida **an** [sic] **talqā** fī al-māʾ al-bārid fa-yakūnu ka-annahu yakhruju al-jamd ʿanhā wa-yantasiju ʿalayhā fa-talīnu wa-tastawī*	[3]	***wa-yuwakkidu dhālika** al-fākiha al-jāmida **idhā wuḍiʿat fī** al-māʿ al-bārid yakhruju al-jamd ʿanhā wa-tazhū wa-yaḥsunu ṭaʿmuhā*
wa-law annahā quribat min al-nār fasadat	[4]	–

The next type of affliction in Ibn al-Amshāṭī's discussion is when the limb turns dull-coloured. It is only Ibn Sīnā who uses this particular expression, and the treatment offered by him and by Ibn al-Amshāṭī concurs with the treatment the rest of the physicians prescribe for a limb which turned green or black. This is, following Ibn al-Amshāṭī's words, a deep incision of the limb, then putting it into hot water to avoid clotting and to let the blood flow freely before it stops on its own accord. Then it is to be coated with Armenian bole soaked in vinegar and rose water. This coating is to be changed after a day and a night. Besides Armenian bole, tar is also useful on its own. On closer inspection, it becomes

80 Ibn Sīnā, *al-Qānūn*, 1/324.
81 Ibn al-Amshāṭī, *al-Isfār*, 136:7–9.

apparent that Ibn al-Amshāṭī borrowed this expression of dullness from Ibn Sīnā but relied on al-Majūsī for changes compared to Ibn Sīnā's treatment. It seems that Ibn al-Amshāṭī combined the two sources organically instead of sticking to his sources more exactly. The relationship of the three texts is illustrated again in a side-by-side comparison, with the differences in bold, the omissions in red, and the addenda in green.

al-Majūsī [M][82] / Ibn Sīnā [IS][83]		**Ibn al-Amshāṭī[84]**
[IS] ***fa-ammā** idhā akhadha al-ṭaraf yakmudu fa-**yajibu** an* ([M] *fa-in kānat al-aṣābiʿ qad akhḍarrat aw aswaddat fa-yanbaghī an*)	[1]	***wa**-idhā akhadha al-ṭaraf yakmadu fa-**ṭarīq ʿilājihi** an*
[M] *yashruṭa sharṭan ʿamīqan **wa-yatruka** fī al-māʾ al-ḥārr ḥattā **yakhruju** minhā al-dam* (*wa-yatruku ḥattā yanqaṭiʿu min dhātihi*) [IS] (*yashruṭa wa-yasīlu minhu al-dam wa-al-ʿuḍw*) ***mawḍūʿ** fī al-māʾ al-ḥārr li-allā yajmuda shayʾ min al-dam fī fūhāt al-sharṭ, fa-lā yukhraju bal yutraku ḥattā **yaḥtabisu** min nafsihi*	[2]	*yashruṭa ʿamīqan wa-**yūḍaʿa** fī al-māʾ al-ḥārr ḥattā **yarqā** al-dam li-allā yajmuda shayʾ min al-dam fī fūhāt al-sharṭ fa-yanḥabisu*
[IS] *thumma yuṭlā bi-al-ṭīn al-armanī* (*wa-al-khall al-mamzūj, fa-inna dhālika yamnaʿu fasādahu*) [M] *fa-idhā inqaṭaʿa khurūjuhu wa-qalla* (*fa-yuṭlā bi-al-armanī*) ***maʿjūnan bi**-khall wa-mā ward wa-yashuddu yawman wa-layla thumma **yughsila** bi-sharāb wa-yuʿādu ʿalayhā al-**ṭalāʾ** ilā an yanbuta al-laḥm fī dhālika al-mawḍiʿ wa-yaṣlubu wa-tajiffu al-qarḥa*	[3]	*thumma yuṭlā bi-al-ṭīn al-armanī manqūʿan **fī** al-khall wa-māʾ al-ward wa-yashuddu yawman wa-layla thumma **yazālu ʿanhu** wa-yuʿādu al-**ṭaly***

82 Al-Majūsī, *Kāmil al-ṣināʿa*, II/83.
83 Ibn Sīnā, *al-Qānūn*, I/325.
84 Ibn al-Amshāṭī, *al-Isfār*, 136:10–12.

(*cont.*)

al-Majūsī [M] / Ibn Sīnā [IS]		Ibn al-Amshāṭī
[IS] *wa-al-qaṭrān* ***yanfaʿu bidʾan*** *wa-* ***akhīran*** ([M]—)	[4]	*wa-al-qaṭrān* ***nāfiʿ awwalan*** *wa-* ***ākhiran***

The last type of treatment discussed by Ibn al-Amshāṭī is for when the afflicted organ is not only black or green but it is past this stage and the organ starts to putrefy. First and foremost, Ibn al-Amshāṭī instructs to act fast and eliminate the putrid parts so that the healthy tissue next to it does not start to decay. For this, one should boil the outer parts of cabbage and beet, make a mixture from it with clarified butter, and put it onto the organ until it makes the putrid parts fall off. For this first section, Ibn Sīnā is a likely inspiration, as he expresses the same concern but instead of offering a treatment, refers his reader to another chapter of his encyclopaedia.[85] As redirecting the reader is not a possibility for Ibn al-Amshāṭī, he articulates the general instruction in a clearer way and also includes a treatment. Then, Ibn al-Amshāṭī includes another method, namely warm bandages made from the leaf of marshmallow, mallow, and gooseberry in a powdered form and mixed with violet oil. This bandage is to be applied two to three times a day to make the putrid parts fall off, then the rest of the organ is to be treated like ulcers. This second part is a more faithful copy of al-Majūsī's text.[86] This means that for the treatment of putrefied organs, Ibn al-Amshāṭī combines the material from his two sources, being clearer and more inclusive in the first half of this section than Ibn Sīnā but sticking more closely to the text of the treatment recommended by al-Majūsī.

The most prominent feature of this chapter is probably the arrangement of its material. Starting with prevention, Ibn al-Amshāṭī includes protection of the eyes, more precisely the vision, in this chapter. While some other physicians dedicated separate, short chapters to this topic, Ibn al-Amshāṭī discusses only its wintertime protection. Symptoms of the effects of the cold reaching the limbs and an explanation on how the cold actually harms the limbs is mentioned only on one occasion in previous regimens. Including ulcers and their treatments in the regimen is a novelty offered by Ibn al-Amshāṭī's text. While

85 Ibn Sīnā, *al-Qānūn*, I/325.
86 Al-Majūsī, *Kāmil al-ṣināʿa*, II/83.

al-Majūsī and Ibn Sīnā are still obviously the sources for Ibn al-Amshāṭī, he uses their materials in different ways. There is, of course, the method seen before when Ibn al-Amshāṭī rearranges the source material with omissions, addenda, and inclusion of explanations as well as his own material. However, there are examples for more simple copying as well as more complicated combining of the two sources as well.

2.7 *'Sixth Chapter on Preserving the Complexion'*

In this short chapter, Ibn al-Amshāṭī states that the colour of the traveller's skin (his face, hands, and legs) might change due to the hot or cold weather or because of washing himself with costive waters. To avoid this, he offers advice on how to preserve the complexion of the face and treat fissures of the skin caused by the cold, wind, or sun.

For protecting the face, Ibn al-Amshāṭī recommends coating it with something sticky with a glutinous agent, such as mucilage of psyllium seeds, purslane seeds, tragacanth, and gum dissolved in water or egg whites and semolina pastries soaked in water. It is only al-Rāzī and Ibn Sīnā who write about this issue in their travel regimens. As before, al-Rāzī's text was surely not consulted by Ibn al-Amshāṭī when he compiled his own chapter but it is obvious that he used Ibn Sīnā's passage.[87] However, Ibn Sīnā omits any kind of introductory remark and offers this preventive measure only, referring his reader once more to a separate chapter for a treatment of fissures. Focusing on the treatment only, the two texts run parallel to each other neatly. Besides a variation for seamless inclusion in his chapter, Ibn al-Amshāṭī changes mucilage of arfaj plant (*ʿarfaj, Rhanterium epapposum*) to purslane seeds and omits mentioning flat bread loaves (dissolved in water like semolina pastries) and "the recipe of Qrīṭūn".

For treating the fissures, Ibn al-Amshāṭī provides a recipe for a *qayrūṭī* [his own vocalisation], cerate, or recommends oils and greases if preparing the plaster is not possible: four dirhams each of [two kinds of] sandalwood and rose, five dirhams of melilot, two dirhams of saffron, half a dirham of camphor, ten dirhams of wax, and half a *raṭl* of rose oil in winter or four *ūqiya*s in summer mixed well. Ibn Sīnā mentions various cerates in general in his chapter on the fissures of the skin in various places of the body but he does not include a recipe for any of them in these passages.[88]

87 Ibn Sīnā, *al-Qānūn*, I/325.
88 Ibn Sīnā, *al-Qānūn*, IV/224–226.

2.8 *'Seventh Chapter on the Matters of the Waters'*

In this chapter, Ibn al-Amshāṭī discusses the various types of water the traveller encounters on his journey. After a general point he makes, the chapter can be separated into three parts. In the first part, Ibn al-Amshāṭī lists the best and worst kinds of water with their characteristics. In the second part, he discusses prophylaxis. In the third part, he gives some additional advice.

Ibn al-Amshāṭī begins this chapter by stating that the difference in waters makes the traveller sick more often than the difference of food because the constitution needs it more and it is less capable of enduring its lack than a lack of food. While the explanation is Ibn al-Amshāṭī's own, the statement itself likely comes from Ibn Sīnā (Ibn al-Amshāṭī writes *ikhtilāf al-miyāh yūqiʿu al-musāfir fī amrāḍ akthar min ikhtilāf al-aghdhiya*,[89] while Ibn Sīnā writes *inna ikhtilāf al-miyāh qad yūqaʿu al-musāfir fī amrāḍ akthar min ikhtilāf al-aghdhiya.*)[90] Despite this, it is important to point out that based on al-Rāzī's notes in the *Ḥāwī*, not only Ibn Māsawayh wrote this in his *al-Masāʾil* but it can be easily traced back to Aristotle's *al-Masāʾil al-ṭabīʿiyya*. Nevertheless, the content of this statement is the reason Ibn al-Amshāṭī deems it necessary to mention some of the principles regarding waters.

The first part of this chapter starts with the statement of Ibn al-Amshāṭī: "I say that the water does not nourish but refines nourishment."[91] While it can be taken for certain that Ibn al-Amshāṭī is not the first one who actually said this but this remark has its origins in the Hippocratic tradition on water(s) and nourishment,[92] it is obvious that the rest of this part indeed relies on the Hippocratic *Airs, waters, places*. Ibn al-Amshāṭī starts with the best kinds of waters: first are the waters of springs of clayey lands descending from elevated places, abundant and uncovered, far from their source, lightweight, running towards the summer sunrise or north.[93] These are clearly the Hippocratic waters flowing from high places and earthy hills, coming from very deep springs, the best of which are those running towards the summer rising of the sun.[94] After such

89 Ibn al-Amshāṭī, *al-Isfār*, 140:1.

90 Ibn Sīnā, *al-Qānūn*, 1/325.

91 Ibn al-Amshāṭī, *al-Isfār*, 141:7.

92 See Jouanna, *Water, health and disease*. Cf. Ibn al-Dhahabī's (d. 456/1064) treatise "on the lack of nourishment in water (*Maqālah fī anna l-māʾ lā yaghdhū*)", LHOM 13.41. Ibn Sīnā writes elsewhere in the *Qānūn* that water is special (*makhṣūṣ*), *lā li-annahu yaghdū, bal li-annahu yunfidhu al-ghadhāʾ wa-yuṣliḥu qawāmahā* (Ibn Sīnā, *al-Qānūn*, 1/181).

93 Ibn al-Amshāṭī, *al-Isfār*, 140:5–7.

94 Hp. *Aër.* VII; Jones, *Hippocrates*, 1/89. In this section, I use the abbreviation present in the Liddell-Scott Greek-English Lexicon when referencing the work of Hippocrates, the English translation of Ibn al-Amshāṭī's treatise, and the English rendition of the Hippocratic *Airs, waters, places* by W.H.S. Jones.

spring waters, Ibn al-Amshāṭī praises rainwater, since it is of excellent and delicate consistency, especially if it is from plentiful clouds, despite the fact that it putrefies fast, in which case it should be boiled.[95] The Hippocratic text also praises rainwaters as the "lightest, sweetest, finest, and clearest" of waters in addition to discussing its generation in greater detail and warning the reader that "they need to be boiled and purified from foulness".[96]

Still in the first part of this chapter after the two kinds of good waters mentioned in the above paragraph, Ibn al-Amshāṭī moves on to a general discussion of bad waters. He starts with waters of water pits and canals and waters flowing toward west and south, especially if affected by southern winds. He then lists the overall effects of certain waters: tranquil ones burden the stomach, swampy ones produce phlegm, and those with minerals are bad in general with the exception of iron-rich water, which strengthens the bowels. Ammonic water loosens and aluminous water obstructs the bowels, while salty water first relieves then confines them. Hot water corrupts the digestion which can lead to hectic fever and heated fever. Tepid water causes nausea or due to its heat leads to colic. Lastly, ice and snow are harmful for the nerves but useful to cool down oneself with these from the outside. Ibn al-Amshāṭi ends this part with stating that moderately cold water is the most appropriate for a healthy person.[97] Comparing these with the Hippocratic text, the following observations can be made. The discussion of the worst of the waters, namely swampy waters is more detailed in the Hippocratic text but the capacity of swampy waters to cause of phlegm is mentioned. The second-worst are hard, hot, or mineral-rich waters, which are "hard, heating waters, difficult to pass and causing constipation". Interestingly, the Hippocratic text includes iron-rich waters here as well and does not make it an exception, although it is stressed that in some cases, bad waters can be beneficial for certain constitutions and diseases. The orientation of waters is also discussed by the Hippocratic text, describing those facing south as the worst waters, especially with southern winds.[98] Finally, waters from snow and ice are considered bad for all purposes by the Hippocratic text.[99] The differences found in Ibn al-Amshāṭī's text clearly indicate that he utilises the evolving and adapted tradition built on the Hippocratic text.

In the second part of this chapter, Ibn al-Amshāṭī discusses general prophylaxis, then writes about salty and stagnant waters in greater detail and alumic

95 Ibn al-Amshāṭī, *al-Isfār*, 140:7–8.
96 Hp. *Aër.* VII; Jones, *Hippocrates*, I/91, 93.
97 Ibn al-Amshāṭī, *al-Isfār*, 140:8–15.
98 Hp. *Aër.* VII; Jones, *Hippocrates*, I/85–87, 89.
99 Hp. *Aër.* VII; Jones, *Hippocrates*, I/93–95.

and ammonic water briefly. Ibn al-Amshāṭī starts by stating that vaporisation and distillation repel or lessen the harms of the difference of waters as this difference occurs due to the foreign parts mixed into the water. He also briefly explains why these methods and boiling the water are effective.[100] At first, it might be tempting to say that Ibn al-Amshāṭī was inspired by Ibn Sīnā who explained these and an additional filtering method in his travel regimen; on closer inspection, however, it is obvious that this is not the case. Here, Ibn al-Amshāṭī did not consult Ibn Sīnā's text due to a lack of similarities but rather a shared, as of now unidentified, source material or tradition.

For consuming salty water, Ibn al-Amshāṭī recommends mixing it with vinegar and oxymel besides throwing carob and myrtle seeds into it. He explains the negative effects of salty water and lists how the materials he lists protect against these effects.[101] The recommended materials are the same as those mentioned by the other physicians, although Ibn al-Amshāṭī does not list azerole (*zuʿrūr*) and also omits other methods. However, it is only he who explains why the materials he does list work.

Ibn al-Amshāṭī then advises drinking mucilage of psyllium seeds or other similar things making the constitution tender with alumic water and drinking costive things with ammonic water.[102] Ibn Sīnā and Ibn al-Quff mention alumic water but with different materials, therefore it seems that these two kinds of water and their method of consumption relies on Ibn al-Amshāṭī's own knowledge. It can be pointed out that the methods recommended by Ibn al-Amshāṭī oppose the general negative effects listed by him in the previous section.

The last kind of water discussed by Ibn al-Amshāṭī is stagnant water of *wādi*s and swamps. If such a water is putrid, Ibn al-Amshāṭī advises against warm foods as those would facilitate the water's getting through to the organs but recommends costive and cooling fruits and herbs such as quince, apple, and ribes, as these protect against putridity and counteract the loosening effect of swampy waters.[103] While costive things are the general recommendations, previous physicians discuss stagnant waters under the Arabic term *qāʾim* while Ibn al-Amshāṭī uses the term *rākid*. Al-Rāzī and Ibn Sīnā both advise against warm foodstuffs; the sections of these two physicians are, however, not likely to be a source for Ibn al-Amshāṭī, as the first is noticeably different altogether and the second would be even more reworked, changed, and amended than usual. It is

100 Ibn al-Amshāṭī, *al-Isfār*, 140:16–142:3.
101 Ibn al-Amshāṭī, *al-Isfār*, 142:4–8.
102 Ibn al-Amshāṭī, *al-Isfār*, 142:9–10.
103 Ibn al-Amshāṭī, *al-Isfār*, 142:11–15.

more likely in this case, again, that the source is the common tradition rather than an exact passage of another travel regimen.

In the last part of this chapter, Ibn al-Amshāṭī provides additional general advice for the traveller regarding waters. These are bringing water from his country and mixing it into the waters he consumes during his journey, taking clay from his home country and mixing it into the waters then letting it settle before drinking, as well as using something to filter the water for fear of worms or leech being in it. Finally, Ibn al-Amshāṭī recommends mixing sour robs into waters in general. The only author listing all of this advice is Ibn Sīnā. When comparing the two texts, there are some short concurrent sections but for the most part the same concepts are expressed differently by Ibn al-Amshāṭī, in addition to a brief explanation not present in Ibn Sīnā's text. This would mean that such reworking that Ibn Sīnā's text was at most only an inspiration for Ibn al-Amshāṭī.

Ibn al-Amshāṭī's method of compiling this chapter can be characterised by stressing that here he relies on the medical tradition on waters instead of relying on the travel regimens of his predecessors. However, as a scrutiny of the afterlife of the Hippocratic texts and concepts about the different waters in the Arabic-Islamic medical tradition seems to be a *desideratum*, pinpointing the exact state of this tradition Ibn al-Amshāṭī utilised, placing it in time and space, and connecting it to other physicians and texts with certainty are not possible.

2.9 *'Eighth Chapter on the Circumstances of the Traveller on the Sea'*

In the last chapter of the work before the epilogue, Ibn al-Amshāṭī explains how nausea and vomiting occur when travelling on sea. Dizziness and the sensation that everything is turning around someone who is therefore unable to stand firm are the result of the fine humours being stirred up by the movement of the ship. These humours therefore move in a way that is not natural for them, and the spirit tries to oppose it with a contrary natural movement. These two movements then result in a circular movement leading to nausea and vomiting. Vomiting then does not stop until it is so excessive that the stomach becomes depleted. A similar explanation cannot be found in any of the previous travel regimens; it is only Ibn al-Khaṭīb who explains dizziness, however, his explanation is an unlikely antecedent for Ibn al-Amshāṭī's exposition. This either goes back to another source or relies on Ibn al-Amshāṭī's own knowledge.

To prevent vomiting, Ibn al-Amshāṭī recommends consuming costive fruits such as quince, sour pomegranate, sour apple, minted syrups of these, or tamarind. These, taken separately or together, strengthen and empty the stomach while preventing excess materials from flowing to it. Drinking celery seeds and absinthe can calm nausea. Here, Ibn al-Amshāṭī explains that this is due to a characteristic of these materials. Another advice is consuming sour things which strengthen the cardia and prevent vapours rising to the brain, such as lentils with sour grapes and vinegar. The last preventive method is smelling sandalwood and Armenian bole soaked in rose water and vinegar, besides smearing white lead onto the inside of the nose in order to prevent both nausea and vomiting. This section builds on combining al-Majūsī's and Ibn Sīnā's preventive advice: Ibn al-Amshāṭī advises eating the fruits listed by Ibn Sīnā and consuming the drinks mentioned by al-Majūsī, then inserts an explanation not found in either of his sources. Then, Ibn al-Amshāṭī returns to Ibn Sīnā's text and repeats the drinks mentioned there, yet again including an explanation of his own on why exactly those drinks are beneficial. The cardia-strengthening foodstuffs come from Ibn Sīnā, the materials to sniff are, with some changes, from al-Majūsī, and the use of white lead is, again, from Ibn Sīnā. It is important to point out that this is another example of rearranging the source materials and mixing their parts in a way that was probably more logical to Ibn al-Amshāṭī, and besides the rearranging, he omitted certain practices (sucking on sour fruits, general dietary remarks, not looking at the water, and the issue of lice from al-Majūsī; bread cooled in odorous wine or cold water from Ibn Sīnā) and also provided his own insights via short theoretical explanations regarding certain materials. To better illustrate this process, the sources are compared side-by-side, with the differences in bold, the omissions in red, and the addenda in green.

al-Majūsī [M][104]/Ibn Sīnā [IS][105]		**Ibn al-Amshāṭī[106]**
[IS] *bi-an-**yatanāwala** min al-fākiha mithla al-safarjal wa-al-tuffāḥ wa-al-rummān* [M] *fa-l-yastaʿmil sharāb al-ḥiṣrim aw sharāb al-rummān **bi-al-naʿnaʿ** wa-sharāb al-tuffāḥ **wa**-al-tamr hindī*	[1]	***fa-l-tanāwal** min al-fākiha al-qābiḍa mithla al-safarjal wa-al-rummān al-muzz wa-al-tuffāḥ al-muzz aw sharāb al-ḥisrim aw sharāb al-rummān al-muzz **al-munaʿnaʿayn** aw sharāb al-tuffāh al-muzz **aw** al-tamr al-hindī*
–	[2]	[*explanation*]

104 Al-Majūsī, *Kāmil al-ṣināʿa*, II/83.
105 Ibn Sīnā, *al-Qānūn*, I/326.
106 Ibn al-Amshāṭī, *al-Isfār*, 144:7–14.

(*cont.*)

al-Majūsī [M]/Ibn Sīnā [IS]		Ibn al-Amshāṭī
[IS] *wa-idhā* ***shariba*** *bizr al-karafs manaʿa al-ghathayān an-yahīja bihi wa-****sakkanahu*** *idhā hāja wa-al-afsatīn* [*sic*] *ayḍan kadhālika*	[3]	*wa-****yashrab*** *ayḍan min bizr al-karafs li-annahu* ***yusakkinu*** *al-ghathayān ka-mā qīla* [*explanation*] *wa-kadhālika al-afsantīn*
[IS] (*wa-mimmā yamnaʿuhu*) *an yaghtadhī bi-al-ḥumūḍāt al-muqawwiya li-fam al-maʿida al-māniʿa min irtifāʿ al-bukhār ilā al-ra's,* ***wa-dhālika ka****-al-ʿadas bi-al-khall wa bi-al-ḥiṣrim wa-qalīl fūdanaj aw ḥāshā,* […]	[4]	*wa-an yaghtadhī bi-al-ḥumūḍāt al-muqawwiya li-fam al-maʿida wa-al-māniʿa min irtifāʿ al-bukhār ilā al-ra's* ***mithla*** *al-ʿadas bi-al-ḥiṣrim wa-al-khall wa-naḥwahu*
[M] *wa-****yashtamm*** *al-ṣandal wa-al-māward wa-al-ṭīn al-ḥarr* ***mablūlan*** *bi-al-khall aw bi-al-sharāb*		*wa-an* ***yashimma*** *al-ṣandal wa-al-ṭīn al-armanī* ***manqūʿayn*** *fī al-mā' al-ward wa-al-khall*
[IS] *wa-yajibu an yamsaḥa dākhil al-unf bi-al-isfīdāj*		*wa-an yamsaḥa unfahi min dākhil bi-al-isfīdhāj fa-innahu yamnaʿu min al-ghathayān wa-al-qay' bi-khāṣṣiyya fīhi*

To sum up Ibn al-Amshāṭī's method of compilation for this chapter, he starts with his own theoretical explanation, then uses his two sources, al-Majūsī and Ibn Sīnā, to compile a text for which he uses materials from both authors as well as omits from both texts, rearranges the material he chooses to keep, and includes short theoretical remarks in between.

The chapter ends with praising God and a *ṣalwala* for Muḥammad, his family, and his companions as a way to wrap up the eight chapters before moving on to the epilogue.

3 Epilogue: Simple and Compound Medicaments for Travellers

The epilogue (*khātima*) lists all the medicaments the traveller should bring along in two chapters (*faṣl*), one for simple medicaments and one for compound medicaments. Considering the fact that none of the travel regimens discussed in this book contain a list of simples or a mini-pharmacopoeia, I follow two different approaches to offer at least a preliminary study of this material.

First, resorting to simple statistical methods, I survey both the simples and the recipes in relation to one another as well as the previous eight chapters of the *Isfār*, in addition to some aspects of the recipes themselves.

Then, I attempt looking for the possible sources for Ibn al-Amshāṭī's recipes in al-Kūhīn al-ʿAṭṭār's *Minhāj al-dukkān*, Ibn al-Tilmīdh's *Aqrābādhīn*, and Ibn Sīnā's *Qānūn*.

In case of the first chapter of the epilogue on simple medicaments, I survey the simples mentioned in the eight chapters of the treatise as well as those listed in the recipes in the second chapter of the epilogue. The ratio of overlapping simples and those present only in one of the three sample groups ('main text', list of simples, ingredients of recipes) will be an indicator of the interrelatedness of and dialogue between these three parts of the treatise.

For the second chapter of the epilogue, I focus on the recipes themselves while sticking to simple statistics. Besides this method, I also note interesting features of this chapter.

At the end of this section, I present some additional observations regarding the whole of the epilogue and attempt a preliminary evaluation of it based on the data gathered throughout this statistical overview.

For ease of referencing, I refer to Ibn al-Amshāṭī's travel regimen in its edited form and its translation present in this book in the footnotes of this chapter as "Ibn al-Amshāṭī, *al-Isfār*, [page number(s)]:[line number(s)]." For specific recipes of the epilogue, I use their ID code supplied by me in both the Arabic text and the English translation.

3.1 *Statistical Overview*

In case of the first chapter of the epilogue on simple medicaments, I survey the simples mentioned in the eight chapters of the treatise as well as those listed in the recipes in the second chapter of the epilogue. The ratio of overlapping simples and those present only in one of the three sample groups ('main text', list of simples, ingredients of recipes) will be an indicator of the interrelatedness of and dialogue between these three parts of the treatise.

For the second chapter of the epilogue, I focus on the recipes themselves while sticking to simple statistics. Besides this method, I also note interesting features of this chapter.

At the end of this section, I present some additional observations regarding the whole of the epilogue and attempt a preliminary evaluation of it based on the data gathered throughout this statistical overview.

3.1.1 First Chapter of the Epilogue

In the epilogue's first chapter, Ibn al-Amshāṭī lists simple medicaments in two groups, hot and cold ones. In total, he lists 45 hot and 29 cold medicaments. The majority of these are plants and plant-based substances (~96 %), with only one mineral substance (tar) and two animal-based substances (honey and castoreum).

3.1.1.1 *The List of Simples and the 'Main Text'*

To compare the simple medicaments Ibn al-Amshāṭī mentions in the eight chapters of the *Isfār* with those he lists in the epilogue's first chapter, I collected the former in Table 2 (see in the Appendix). I marked each item Ibn al-Amshāṭī listed in the epilogue's first chapter by colouring them red if listed as hot or blue if listed as cold. I marked the items only in case of a perfect match with the exception of mucilage of psyllium seeds and purslane seeds, since the text confirms that the mucilages are cold just like the seeds.[107] To arrive at more precise results, I separated the simples into two groups: the first is foodstuffs, drinks, or their ingredients and the second is medicaments or their ingredients. The basis of this division is Ibn al-Amshāṭī's text, as I listed materials in the first category when he recommends them as foodstuffs or drinks and in the second category when he refers to them as medicaments, mostly for external, but sometimes for internal use.

Based on this comparison, it is stunning how low a percentage of foodstuffs and medicaments of the eight chapters of the *Isfār* are listed in the epilogue's first chapter. From a total of 65 foodstuffs, 21 is listed in the epilogue (~32 %) and from a total of 68 medicaments, 24 are listed in the epilogue (~35 %). If we are to take a look from the point of view of the epilogue's first chapter, 18 of the 45 hot simples (40 %) and 7 of the 29 cold simples (~21 %) appear in chapters 1–8, or in total 27 of the 74 simples (~36,5 %). Those not mentioned in the eight chapters of the *Isfār* are listed in Table 3 (see in the Appendix).

Even if we disregard the foodstuffs, recommending medicaments in the eight main chapters of the work of which only approximately one-third is included in the list of materials the traveller should bring with himself on a journey clearly indicates that the eight chapters and the epilogue are separate parts of the treatise. The main chapters fit into the general tradition of travel

107 Relying on Ibn al-Amshāṭī's list, flower of violet is cold but violet oil is hot. He lists pumpkin seeds as cold but pumpkinseed oil is not listed, therefore I wanted to avoid jumping to conclusions which are not specified in the text as well as asserting the qualities of not listed materials from other sources, as my focus here is an internal analysis.

regimens and the epilogue seems to be a practical addition to the text which does not reflect on the main text.

3.1.1.2 *The List of Simples and the Compound Medicaments*

To compare the simple medicaments of the first chapter of the epilogue to the ingredients of the recipes present in the second chapter of the epilogue, I list the simples and reference the recipes in which they appear in Table 4 (see in the Appendix). If the match is not perfect, it is noted in brackets and accounted for it when calculating percentages.

From the 45 hot simples, 24 are not mentioned as a recipe ingredient (~53%). 6 are not a perfect match (~13%); however, these might still be considered as matches due to the nature of these medicaments. 15 are perfect matches (~33%). This means that either approximately one-third or half of the hot simples appear as ingredients in recipes.

From the 29 cold simples, 10 are not mentioned as a recipe ingredient (~34,5%). 4 are not a perfect match (~13,8%); however, one of them in my opinion is still a match (watermelon seeds as peeled watermelon kernels) and therefore will be counted as such and the other three are not matches. 15 are perfect matches (~51,7%). This means that 16 of the cold simples appear as ingredients in recipes (~55,2%).

In total, either 31 or 37 of the simples listed in the first chapter of the *Isfār*'s epilogue appear as recipe ingredients in the second chapter of the epilogue (~41,9% and 50%, respectively). This ratio undoubtedly suggests that the simples and compounds of the epilogue are to be treated separately. This proposition is further supported by the fact that if we take a look from the point of view of the recipes themselves, there are an additional 94 ingredients not listed in the epilogue's first chapter with variations in some of them, putting their final number above 100. This is illustrated in Table 5 (see in the Appendix), which shows the ingredient list of the recipes of the second chapter of the epilogue, with the hot and cold single medicaments of the first chapter of the epilogue coloured red or blue, respectively.

3.1.1.3 *The List of Simples According to the Numbers*

Based on the data produced by comparing the list of simples to those mentioned in the eight chapters and the recipes of the *Isfār*, it is not an inventory of materials mentioned in the eight chapters of the book, and neither is it a kind of shopping list for the recipes of the second chapter of the epilogue. Moreover, there are some medicaments in it which do not appear anywhere else in the work, 24 from the 74 simples (~36,5%), listed in Table 6 (see in the Appendix).

Nevertheless, it can be a useful addition to the 'classical' travel regimen, that is the eight main chapters of the *Isfār*, as a list of 'what he [the traveller] should bring with him from the simple medicaments'[108] on the journey. This is due to the fact that the regimen itself generally mentions the characteristics of the afflictions or that of the medicaments to use (hot or cold), therefore it can function as a handy list of substitutes, even if the moistening or drying property of the medicaments is not disclosed in the list and the degree of hotness or coldness varies between the medicaments. In some cases, the regimen recommends warming or cooling remedies in general, or names a few and advises 'similar' medicaments; for both type of instructions, the list of simples can also be useful.

3.1.2 Second Chapter of the Epilogue

In the second chapter of the epilogue, Ibn al-Amshāṭī lists compound medicaments to use for certain ailments, organised according to the type of the medicaments. In total, he provides 57 recipes for his reader. In some cases, he also includes shorter or longer theoretical remarks, additional information, and instructions besides the recipes.

In addition to the recipes of the epilogue, Ibn al-Amshāṭī includes two more recipes in the treatise, namely a recipe for a thirst-quenching pastille[109] in his first chapter and a *qayrūṭī* [his own vocalisation], cerate, for fissures of the skin[110] in his sixth chapter. Since these were discussed with the chapters they are in, these two recipes are not counted and accounted for in this analysis of the epilogue.

3.1.2.1 *Forms or Types of Preparation*

The types of compound medicaments and the names of recipes are as follows. For ease of referencing them, I supplied each recipe with an ID code based on its type and number both in the Arabic text and the English translation and listed those here in addition to an approximate percentage of each type of medicament compared to the total of 56 recipes.

- syrups: 9 in total (~16%), SY1–9 (pure oxymel, honey oxymel, mint-infused pomegranate syrup, sour grape syrup, rose syrup, violet syrup, water lily syrup, borage syrup, sandalwood syrup),
- robs: 6 in total (~10,7%), R1–6 (robs of: sour apple, quince, sour grapes, pomegranate, lemon, barberry),

108 Ibn al-Amshāṭī, *al-Isfār*, 147:2–3.
109 Ibn al-Amshāṭī, *al-Isfār*, 124:10–14.
110 Ibn al-Amshāṭī, *al-Isfār*, 138:7–10.

- electuaries: 5 in total (~8,9%), E1–5 (triphala, electuary of purging cassia, quadruple theriac, electuary of ajowan, electuary for ripe phlegmatic cough),
- purgative pills: 4 in total (~7,1%), PP1–4 (pill for purification of the body, pill for purging black bile and phlegm, pill to make the breath pleasant, pill of kings against diarrhoea),
- suppositories: 2 in total (~3,6%), SU1–3 (suppository of violet, warm suppositories for cold colic, warming the back, and purging black bile),
- pastilles: 3 in total (~5,4%), PA1–3 (camphor pastille, aloeswood pastille, rose pastille),
- medicinal powders: 3 in total (~5,4%), MP1–3 (*muqliyāthā* powder, seed powder against burning urine, powder against incontinence of urine),
- collyriums and eye remedies: 3 in total (~5,4%), C1–3 (remedy for inflammation, collyrium for warmness and roughness of the eye and tears, antimony),
- oils: 13 in total (~23,2%), O1–13 (oils of: violet, rose, poppy, lettuce, pumpkin, iris, jasmine, lemon balm, castor bean, chamomile, cucumber, myrtle, quince),
- liniments and powders: 2 and 2 in total, respectively (~3,6% and ~3,6%), L1–2 and PO1–2 (liniment for tissue growth, basilicon liniment, soldering powder, drying powder),
- haemostatics: 2 in total (~3,6%), H1–2 (Cyprian vitriol, burnt alum),
- dentifrices: 2 in total (~3,6%), D1–2 (dentifrice for clearing the teeth, dentifrice for strengthening the gums and the teeth).

In pharmacopoeias, the "most common form" of arrangement is when "each chapter is devoted to a particular form of preparation".[111] The 'mini-pharmacopoeia' of the *Isfār* follows this common arrangement method.

3.1.2.2 *Some Statistics Based on the Recipes*

"A typical recipe would be composed of the following elements, not necessarily always in this order: The heading or title of the drug; its indications; the ingredients and their quantities; the manner of preparation; recommended dosage or application. Often the expression *mujarrab* (tried) or *nāfiʿ* (effective, beneficial) would appear at the end of the recipe, sometimes together with the pious hope of *in shāʾa allāh taʿālā*, 'God willing.'"[112]

In Table 7 (see in the Appendix), I noted whether a recipe contains (y) or lacks (n) most of these elements, namely the title, use, ingredients, quantit-

111 Chipman, *The world of pharmacy*, 13.
112 Chipman, *The world of pharmacy*, 13.

ies, preparation, and recommended dosage or application. A dash (–) marks quantities, preparation, and dosage for recipes H1–2, since those are, in fact, not actual recipes. A tilde (~) indicates when an element is not included in a recipe, only some information related to it. On two occasions, the affirmative y letter is in parentheses, as in these cases those elements are not in the actual recipe but rather in an explanation right before the recipe. From this examination, the following data can be gathered.

43 recipes have a title (~76,9%). Only 33 recipes include a description on what they are to be used for (~58,9%). Not counting recipes H1–2, 24 include quantities (either specific or nonspecific; ~44,4%) and one some guidelines for quantities. 49 contain more or less detailed instructions for preparation (~90,7%), again disregarding recipes H1–2 when calculating the percentages. As for dosage or application, without recipes H1–2, only 11 recipes provide some information (~20,4%) and 3 contain some guidelines (~5,6%).

None of the recipes is marked as tried (*mujarrab*) or effective (*nāfiʿ*). While at first this might make the recipe collection seem more theoretical than practical, in my opinion it indicates the exact opposite. As this 'mini-pharmacopoeia' is not an integral part of travel regimens but a unique addition to a regimen, Ibn al-Amshāṭī was completely free to choose whatever recipes he wished to include. Therefore, it is logical to assume that he would only choose recipes which he either knew and trusted (and this way all were tried or effective by default) or which seemed to be effective based on the recipes themselves.

When inspecting the ingredients of the recipes (see Table 5 in the Appendix), it is apparent that none of them give substitutes for certain ingredients.[113] Likewise, synonyms are not provided for any ingredient of the recipes.[114]

3.1.2.3 *Theory Mixed with Recipes*

Moving away from statistics and taking under scrutiny the recipes once more, it becomes apparent that in some cases, there are inserts in the text which pertain to medical theory and are not essential for the recipes at all.

We find such a theoretical explanation right at the beginning of the second chapter of the epilogue, where Ibn al-Amshāṭī states that the simple syrups which are plain as clear water are the best and then proceeds to explain why this is so. The next lengthy bit of additional information is in the recipe of the triphala electuary (E1), where we get an exposition on the benefits of honey.

---

113 The only variations in the recipes are as follows: either leaves or peels of citron (SY3, SY4); clarified butter or almond oil depending on the desired shelf-life (E1).

114 A synonym is given in the list of hot simples: *barsāwushān* is *kuzbarat al-biʾr*, maidenhair. See Ibn al-Amshāṭī, *al-Isfār*, 146:4 and 147:6.

Regarding suppositories, Ibn al-Amshāṭī gives some instructions on how to shape them according to the application.

In some other cases, where the preparation can be made in different ways or with different ratios of ingredients to better suit the needs of the patient, Ibn al-Amshāṭī is also a bit lengthier and notes this, such as in case of recipes SY1, SY2, E1. In case of oils, he offers two different methods of preparation and compares those, noting which method is more appropriate for what kinds of oils.

3.1.3 Additional Observations regarding the Epilogue

As shown throughout the analysis of the epilogue, the epilogue is a separate unit of the treatise, independent of the 'main body' of the travel regimen, meaning the first eight chapters of the *Isfār*. Moreover, the two chapters of the epilogue are also independent components of the epilogue. Nevertheless, the codicological evidence of the manuscripts of the *Isfār* and the existence of a similar epilogue at the end of another medical treatise, the *Taʾsīs al-itqān* of Ibn al-Amshāṭī leaves no doubt that the epilogue is an original part of the *Isfār*. Also, as has been mentioned, both the list of simples and the recipes are useful additions to the travel regimen. For the simples, the knowledge of their properties can help the reader or traveller when choosing a simple medicament to treat an affliction or alleviate certain symptoms, while for the recipes, more than half of them include what they are used for and almost all of them contain instructions for preparation.

The intended purpose of the epilogue, however, is still not clear. This 'mini-pharmacopoeia' is written by a physician for a layman, at least according to the dedication of the *Isfār*. Therefore, it is interesting to inspect what is included in such, albeit much longer texts which are written by physicians to physicians and by pharmacists to pharmacists, in order to arrive at a rough estimation of the epilogue's place on the spectrum between a theoretical or practical approach.

The epilogue is clearly a list of simples and a list of recipes. We do not find any additional information on why the simples might not suffice, how to gather, examine, or store the ingredients, what certain preparation methods mean exactly, nor is there a section on the weights and measures used in the recipes. Therefore, we lack sections typical of pharmacopoeias of medical encyclopaedias but also do not have at our disposal enough practical instruction to assume that a non-practitioner could necessarily prepare each and every recipe on his own, provided he has the ingredients and utensils needed. Assuming the knowledge of a pharmacist, however, the instructions can sometimes seem superfluous. Considering all these factors, it is a possibility that this epilogue could function as a checklist when a well-off layman travels with an entourage which includes a physician who could then rely on this epilogue besides his own knowledge when sourcing the simples or compounds from pharmacists on way stations. Bearing in mind the inclusion of theoretical bits in between the recipes, it is also possible that Ibn al-Amshāṭī illustrates and underlines the broadness of his knowledge by including pharmacological material at the end of his travel regimen, while also attempting to remain entertaining through educating with these theoretical snippets which break up the monotony of a recipe list, at least throughout the first half of the recipes.

While we will likely never know for sure the reasons Ibn al-Amshāṭī decided to include the epilogue, a list for a 'travel medicine kit' of simple drugs and compound remedies, in his travel regimen, it is the most significant innovation of the *Isfār* if we look at the whole of the medical tradition of medieval Arabic travel regimens. While it is true that al-Rāzī provides some recipes in his regimen in the *Manṣūrī* for specific afflictions, this singular example is rather partial and ad hoc compared to a dedicated epilogue. The epilogue of the *Isfār* is most definitely a novelty, one which provides material for many future analyses.

3.2 *Comparative Analysis*

Comparing the first eight chapters of Ibn al-Amshāṭī's *Isfār* to earlier examples of travel regimens shows quite clearly how the author used and engaged with his sources when compiling his treatise and how he expanded on them. However, a similar treatment of the epilogue of the *Isfār* is in a sense less straightforward, considering the fact that none of the texts in the corpus of travel regimens we are aware of contains a similar 'mini-pharmacopoeia'. Thus, the material to contrast the epilogue with seems to be, out of necessity, pharmacopoeias in general.

Ibn al-Amshāṭī's mini-pharmacopoeia is arranged according to the types of preparations following the most common form of arrangement. For comparing the particular order of the preparations to other standalone pharmacopoeias, Chipman's survey is especially informative.[115] Ibn al-Amshāṭī's order is syrups, robs, electuaries, purgative pills, suppositories, pastilles, medicinal powders, collyriums and eye remedies, oils, liniments and powders, haemostatics, and dentifrices. While the order of the types of preparations is not exactly the same as that in al-Kūhīn al-ʿAṭṭār's *Minhāj al-dukkān*, a manual for pharmacists, it is mostly similar when only the preparations mentioned by Ibn al-Amshāṭī are

115 Chipman, *The world of pharmacy*, 15–18.

investigated. Notably, Ibn al-Amshāṭī's order does not correspond at all with that of al-Majūsī and Ibn Sīnā, despite the fact that their texts were the main sources for Ibn al-Amshāṭī's travel regimen.

3.2.1 Al-Kūhīn al-ʿAṭṭār (d. after 658/1260): *Minhāj al-dukkān*

The similarity in arrangement with al-Kūhīn al-ʿAṭṭār's *Minhāj al-dukkān* prompts a closer study of its recipes as potential sources of Ibn al-Amshāṭī's collection of recipes. Although the *Minhāj al-dukkān*'s date and place of composition (658/1260, Cairo) make the work a quite early Mamluk work, Chipman shows its continuous popularity and use throughout the entire Mamluk era.[116]

Following Ibn al-Amshāṭī's order of preparations, syrups are the first to be examined. The most striking in this regard is how the two authors begin their discussion of these preparations. Al-Kūhīn al-ʿAṭṭār starts with a discussion of *julāb* and detailed instructions on its preparation, as it is the basis of all syrups (its ingredients are pure sugar, egg whites, and water).[117] In comparison, Ibn al-Amshāṭī never mentions the term *julāb*, moreover, he forms his introductory discussion of syrups in a way that leads to oxymels (syrups made from vinegar and sugar or honey) occupying the most distinguished place amongst the syrups he lists. While at first we might assume that using *julāb* as a basis of syrups was considered common knowledge and thus it was not mentioned by Ibn al-Amshāṭī, a closer look at his syrups reveals that he always instructs to add sugar to the liquids needed in each recipe and to apply the appropriate heat treatments but he never mentions egg whites separately. Moreover, when looking for possible parallels between the recipes of the two authors based on similar 'active ingredients', it seems there is none to be found. The only tempting option would be Ibn al-Amshāṭī's sandalwood syrup (SY9) and al-Kūhīn al-ʿAṭṭār white sandalwood syrup,[118] for the sole fact of requiring rasped *Maqāsīrī* sandalwood to be soaked for a while; which is to be discarded rather, due to the different uses, quantities, soaking materials, additional ingredients and preparation methods.

Moving forward, Ibn al-Amshāṭī's rose pastille (PA3) seems to be fundamentally the same as al-Kūhīn al-ʿAṭṭār's recipe for rose pastilles.[119] Although al-Kūhīn al-ʿAṭṭār lists more uses for the preparation, he also recommends it

---

116 Chipman, *The world of pharmacy*, 1–3.

117 Its ingredients are pure sugar, egg whites, and water; al-Kūhīn al-ʿAṭṭār, *Minhāj al-dukkān*, 6; Chipman, *The world of pharmacy*, 159–160.

118 Al-Kūhīn al-ʿAṭṭār, *Minhāj al-dukkān*, 14.

119 Al-Kūhīn al-ʿAṭṭār, *Minhāj al-dukkān*, 69.

for strengthening the stomach, just like Ibn al-Amshāṭī. For the ingredients, both authors list rose, liquorice, spikenard, and mastic. Ibn al-Amshāṭī calls for rob of liquorice, while al-Kūhīn al-ʿAṭṭār also lists chalk. As for the quantities, both authors call for 10 dirhams of rose but recommend different quantities from all the rest of the ingredients. After pulverising, the materials are to be kneaded into pastilles. Al-Kūhīn al-ʿAṭṭār calls for rose water to do this, unlike Ibn al-Amshāṭī, in whose recipe the liquorice rob likely makes up for the lack this ingredient. Altogether, it seems that these rose pastille recipes are slight variants of the same recipe.

Mention must be made of the various oil recipes of Ibn al-Amshāṭī and al-Kūhīn al-ʿAṭṭār. Ibn al-Amshāṭī describes two methods of preparation. The first is to boil the 'active ingredient' in water, clean the water which this way took the power of the indgredient, mix this into the kind of oil one wishes to use, then boil it once more to evaporate the water and thus leave the power of the 'active ingredient' in the oil. The second is to throw the fresh 'active ingredient' into the oil and then this is left in the sun, repeating this process some times so that the kernels [from the 'active ingredient'] collect the power and odour of the medicament, and when needed, the oil squeezed out from these kernels are used. The second method results in a weaker medicament but it is more appropriate for cold and moist oils, since it does not require additional heat treatments which might counteract the desired cooling and moistening effects of the end product. The general methods of preparation presented by al-Kūhīn al-ʿAṭṭār are quite different for flowers.[120] For oils of warm flowers, he recommends adding four *ūqiya*s of flowers to one *raṭl* of olive oil and leaving it in a glass vial in the sun for 40 days. For oils of cold flowers, he instructs to add four *ūqiya*s of flowers to one *raṭl* of sesame oil and leaving it in a glass vial in the sun for 20 days before straining and storing the finished product. To compare, Ibn al-Amshāṭī recommends repeating the process without providing his reader with precise timeframes, deems this method to result in a weaker end product, and altogether recommends it only for cool and moist oils. However, looking at al-Kūhīn al-ʿAṭṭār's instructions for oils of seeds and roots,[121] Ibn al-Amshāṭī's first method is identical to it, although of course worded differently and with more explanations on what happens during the process. Altogether, due to these methodological differences, there are no actual oil recipes by the two authors that would correspond to each other.

120 Al-Kūhīn al-ʿAṭṭār, *Minhāj al-dukkān*, 121.
121 Al-Kūhīn al-ʿAṭṭār, *Minhāj al-dukkān*, 122.

Even though it seems that for the preparation forms there are no similar recipes or similar marked methodological differences to point out, mention must also be made of two instances when al-Kūhīn al-ʿAṭṭār quotes recipes from Ibn al-Tilmīdh. The first of these is a medicinal powder for urine and the second is an eye remedy prepared from sour grapes,[122] both of which can be connected to certain recipes by Ibn al-Amshāṭī.

3.2.2 Ibn al-Tilmīdh (d. 560/1165): *al-Aqrābādhīn*

Combing through the pharmacopoeia of Ibn al-Tilmīdh based on Ibn al-Amshāṭī's order of preparations, we find two additional 'matches' besides the recipes quoted by al-Kūhīn al-ʿAṭṭār.

Ibn al-Tilmīdh's rose pastille against phlegmatic fevers and stomach pain calls for roses, spikenard, and liquorice rob kneaded with wine boiled down to one third to be formed into pastilles.[123] Ibn al-Amshāṭī's rose pastilles for strengthening the stomach is similarly made up of roses, spikenard, and liquorice rob, but we find mastic instead of the reduced wine. The ratio of the ingredients changes from 2:1:1: (not specified) to 10:2:1:1, making one wonder about the consistency of the end product. Regardless, the two recipes are still related in some way.

As for the powder against incontinence mentioned by al-Kūhīn al-ʿAṭṭār, Ibn al-Tilmīdh's ingredients are acorn, bark of frankincence(-tree), myrrh, and elecampane (*rāshin*) in equal parts pounded together, though for its usage, consuming wine boild down to one quarter and sumac is possible after taking the powder.[124] Although only the first two ingredients, namely acorn kernels and frankincense are a match in Ibn al-Amshāṭī's recipe (MP3), this is the only instance for urinary powders and uses of acorn that bear resemblance to Ibn al-Amshāṭī's recipe amongst those presented by al-Kūhīn al-ʿAṭṭār and Ibn al-Tilmīdh.

Ibn al-Tilmīdh provides recipes for a "smaller *iṭrīfal*" and a "larger *iṭrīfal*".[125] Taking a closer look at the former, the basic ingredients and their equal ratio together with the basic preparation menthods are the same as in Ibn al-Amshāṭī's triphala recipe (E1). It must be noted, however, that Ibn al-Tilmīdh provides a straightforward recipe while Ibn al-Amshāṭī presents a way more complex description laden with explanations and also offers some alternatives to meet the desired shelflife of the final product.

---

122 Al-Kūhīn al-ʿAṭṭār, *Minhāj al-dukkān*, 64 and 104, respectively.

123 Ibn al-Tilmīdh, *Dispensatory*, 56 (Arabic), 186 (English translation) (no. 25).

124 Ibn al-Tilmīdh, *Dispensatory*, 72, 203 (no. 81).

125 Ibn al-Tilmīdh, *Dispensatory*, 79, 211 (no. 106).

Lastly, Ibn al-Tilmīdh describes a coolant prepared by steeping tutty (a crude zinc-oxide) in filtered water of fresh unripe grapes for seven days.[126] Ibn al-Amshāṭī's collyrium for the warmness of the eye, the roughness of the eyelids, and tears is the same preparation with quite some extra steps, as he instructs to cook finely pulverised zinc oxide with juice squeezed from unripe sour grapes into a jam-like consistency, put it in the sun for a few days, clear it and cook it once more, and once dried out, pulverise it to colour the eyelids with it. Still, as the basic idea of the two recipes is the same. Supposedly, the method of preparation is not more involved in Ibn al-Amshāṭī's case just for the sake of complexity but hopefully due to it being more effective this way or for ease of storage.

3.2.3 Ibn Sīnā: *al-Qānūn fī al-ṭibb*

Considering the fact that Ibn Sīnā's travel regimen incorporated into the *Qānūn* is one of Ibn al-Amshāṭī's source for his regimen, one might expect to perhaps find more similarities between the recipes of the *Qānūn* and the *Isfār*. Unfortunately, this is not the case with only three related recipes to be found.

In case of the recipe of quadruple theriac, speaking of an exact match is not much of a stretch. Ibn al-Amshāṭī's recipe (E3) uses the same ingredients (but Meccan myrrh instead of simply myrrh) in the same quantities with the same preparation and dosage as Ibn Sīnā.[127] In this case, it is Ibn Sīnā who records two alternative ingredients and while Ibn al-Amshāṭī starts with the uses of the recipe, Ibn Sīnā mentions it at the end.

Ibn Sīnā's recipe for rose pastilles is also worthy of mention,[128] though it is the same as Ibn al-Tilmīdh's rose pastilles. It is only the relative measurments being changed to exact ones (still, the ratio remains the same), though Ibn Sīnā mentions that some physicians use liquorice rob instead of its roots and also to dry the pastilles in the shade, details left ouf from the recipes of both Ibn al-Tilmīdh and Ibn al-Amshāṭī.

The basilicon liniment of Ibn Sīnā[129] is also obviously related to Ibn al-Amshāṭī's recipe, as the latter calls for the same ingredients and preparation with one additional ingredient, galbanum.

It might be worth noting that some of Ibn Sīnā's syrups that we can find parallels for by Ibn al-Amshāṭī are prepared in a different manner (these are: minted pomegranate syrup, sour grape syrup, rose syrup, and the oxymels).

---

126 Ibn al-Tilmīdh, *Dispensatory*, 126, 260 (no. 255).

127 Ibn Sīnā, *al-Qānūn*, IV/265.

128 Ibn Sīnā, *al-Qānūn*, IV/375–376.

129 Ibn Sīnā, *al-Qānūn*, IV/416.

3.2.4 Further Questions regarding the Epilogue

Comparing Ibn al-Amshāṭī's 'mini-pharmacopoeia' with al-Kūhīn al-ʿAṭṭār's *Minhāj al-dukkān* based on the popularity of the latter throughout the Mamluk period and the structural similarity of the two, Ibn al-Tilmīdh's *Aqrābādhīn* due to the presence of similar recipes also quoted by al-Kūhīn al-ʿAṭṭār, as well as the relevant parts of Ibn Sīnā's *Qānūn* on account of it being one of the main sources for the rest of Ibn al-Amshāṭī's travel regimen does provide some results but all things considered, it results to more questions than it manages to answer.

The methodological differences between al-Kūhīn al-ʿAṭṭār and Ibn al-Amshāṭī regarding the preparation of certain types of medicaments might be one of the most disconcerting issue raised by this comparison. A possible solution would be that Ibn al-Amshāṭī relies on an alternate pharmacological school in the case of syrups and oils but this would presuppose the prevalence of multiple parallel 'schools' or 'traditions' of pharmacy existing side by side. Another explanation would be that by the late Mamluk period, the methodology of certain pharmacological preparations changed. Probing other late Mamluk sources (pharmacopoeias, shorter collections like Ibn al-Amshāṭī's, or even *ḥisba* manuals) might support or dismiss these or similar speculations. After all, it is also possible that these deviations are Ibn al-Amshāṭī's own.

Still, the low number of same or similar recipes in the three sources examined here also pose the question whether there is another pharmacological work that was popular and circulated in Ibn al-Amshāṭī's time. Even after seeing how much original material is found in the *Isfār*, one would expect more than 6 out of 56 recipes to have parallels in the works of Ibn Sīnā, Ibn al-Tilmīdh, or al-Kūhīn al-ʿAṭṭār. This is even more curious when considering that recipes with unique ingredients or names either lack parallels in these works or they are too different to be considered for comparison.

Concluding Remarks

The present book had two major undertakings, the first being a study of the travel regimens of the medieval Arabic medical tradition and the second being an edition, translation, and analysis of Ibn al-Amshāṭī's travel regimen entitled *al-Isfār ʿan ḥikam al-asfār*.

The discussion of medieval Arabic travel regimens presented in this book is preliminary due to the scope and limitations of my research in addition to the fact that the corpus of travel regimens even within these limitations is surely far from being final or definitive. Nevertheless, it provided some details worth further inquiry and consideration.

It seems quite curious that the classification of topics present in Qusṭā ibn Lūqā's regimen of the pilgrims, however well-articulated, has not had a distinct impact on other works of this genre. Additionally, later physicians did not copy al-Ṭabarī's regimen. Similarly, Ibn al-Jazzār's *Zād al-musāfir* does not seem to be an integral part of this tradition. While the latter not belonging to the genre of travel regimens despite its misleading title, and perhaps even more misleading title in its Latin translation, there is no such palpable explanation for Qusṭā's and al-Ṭabarī's case. It would be interesting to see whether the manuscript tradition of these regimens or some other reasons might offer a solution.

The relationship between the various specimens of travel regimens shows that the physicians in general engaged with other texts in a meaningful way. Some of them copied verbatim, while others reworked their sources more. Still, even those belonging to the former group provided some unique material or twists in their regimens. Thus, it seems that the tradition of travel regimens cannot, at any point in time, be dismissed as motionless and be accused of simply repeating what the predecessors had to say on the topic.

Looking for the sources of some of the material present in the various travel regimens as well as attempting to look at these sections as a part of the wider medical tradition reveals that there are additional topics lacking and deserving of closer studies, for example purging or the issue of waters. Such work can even be considered fitting the current research trends if we take a step back view it as necessary groundwork to uncover pieces of a puzzle from which a whole picture can emerge later on that in turn allows for broader observations and conclusions later on.

As for Ibn al-Amshāṭī, there are still some unanswered questions regarding his life or points in need of further evidence. Especially the fact that only one of his biographers mentions his chief physicianship is baffling. In case no fur-

 | DOI:10.1163/9789004708204_005

ther biographies or documents pertaining to this issue come to light, perhaps a prosopography of the Cairene chief physicians might come to our aid. Unfortunately, I am unaware of such works or studies.

Regardless, the life and career of Ibn al-Amshāṭī shows that he was not only a scholar of jurisprudence: his participation in *jihād*, some military campaigns also contributed to his religious or pious image, as this fact is recorded by his biographers.

Ibn al-Amshāṭī as physician also shows us that thinking of oneself rather as a physician than a jurisprudent is acceptable. He is still included in the biographies of the scholarly elite and this preference is not concealed either. His medical education shows that he not only sought knowledge in Cairo, his hometown, but also sojourned in Mecca to study, amongst other subjects, medicine. Although the biographers do not record which books he studied exactly, we can gather some authors and titles he was familiar with based on what he mentions in his works. (Not to mention, their meticulous analysis might also uncover additional anonymous sources.) These authors and titles are most likely indicative of the education and erudition of the physicians of this time.

How he engages with his source material in his travel regimen, the *Isfār*, is also surely indicative of the expectations of his time and not only a product of his personal whims. It is also interesting to note that even the same author throughout one work can employ distinctly different methods for dealing with the same sources. The fact that these sources turned out to be al-Majūsī's regimen in the *Kāmil al-ṣināʿa al-ṭibbiyya/Kitāb al-malakī* and Ibn Sīnā's regimen in the *Qānūn* might raise a further question. On account of Ibn al-Qifṭī's *Tārīkh al-ḥukamāʾ*, we find the remark that al-Majūsī's encyclopaedia was overshadowed by Ibn Sīnā's *Qānūn*. Using the two works to complement each other is, then, either a personal decision and preference of Ibn al-Amshāṭī or an indication that the possibility of this statement being in need of some refinement might be worth exploring.

The *Isfār* as a text within the corpus of travel regimens is apparently a comprehensive work. Taking inventory of the topics Ibn al-Amshāṭī discusses in it, only the treatment of the eyes and fatigue are omitted, not counting the unique topics; while there is no separate section with instructions for armies, elements of the content of these appear in Ibn al-Amshāṭī's regimen. Besides his two sources mentioned in the above paragraph, it is obvious that he also relied on the wider medical tradition when introducing new material into the corpus and when discussing topics already present in the corpus. Connected to this point are Ibn al-Amshāṭī's methods of compilation, already referred to in the above paragraph. The least attested of these is copying with minuscule variations made to fit the quoted parts into the new text. The most frequent method is a kind of dissection of the source text, with changes, omissions, and either practical or theoretical addenda which cannot be found elsewhere in the corpus. Additionally, there are examples of Ibn al-Amshāṭī carefully merging his two sources, also with omissions, changes, and addenda. Moreover, it is apparent that Ibn al-Amshāṭī paid more attention to theory, explanations, and elaborating certain ideas than any of his predecessors had. Only approximately one fourth of the text can be directly linked to specific passages of al-Majūsī's or Ibn Sīnā's travel regimen, meaning that a bit more than three fourths of the *Isfār*'s text is the work of Ibn al-Amshāṭī, or even more if we count the epilogue as well. Besides this 'ratio of originality', a complete inventory of all novel details of the *Isfār* would be quite lengthy; deserving special mention regarding originality and novelty is the fact that including a list of simple medicaments and recipes is a feature unparalleled in other travel regimens. This 'mini-pharmacopoeia' is especially promising for further studies in terms of its potential practical use. Even though it is quite unlikely that a chronicle would mention that the patron of the treatise indeed had a copy of the work with him in his patronage, perhaps some documents akin to Abraham Ben Yiju's luggage list or the prescriptions of the Cairo Geniza will indicate actual uses of this epilogue. Alternatively, even better, this 'mini-pharmacopoeia' will perhaps someday provide the key to understanding some details in other types of sources.

The fact that Ibn al-Amshāṭī's travel regimen was copied in 976/1568 and 1083/1672 based on its surviving manuscript copies not only illustrates the interest in this specific work but also underlines the fact that the tradition of Arabic-language travel regimens continues even after the temporal limits set in the beginning of the present book. Thus, expanding the temporal limits of the research would likely provide more results, especially if the linguistic scope could include Persian or Ottoman Turkish. In that case, Ibn al-Amshāṭī's *Isfār* would not end the list of texts in the corpus but could potentially serve as a source for the works of later authors.

Attempting to write a comprehensive history of travel regimens through an even longer period and numerous cultures and the languages in which they produced literature is likely an impossible undertaking as of now, considering that there is not much on the singular histories of travel regimens. The brief overview of previous scholarly literature pertaining to medieval Arabic travel regimens showed that there is such a material in the Graeco-Roman, Byzantine, and various medieval European medical traditions. Syriac, Persian, Sanskrit, and Hebrew are frequently mentioned languages in the history of Islamic, as in Islamicate medicine and so one has to wonder whether the medical traditions written in those languages also contain regimens or at least scattered instructions for travellers. It is my sincere hope that the present book illustrates that it can be worthwhile to start examining even limited parts of a single tradition looking for specimens of this literature. Once similar studies become available, it will be possible to truly compare these traditions and trace the life of certain ideas throughout time, space, and cultures.

Appendix

The following table lists the works contained in MS Cairo, Dār al-Kutub, majāmīʿ 210/16 based on the Khedivial Library's catalogue[1] and the Egyptian National Library's catalogue of its collections,[2] in addition to my observations when examining the codex. Only information related to dating is listed here. The names of authors, names of copyists, and titles follow the text of the catalogues.

TABLE 1 List of the contents of MS Cairo, Dār al-Kutub, majāmīʿ 210/16

No.; ff.	Field	Author	Title	Dating
1.; 1r–11v	*uṣūl al-fiqh*	ʿAlā al-Dīn al-Bukhārī, Muḥammad ibn Muḥammad ibn Muḥammad (d. 841/1437–1438)	*Risāla fī al-radd ʿalā Iʿtirāḍāt Saʿd al-Dīn al-Taftazānī fī al-Talwīḥ*	–
2.; 12v–22v	*ḥadīth*	al-Sakhāwī, Muḥammad ibn ʿAbd al-Raḥmān ibn Muḥammad (d. 902/1497)	*Risāla fi istishkāl al-jamʿ bayna duʿā al-Nabī li-Anas b. Mālik …*	–
3.; 23r–47v	*uṣūl al-fiqh*	Ibn Quṭlūbughā, Qāsim ibn Quṭlūbughā (d. 879/1474)	*Sharḥ ʿalā Mukhtaṣar al-Ḥalabī ʿalā Manār al-anwār fī uṣūl al-fiqh*	copyist: ʿAbd al-ʿAzīz ibn ʿAbd al-Raḥmān ibn Abī Bakr al-Ḥanafī date of copying: 18 Rajab 862/1 June 1458
4.; 48r–52v	*uṣūl al-fiqh*	Ẓahīr al-Dīn Abū al-ʿAlāʾ al-Qalānisī	*Iʿjāz al-munāẓirīn*	date of copying: 721/1321
5.; 53r–57v	*sharḥuhu / uṣūl al-fiqh*	–	*Ḥāshiya ʿalā Sharḥ Kitāb fī uṣūl al-fiqh*	–
6.; 58r–63v	*tawḥīd / ʿilm al-kalām*	–	*Risāla fī al-radd ʿalā man iʿtaraḍa ʿalā qawl al-Ghazālī …*	–

1 *Fihrist al-kutub al-ʿarabiyya*, VII–1/258–261.

2 The list of the entries in al-Halwaji, *Catalogue*, listed in order of the treatises: 1: II/493–494 (no. 748); 2: II/421–422 (no. 632); 3: III/270–271 (no. 395); 4: I/206–207 (no. 303); 5 [labelled as treatise number 6]: II/108 (no. 150); 6 [labelled as treatise number 7]: II/495 (no. 750); 7 and 8 [labelled as treatise number 8]: I/44–45 (no. 63); 9: I/466–467 (no. 692); 10: II/203 (no. 297); 11: IV/195–196 (no. 291); 12: III/281–282 (no. 411); 13: IV/356 (no. 527); 14: I/129 (no. 188); 15: III/376 (no. 546); 16: I/154 (no. 225).

 DOI:10.1163/9789004708204_006

TABLE 1 List of the contents of MS Cairo, Dār al-Kutub, majāmīʿ 210/16 (*cont.*)

No.; ff.	Field	Author	Title	Dating
7.; 64r–67v	*sāʾiruhu / muṣṭalaḥ al-ḥadīth, al-ijāzāt*	from: ʿAbd Allāh ibn Shihāb al-Dīn Aḥmad, known as Ibn Kathīr al-Ḥaḍramī al-Shāfiʿī al-Kindī to: Qāsim ibn Muḥammad ibn Qāsim al-Manūfī al-Azharī	*Ijāza*	with inscription from Ibn Kathīr at the end
8.; 68r–76r	*muṣṭalaḥ / muṣṭalaḥ al-ḥadīth, al-ijāzāt*	from: – to: –	*Ijāza*	dating: 7 Shaʿbān 843/13 January 1440
9.; 77r–103v	*ḥadīth / al-ḥadīth, al-siyar wa-al-tarājim*	Ibn Jamāʿa, Badr al-Dīn Muḥammad ibn Ibrāhīm ibn Saʿd Allāh al-Kinānī al-Ḥamawī (d. 733/1333)	(*Mukhtaṣar fī munāsabāt*) *Tarājim al-Bukhārī*	autograph
10.; 104r–138v	*ḥadīth*	Abū Isḥāq Ibrāhīm al-Nājī	(*Risāla fī al-kalām ʿalā aḥādīth faḍāʾil al-Qurʾān wa-*) *Khatm Ṣaḥīḥ al-Bukhārī*	–
11.; 139r–186v	*sharḥuhu / al-ḥadīth, al-zuhd wa-al-raqāʾiq*	al-Kharāʾiṭī, Abū Bakr Muḥammad ibn Jaʿfar ibn Muḥammad ibn Sahl al-Sāmirī (d. 326/939)	*Makārim al-akhlāq wa-maʿālīhā wa-maḥmūd ṭarāʾiqihā wa-marḍīhā*	copyist: Ibrāhīm ibn Muḥammad ibn al-Azhar date of copying: Rabīʿ I 607/August or September 1210 place of copying: Damascus
12.; 187r–204v	*adab / al-madāʾiḥ al-nabawiyya, al-shiʿr al-ʿarabī—dawāwīn wa-qaṣāʾid*	—(*baʿḍ fuḍalāʾ al-qarn al-tāsiʿ*)	*Sharḥ qaṣīdat Umm al-Qurā aw al-hamziyya*	date of composing: 870/1465 place of composing: Cairo
13.; 205r–242r	*ṭibb*	Ibn al-Kirmānī, Yaḥyā ibn Shams al-Dīn Muḥammad ibn Yūsuf al-Baghdādī (d. 833/1430)	*Mukhtaṣar khawāṣṣ Abī al-ʿAlāʾ ibn Zuhr*	date of composing: 8 Jumādā al-ākhar 833/4 March 1430
14.; 242v–244v	*sharḥuhu / al-ṭibb*	ʿAbd al-ʿAzīz ibn Aḥmad al-Damīrī (d. 694/1295)	*Urjūza fī al-ṭibb*	–
15.; 245r–253v	*sharḥuhu / al-ṭibb al-nabawī*	Abū al-Qāsim al-Nīsābūrī (d. 826/1423)	(*Risāla fī*) *al-ṭibb al-nabawī*	date of copying: 882/1477
16.; 254r–269v	*sharḥuhu / al-ṭibb*	—(*baʿḍ al-afāḍil*)	*al-Isfār ʿan ḥikam al-asfār*	–

Table 2 presents the simple medicaments mentioned by Ibn al-Amshāṭī in chapters 1–8 of the *Isfār*. They are separated according to the chapter in which they appear. Additionally, they are in two groups based on how Ibn al-Amshāṭī refers to them in his text: as a foodstuff, drink, or its ingredient or as a medicament or its ingredient. To compare them to the simple medicaments listed by Ibn al-Amshāṭī in the epilogue's first chapter, those listed as hot simples are coloured red, while those listed as cold simples are coloured blue; the items in black do not appear in the epilogue's first chapter. Only perfect matches are coloured, expect for mucilage of psyllium and purslane seeds, since here the text confirms that the mucilages are cold just like the seeds.

TABLE 2 Simple medicaments in the *Isfār*: chapters 1–8 and the epilogue's first chapter

Ch.	As foodstuff or its ingredient	As medicament or its ingredient
1	liver, fat of cattle, almond, almond oil, fatty tail of sheep, violet oil, wax, barley *sawīq*, sugar, vinegar, Indian watermelon, pumpkin, mung bean, sour grape, *dūgh*, mucilage of psyllium seeds, mucilage of purslane seeds, sour pomegranate juice, pumpkinseed oil, quince seeds, fish, cheese, fava beans	thirst-quenching pill (pumpkin seeds, Armenian cucumber seeds, purslane seeds, cornstarch, tragacanth, chalk, mucilage of psyllium seeds)
2	barley *sawīq*	rose oil, violet oil, vinegar
3	onion, *dūgh*, spinach, purslane, pumpkin, lettuce, milk, rose oil, limbs of young goats, sour grape juice, vinegar	rose oil, pumpkinseed oil, vinegar, sap of houseleek tree
4	garlic, walnut, mustard seed, assafetida, onion, pepper, cinnamon, long pepper, ginger	Egyptian willow oil, lily oil, olive oil, bay laurel oil, iris oil, castor oil, chamomile oil
5	–	Egyptian willow oil, iris oil, olive oil, pellitory, pepper, assafetida, jasmine oil, garlic, tar, gallnut, pomegranate peel, red anemones, basilicon liniment, honey, rapeseed, fig, cabbage, dill, chamomile, Armenian bole, vinegar, rose water, cabbage, beet, clarified butter, warm bandage (leaf of marshmallow, mallow, gooseberry, violet oil)
6	–	mucilage of psyllium seeds, mucilage of purslane seeds, tragacanth, gum, egg white, semolina pastry, *qayrūṭī* (sandalwood, rose, melilot, saffron, camphor, wax, rose oil), solid fat
7	vinegar, oxymel, carob, myrtle seeds, mucilage of psyllium seeds, quince, costive apple, ribes, rob of sour grape, rob of sour pomegranate	–
8	quince, sour pomegranate, sour apple, minted sour grape syrup, minted sour pomegranate syrup, sour apple syrup, tamarind, [juice of] celery seeds, lentils, sour grapes, vinegar	sandalwood, Armenian bole, rose water, vinegar, white lead

TABLE 3 Simple medicaments in the *Isfār*: simples of the epilogue's first chapter not mentioned in chapters 1–8

Hot simple medicaments:	Cold simple medicaments:
true cardamom, fragrant nutmeg, fennel, anise, caraway, liquorice, maidenhair, marjoram seeds, garden cress seeds, sesame oil, senna, mastic, rue, beaver testicle, scammony, turpeth, agaric, ajowan, jujube, manjack, borage, purging cassia, date, raisin, pistachio, aloe, bdellium	marshmallow seeds, mallow seeds, bladder dock seeds, lettuce seeds, basil seeds, watermelon seeds, tall marshmallow tree, Egyptian spinach seeds, endive seeds, flax dodder seeds, flower of violet, peach, cherry, barberry, quince seeds, chebulic myrobalan, yellow myrobalan, black myrobalan, Indian myrobalan, beleric myrobalan, amla, opium

The simple medicaments listed in Table 3 appear only in the epilogue's first chapter; they are not mentioned in chapters 1–8 of the *Isfār*.

Table 4 lists the hot and cold simple medicaments of the epilogue's first chapter and notes the recipes of the epilogue's second chapter in which each simple appears as an ingredient. If the match is only partial or not perfect, it is noted in parentheses.

TABLE 4 Simple medicaments in the *Isfār*'s epilogue as ingredients in the recipes

Hot simple medicament	Ingredient in recipe(s)
pepper	C3 (as white pepper)
long pepper	C3
cinnamon	PP3
ginger	PP1, PP2, SU2
true cardamom	–
fragrant nutmeg	PP3
assafetida	–
pellitory	–
fennel	E2 (seeds of)
anise	E2 (seeds of)
caraway	–
liquorice	E2 (rob of), PA3 (rob of), MP2 (rob of)
maidenhair	–

TABLE 4 Simple medicaments in the *Isfār*'s epilogue as ingredients in the recipes (*cont.*)

Hot simple medicament	Ingredient in recipe(s)
marjoram seeds	MP1
garden cress seeds	–
celery seeds	–
onion	–
garlic	–
tar	–
olive oil	SU2 (soap made of), O1–13, L1, L2
sesame oil	–
violet oil	–[O1 is its recipe]
senna	–
mastic	E2, PP1, PP4, PA2, PA3
dill	–
chamomile	O10
melilot	–
rue	–
beaver testicle	SU2
scammony	E2, PP2, PP4 (Antiochian), SU1, SU2
turpeth	E2, PP1, PP2, PP4, SU1, SU2
agaric	PP1, PP2, PP4
ajowan	–
jujube	–
manjack	–
borage	SY8
purging cassia	E2 (scales of, kernels of)
honey	SY2, E1, E2, E3, E4, E5
date	–
raisin	–
fig	–
carob	–
pistachio	SY3 (shell of)
aloe	–
bdellium	PP1, PP2
psyllium seeds	MP1
marshmallow seeds	–
mallow seeds	–
bladder dock seeds	MP1

TABLE 4 Simple medicaments in the *Isfār*'s epilogue as ingredients in the recipes (*cont.*)

Cold simple medicament	**Ingredient in recipe(s)**
lettuce seeds	PA1 (as lettuce), O4 (as lettuce)
purslane seeds	PA1 (as purslane), MP2
Armenian cucumber seeds	PA1 (as seeds of cucumber [?]), MP2 (as peeled cucumber kernel), O11 (as cucumber)
basil seeds	–
pumpkin seeds	MP2 (as pumpkin), O5 (as pumpkin)
watermelon seeds	MP2 (as peeled watermelon kernel)
tall marshmallow tree	–
Egyptian spinach seeds	–
endive seeds	PA1
flax dodder seeds	–
flower of violet	SY2, E2 (as Isfahanian violet), SU1, MP2 (syrup of), O1
peach	–
cherry	–
barberry	R6
quince seeds	R2, MP1 (rob of), O13 (as quince)
tamarind	SY9 (juice of)
chebulic myrobalan	E1
yellow myrobalan	E1, PP1, PP4, D2
black myrobalan	E1, PP4
Indian myrobalan	–
beleric myrobalan	E1, PO2 (peels of)
amla	E1
myrtle seeds	MP1, MP1 (rob of), O12
opium	–
vinegar	SY1, SY2, SY9

Table 5 summarises the ingredients of the recipes present in the epilogue's second chapter. If a specific version of an ingredient is mentioned, it is included in parentheses. Ingredients not written explicitly but referred to in the recipes are given in square brackets. Slashes separate ingredients when multiple recipes are accounted for in the same row of the table. The word 'or' indicates that the recipe itself offers variable ingredients based on the application of the medicament. The ingredients listed in the epilogue's first chapter as hot simples are coloured red, while those listed as cold simples are coloured blue; those in black are not listed in the epilogue's first chapter.

TABLE 5 The recipes of the *Isfār*: ingredient list

Recipe	Ingredients
SY1	vinegar, sugar (truly white and tender or red)
SY2	vinegar, honey
SY3	sour pomegranate, sugar, juice of mint, outer shell of pistachio, leaves or peel of citron
SY4	sour grape [, sugar, juice of mint, outer shell of pistachio, leaves or peel of citron]
SY5–8	[rose / violet / water lily / borage], sugar
SY9	Maqāsīrī sandalwood, vinegar, sour pomegranate juice, tamarind juice, sugar (solid white), chalk, powdered sandalwood, camphor, saffron
R1–6	sugar, juice of sour apple / quince / sour grapes / pomegranate / lemon / barberry
E1	chebulic myrobalan, beleric myrobalan, amla, yellow myrobalan, black myrobalan, clarified butter or almond oil, honey
E2	Isfahanian violet, turpeth, Indian salt, fennel seeds, anise seeds, mastic, liquorice rob, scammony, scales of purging cassia, purging cassia kernels, pulled taffy, honey
E3	Byzantine gentian, bay kernels, Meccan myrrh, long aristolochia, honey
E4	ajowan, honey
E5	flaxseed, honey
PP1	turpeth, yellow myrobalan, dodder, agaric, colocynth pulp, ginger, mastic, bdellium, tragacanth, rose (red)
PP2	turpeth, hiera picra, lavender, agaric, scammony, ginger, rose (red), bdellium
PP3	musk, clove, cinnamon, fragrant nutmeg, cyperus, spikenard, citron peel, apricot rob
PP4	turpeth, agaric, yellow [myrobalan], black myrobalan, wormwood, mastic, lemon balm, Antiochian scammony, saffron, chalk, rose (red), julep
SU1	violet, sugar (red), whey, scammony, turpeth, borax, Indian salt
SU2	soap made from olive oil, pulled taffy, honey, powdered salt, borax, turpeth, ginger, colocynth pulp, scammony, nigella, cumin, beaver testicles, opopanax, sagapenum
PA1	chalk, rose, white sandalwood, seeds of cucumber [?], endive seeds, lettuce, purslane, barley, camphor, apple juice

TABLE 5 The recipes of the *Isfār*: ingredient list (*cont.*)

Recipe	Ingredients
PA2	frankincense, rose, aloeswood, clove, musk, spikenard, Naysābūr clay, chalk, mastic, pomegranate seed stems
PA3	rose (red), liquorice rob, sweet-scented spikenard, mastic
MP1	psyllium seeds, marjoram seeds, white poppy seeds, bladder dock seeds, seeds of *qarfaḥ*, myrtle seeds, gum arabic, Armenian bole, quince rob or myrtle rob
MP2	peeled watermelon kernel, peeled cucumber kernel, pumpkin, purslane seeds, poppy, cornstarch, tragacanth, liquorice rob, henbane seeds, sugar, violet syrup or julep syrup
MP3	acorn kernels, frankincense, dry coriander, Armenian bole, gum Arabic
C1	cleaned hematite, burnt copper, coral, pearl, amber, red lead, gum Arabic, tragacanth, dragon's blood, saffron, rose water or sour grape juice
C2	zinc oxide, sour grape juice
C3	saffron, sweet-scented spikenard, long pepper, white pepper, ammonia, gallnuts, camphor
O1–13	[violet / rose / poppy / lettuce / pumpkin / iris / jasmine / lemon balm / castor bean / chamomile / cucumber / myrtle / quince,] olive oil
L1	litharge, olive oil, frankincense, anzerot, dragon's blood, galbanum, dry pitch
L2	pitch, resin, wax, galbanum
PO1	frankincense, anzerot, Meccan myrrh, dragon's blood
PO2	litharge, iris leaves, beleric myrobalan peels, gallnuts, pomegranate peel
H1–2	Cyprian vitriol / burnt alum
D1	burnt sea foam, seashell ashes, Persian sugarcane trunk ashes, smearwort
D2	burnt antler of red deer, burnt Andarānī salt, yellow myrobalan, rose, pomegranate flowers

Table 6 offers an overview of the simples of the epilogue's first chapter according to where they appear in the work. The hot simples are in red, while the cold simples are in blue.

Table 7 notes whether a recipe contains (y) or lacks (n) certain formal elements. A dash (–) marks elements for recipes H1–2 which are not actual recipes. A tilde (~) indicates that an element is only partially included in a recipe. The affirmative y letter is in parentheses when an element is not in the actual recipe but in an explanation right before the recipe.

TABLE 6 Simple medicaments in the *Isfār*: a summary of the simples in the epilogue's first chapter

Simples mentioned in both chapters 1–8 and the second chapter of the epilogue
pepper, long pepper, cinnamon, ginger, olive oil, chamomile, honey, psyllium seeds, purslane seeds, myrtle seeds, vinegar

Simples mentioned only in chapters 1–8
assafetida, pellitory, celery seeds, onion, garlic, tar, violet oil, dill, melilot, fig, carob, Armenian cucumber seeds, pumpkin seeds, tamarind

Simples mentioned only in the second chapter of the epilogue
fragrant nutmeg, fennel, anise, liquorice, marjoram seeds, mastic, beaver testicle, scammony, turpeth, agaric, ajowan, borage, purging cassia, pistachio, bdellium, bladder dock seeds, watermelon seeds, endive seeds, flower of violet, barberry, chebulic myrobalan, yellow myrobalan, black myrobalan, beleric myrobalan, amla

Simples listed only in the first chapter of the epilogue
true cardamom, caraway, maidenhair, garden cress seeds, sesame oil, senna, rue, jujube, manjack, date, raisin, aloe, marshmallow seeds, mallow seeds, lettuce seeds, basil seeds, tall marshmallow tree, Egyptian spinach seeds, flax dodder seeds, peach, cherry, quince seeds, Indian myrobalan, opium

TABLE 7 The recipes of the *Isfār*: an account of the elements of the recipes

Recipe	Title	Use	Ingredients	Quantities	Preparation	Dosage or application
SY1	y	y	y	y	y	n
SY2	y	y	y	~	n	n
SY3	y	y	y	n	y	~
SY4	y	y	y	n	y	~
SY5–8	y	n	y	n	y	n
SY9	y	y	y	y	y	n
R1–6	y	n	y	n	y	n
E1	y	y	y	y	y	n
E2	y	y	y	y	y	y
E3	y	y	y	y	y	y
E4	y	y	y	n	y	y

TABLE 7 The recipes of the *Isfār*: an account of the elements of the recipes (*cont.*)

Recipe	Title	Use	Ingredients	Quantities	Preparation	Dosage or application
E5	n	y	y	n	y	n
PP1	n	y	y	y	y	y
PP2	n	y	y	y	y	n
PP3	n	y	y	y	y	y
PP4	y	y	y	y	y	n
SU1	y	(y)	y	y	y	(y)
SU2	n	y	y	n	y	n
PA1	y	y	y	y	y	y
PA2	y	y	y	y	y	n
PA3	y	y	y	y	y	n
MP1	y	y	y	y	y	~
MP2	y	y	y	y	n	y
MP3	n	y	y	y	n	y
C1	y	y	y	y	y	n
C2	n	y	y	n	y	y
C3	y	y	y	y	y	y
O1–13	y	n	y	n	y	n
L1	n	y	y	y	y	n
L2	y	y	y	y	y	n
PO1	n	y	y	y	n	n
PO2	n	y	y	y	y	n
H1–2	n	y	y	–	–	–
D1	n	y	y	y	n	n
D2	n	y	y	y	n	n

Glossaries

1 Weights and Measures

The metric equivalents of the standard weights and measures used in the recipes vary according to the historical period and geographical location of the source text. In some cases, the amount signified by a measure is well documented in a certain period and location, while in other cases, only estimations are available.

The following approximate conversions follow the standard work of Walther Hinz, *Islamische Masse und Gewichte*.[1] The nonspecific measures used in the treatise are collected as well.

Specific weights:

raṭl	=	450 g	(= 12 ūqiya = 1/100 qinṭār)[2]
ūqiya	=	37,5 g	(= 1/12 raṭl)[3]
mithqāl	=	4,68 g[4]	
dirham	=	3,125 g	(= 2/3 mithqāl)[5]
dāniq	=	0,52 g or 0,78 g	(= 1/6 dirham or 1/6 dīnār-mithqāl)[6]
ṭassūj	=	0,195 g	(= 1/24 mithqāl)[7]
qīrāṭ	=	0,195 g	(= 1/24 mithqāl or 1/16 dirham)[8]

Nonspecific measures:

juzʾ (*ajzāʾ*)	part(s)
mithl (*amthāl*)	as much [e.g. *thalāthat amthālihi*, 'thrice as much']
miqdār	amount
sawīya	equal amount

1 Hinz, *Islamische Masse*.
2 Hinz, *Islamische Masse*, 28–29.
3 Hinz, *Islamische Masse*, 35.
4 Hinz, *Islamische Masse*, 4.
5 Hinz, *Islamische Masse*, 3.
6 Hinz, *Islamische Masse*, 11.
7 Hinz, *Islamische Masse*, 34.
8 Hinz, *Islamische Masse*, 27.

 | DOI:10.1163/9789004708204_007

2 *Materia medica*

For identification of the *materia medica* mentioned in Ibn al-Amshāṭī's *al-Isfār ʿan ḥikam al-asfār*, the following works were consulted. The basis of identification was Albert Dietrich's *Dioscurides triumphans*[9] whenever it was possible. The indices *The Dispensatory of Ibn at-Tilmīḏ*[10] and *Sābūr ibn Sahl's Dispensatory*,[11] both edited by Oliver Kahl, were also used. Additionally, two cookbooks, one from the 10th century, another from the 14th century, both edited by Nawal Nasrallah,[12] proved to be useful in many cases. Whenever additional literature was used for identification, it is included in a footnote.

The entries are arranged according to the Arabic names and they are separated into four categories, medicinal plants, medicinal substances of plant origins, medicinal substances of animal origin, and mineral substances.

2.1 *Medicinal Plants*

Scientific name	Common name	Transliteration	Arabic name
Citrus medica	citron	*utrujj*	أترّج
Pyrus sp.	pear	*ijjās*	إجاص
Prunus domestica	plum		
Myrtus communis	myrtle	*ās*	آس
Spinacia oleracea	spinach	*isfānākh*	اسفاناخ
Lavandula sp.	lavender	*usṭūkhūdūs*	أصطوخودوس
Cuscuta epithymum	dodder	*afitīmūn*	افتيمون
Artemisia absinthium	absinthe	*afsantīn*	افسنتين
Melilotus officinalis	melilot	*iklīl al-malik*	اكليل الملك
Phyllanthus emblica	amla	*amlaj*	أملج
Berberis vulgaris	barberry	*amīrbārīs*	أميرباريس
Pimpinella anisum	anise	*ānīsūn*	آنيسون
Chamaemelum nobile	chamomile	*bābūnaj*	بابونج
Melissa officinalis	lemon balm	*bādiranbūya*	بادرنبوية
Vicia faba	fava beans	*bāqillā*	باقلّاء

9 Dietrich, *Dioscurides triumphans*.
10 Ibn al-Tilmīdh, *Dispensatory*, 313–349.
11 Sābūr ibn Sahl, *Sābūr ibn Sahl's dispensatory*, 231–265.
12 Ibn Sayyār al-Warrāq, *Annals*; Nasrallah, *Treasure trove*.

(*cont.*)

Scientific name	Common name	Transliteration	Arabic name
Salix aegyptica	Egyptian willow	*bān*	بان
Adiantum capillus-veneris	maidenhair	*barshiyāwushān*	برشياوسان
Citrullus lanatus	watermelon	*biṭṭīkh*	بطّيخ
?	watermelon (?)	*biṭṭīkh ʿabdī*	بطّيخ عبدي
?	Indian watermelon	*biṭṭīkh hindī*	بطّيخ هندي
Allium cepa	onion	*baṣal*	بصل
Portulaca oleracea	purslane	*baqla ḥamqāʾ*	بقلة حمقاء
Melissa officinalis	lemon balm	*balasān*	بلسان
Terminalia bellirica	beleric myrobalan	*balīlaj*	بليلج
Hyoscyamus niger	henbane	*banj*	بنج
Viola odorata	violet	*banafsaj*	بنفسج
Operculina turpethum	turpeth	*turbad*	تربد
Malus pumila	apple	*tuffāḥ*	تفّاح
Tamarindus indica	tamarind	*tamr hindī*	تمر هندي
Ficus carica	fig	*tīn*	تين
Allium sativum	garlic	*thawm*	ثوم
Gentiana lutea	gentian	*janṭiyānā*	جنطيانا
Juglans regia	walnut	*jawz*	جوز
Myristica fragrans	fragrant nutmeg	*jawzbawā*	جوزبوا
Opopanax chironium	opopanax	*jāwshīr*	جاوشير
Ferula assa-foetida	assafetida	*ḥiltīt*	حلتيت
Rumex vesicarius	bladder dock	*ḥummāḍ*	حماض
Cicer arietinum	chickpea	*ḥummuṣ*	حمّص
Lawsonia inermis	henna	*ḥinnāʾ*	حنّاء[13]
Citrullus colocynthis	colocynth	*ḥanẓal*	حنظل
Aeonium arboretum	houseleek tree	*ḥayy al-ʿālam*	حي العالم
Malva sp.	mallow	*khubbāzī*	خبازي
Ceratonia siliqua	carob	*khurnūb*	خرنوب
Ricinus communis	castor bean	*khirwaʿ*	خروع
Lactuca sativa	lettuce	*khass*	خس
Papaver sp.	poppy	*khashkhāsh*	خشخاش
Althaea officinalis	marshmallow	*khaṭmī*	خطمي

13 It only appears once in the text of MS C, where M and T have خيار, cucumber.

(*cont.*)

Scientific name	Common name	Transliteration	Arabic name
Cucumis sativus	cucumber	*khiyār*	خيار
Cassia fistula	purging cassia	*khiyār shanbar*	خيار شنبر
Cinnamomum verum, Cinnamomum zeylanicum	cinnamon	*dār ṣīnī*	دار صيني
Piper longum	long pepper	*dār fulful*	دار فلفل
Foeniculum vulgare	fennel	*rāziyānj*	رازيانج
Lepidium sativum	garden cress	*rashād*	رشاد
Punica granatum	pomegranate	*rummān*	رمّان
Rheum ribes	ribes	*rībās*	ريباس
Ocimum basilicum	basil	*rayḥān*	ريحان
Aristolochia rotunda	smearwort	*zarāwand mudaḥraj*	زراوند مدحرج
Aristolochia longa	long aristolochia	*zarāwand ṭawīl*	زراوند طويل
Crocus sativus	saffron	*zaʿfarān*	زعفران
Lilium sp.	lily	*zanbaq*	زنبق
Zingiber officinale	ginger	*zanjabīl*	زنجبيل
Cordia sp.	manjack	*sabistān*	سبستان
Ruta graveolens	rue	*sadāb*	سداب
Cyperus rotundus	cyperus	*suʿd*	سعد
Cydonia oblonga	quince	*safarjal*	سفرجل
Convolvulus scammonia	scammony	*saqamūniyā*	سقمونيا
Ferula scowitziana DC. and var.	sagapenum	*sakbīnaj*	سكبينج
Brassica napus	rapeseed	*saljam*	سلجم
Beta vulgaris	beet	*silq*	سلق
Senna sp.	senna	*sanā*	سنا
Glycyrrhiza glabra	liquorice	*sūs*	سوس [14]
Iris sp.	iris	*sawsan*	سوسن
Anethum graveolens	dill	*shibithth*	شبّث
Hordeum sp.	barley	*shaʿīr*	شعير
Anemone coronaria	poppy anemone	*shaqāʾiq al-nuʿmān*	شقائق النعمان

14 It always appears as *duhn/rubb al-sūs*, 'oil/rob of liquorice'. Therefore, its interpretation as wormwood was rejected for this text and glossary.

(*cont.*)

Scientific name	Common name	Transliteration	Arabic name
Nigella sativa	nigella	*shūnīz*	شونيز
Aloe sp.	aloe	*ṣabir*	صبر
Santalum sp.	sandalwood	*ṣandal*	صندل
?	Maqāsīrī sandalwood	*ṣandal maqāṣīrī*	صندل مقاصيري
Anthemis pyrethrum	pellitory	*ʿāqir qarḥā*	عاقر قرحا
Glycyrrhiza glabra	liquorice	*ʿirq al-sūs*	عرق السوس
Ziziphus vulgaris	jujube	*ʿunnāb*	عنّاب
Ribes uva-crispa	gooseberry	*ʿinab al-thaʿlab*	عنب الثعلب
Laurus nobilis	bay laurel	*ghār*	غار
Polyporus officinalis	agaric	*ghārīqūn*	غاريقون
Pistacia vera	pistachio	*fustuq*	فستق
Piper nigrum	pepper	*fulful*	فلفل
Cucumis melo	Armenian cucumber	*qiththā'*	قثّاء
~ var. *flexuosus*	serpent melon		
Cucurbida sp.	pumpkin	*qarʿ*	قرع
Syzygium aromaticum	clove	*qaranful*	قرنفل
Saccharum sp.	sugarcane	*qaṣab*	قصب
Plantago sp.	psyllium	(*bizr*) *qaṭūnā*	(بزر) قطونا
Ferula galbaniflua	galbanum	*qinnā*	قنّا
Linum usitatissimum	flax	*kattān*	كتّان
Astragalus gummifer, Astragalus tragacantha	tragacanth	*kathīrā'*	كثيراء
Carum carvi	caraway	*karāwiyā*	كراويا
Alium graveolens	celery	*karafs*	كرفس
Crambe sp. *Brassica oleracea*	cabbage	*kurunb*	كرنب
Coriandrum sativum	coriander	*kuzbara*	كزبرة
Adiantum capillus-veneris	maidenhair fern	*kuzbarat al-bi'r*	كزبرة البئر
Cuscuta epilinum	flax dodder	*kashūth*	كشوث
Cuminum cyminum	cumin	*kammūn*	كمّون
Borago officinalis	borage	*lisān al-thawr*	لسان الثور
Citrus limon	lemon	*līmūn*	ليمون
Nymphaea sp.	water lily	*līnūfar*	لينوفر
Vigna radiata	mung bean	*māsh*	ماش
Commiphora myrrha	myrrh	*murr*	مرّ

(*cont.*)

Scientific name	Common name	Transliteration	Arabic name
Origanum majorana	marjoram	*marw*	مرو
Prunus armeniaca	apricot	*mishmish*	مشمش
Corchorus olitorius	Egyptian spinach	*mulūkhiyya*	ملوخية
Trachyspermum ammi	ajowan	*nānakhwāh*	نانخواه
Elettaria cardamomum	true cardamom	*hāl*	هال
Terminalia chebula	chebulic myrobalan	*halīlaj kābulī*	هليلج كابلى
Terminalia citrina Roxb.[15]	yellow myrobalan	*halīlaj aṣfar*	هليلج أصفر
[unripe fruit of] *Terminalia chebula*[16]	black myrobalan	*halīlaj aswad*	هليلج أسود
Terminalia horrida Stend.[17]	Indian myrobalan	*halīlaj hindī*	هليلج هندي
Cichorium endivia	endive	*hindabāʾ*	هندباء
Rosa sp.	rose	*ward*	ورد
Jasminum officinale	jasmine	*yāsamīn*	ياسمين

2.2 *Medicinal Substances of Plant Origin*

Common name	Transliteration	Arabic name
triphala	*iṭrīfal*	إطريفل
opium	*afyūn*	أفيون
anzerot	*anzarūt*	أنزروت
hiera picra	*iyāraj fīqrā*	إيارج فيقرا
acorn, oak nut	*ballūṭ*	بلوط
gum resin of opopanax (*Opopanax chironium*)	*jāwshīr*	جاوشير
rose water, julep	*julāb*	جلاب
flower of pomegranate	*jullanār*	جلنار
unripe and sour grapes	*ḥiṣrim*	حصرم
mustard seeds	*khardal*	خردل
vinegar	*khall*	خل

15 Shem Tov ben Isaac, *Sefer ha-Shimmush*, 184–185.
16 Dietrich, *Halīladj*, 349.
17 Shem Tov ben Isaac, *Sefer ha-Shimmush*, 186.

(*cont.*)

Common name	Transliteration	Arabic name
dragon's blood; red resin of the *Dracaena cinnabari* or the *Dracaena draco* tree; or the plant itself[18]	*dam al-akhawayn*	دم الأخوين
pine resin	*rātīnaj*	راتينج
raisin	*zabīb*	زبيب
pitch	*zift*	زفت
olive oil[19]	*zayt*	زيت
gum resin of sagapenum (*Ferula scowitziana* DC. and var.)	*sakbīnaj*	سكبينج
sugar	*sukkar*	سكّر
red sugar, produced from the first boiling of pressed sugarcane juice[20]	*sukkar aḥmar*	سكّر أحمر
solid white sugar	*sukkar ṭabarzad*	سكّر طبرزد
semolina	*samīd*	سميد
spikenard [oil]	*sunbul*	سنبل
sesame oil	*shīraj*	شيرج
gum	*ṣamgh*	صمغ
gum arabic	*ṣamgh ʿarabī*	صمغ عربي
chalk, obtained from certain bamboo stems[21]	*ṭabāshīr*	طباشير
lentil	*ʿadas*	عدس
gallnut	*ʿafṣ*	عفص
aloeswood	*ʿūd*	عود
pulled taffy, sugar-candy[22]	*fānīdh*	فانيذ
cherry	*qarāṣiyā*	قراصيا
cinnamon	*qirfa*	قرفة
sugarcane, 'Persian cane'	*qaṣab fārisī*	قصب فارسي
tar	*qaṭrān*	قطران
camphor	*kāfūr*	كافور

18 *Dracaena cinnabari* is endemic to Socotra, *Dracaena draco* is native to Morocco. For an analysis of the various sources of dragon's blood and their chemical constituents and uses, see Gupta et al., *Dragon's blood*.

19 See Ibn Sayyār al-Warrāq, *Annals*, 622; Nasrallah, *Treasure trove*, 504–505.

20 Sato, *Sugar*, 186, 188.

21 See Nasrallah, *Treasure trove*, 567.

22 On the preparation and different types of *fānīdh*, see Ibn Sayyār al-Warrāq, *Annals*, 596–597 and Nasrallah, *Treasure trove*, 482–483.

(*cont.*)

Common name	Transliteration	Arabic name
frankincense	*kundur*	كندر
amber	*kahrabāʾ*	كهرباء
almond	*lawz*	لوز
rose water	*māward*	ماورد
mastic	*maṣṭakāʾ*	مصطكاء
bdellium	*muql azraq*	مُقْل أزرق
date palm [translated as: date]	*nakhl*	نخل
cornstarch	*nashā*	نشا

2.3 *Medicinal Substances of Animal Origin*

Common name	Transliteration	Arabic name
fat tail of sheep[23]	*alya* (*alayāt*)	ألية (أليات)
coral[24]	*bussadh*	بسّذ
cattle [fat]	*baqar*	بقر
egg	*bayḍ*	بيض
cheese	*jubn*	جبن
young goat [meat]	*jady* (*jidāʾ*)	جدى (جداء)
castoreum	*jundbīdastar*	جندبيدستر
buttermilk	*dūgh*	دوغ
whey	? (in recipe S2)	رجبين (ماء اللبن)
sea foam[25]	*zabad al-baḥr*	زبد البحر
fish [meat]	*samak*	سمك
clarified butter[26]	*samn*	سمن
wax	*sahmʿ*	شمع
solid fat (tallow, suet)[27]	*shaḥm* (*shuḥūm*)	شحم (شحوم)

23 See Ibn Sayyār al-Warrāq, *Annals*, 621; Nasrallah, *Treasure trove*, 503.
24 I would like to thank Shahrzad Irannejad for this identification.
25 See Dietrich, *Dioscurides triumphans*, II/94–96, esp n. 3.
26 See Ibn Sayyār al-Warrāq, *Annals*, 622; Nasrallah, *Treasure trove*, 503.
27 See Ibn Sayyār al-Warrāq, *Annals*, 622; Nasrallah, *Treasure trove*, 503.

(*cont.*)

Common name	Transliteration	Arabic name
sea shell	*ṣadaf*	صدف
honey	*ʿasal*	عسل
antler of red deer (*Cervus elaphus*) stag[28]	*qarn ayyil/uyyal*	قرن أيل
liver	*kabid* (*kubūd*)	كبد (أكباد)
pearl	*luʾluʾ*	لؤلؤ
milk	*laban*	لبن
musk; gland secretion of the male musk deer	*misk*	مسك

2.4 *Mineral Substances*

Common name	Transliteration	Arabic name
antimony	*ithmid*	إثمد
lead	*usrub*	اسرب
red lead	*usrunj*	اسرنج
white lead	*isfīdhāj*	اسفيذاج
borax	*bawraq*	بورق
zinc oxide	*tūtiyā*	توتيا
Cyprian vitriol	*zāj qubruṣī*	زاج قبرصي
hematite	*shādanaj*	شادنج
alum	*shabb*	شب
clay	*ṭīn*	طين
Armenian bole	*ṭīn armanī*	طين ارمني
Naysābūr clay	*ṭīn al-akl*	طين الأكل
Lemnian earth[29]	*ṭīn makhtūm*	طين مختوم
kohl, antimony	*kuḥl*	كحل
litharge	*mardāsanj*	مرداسنج
salt	*milḥ*	ملح

28 Bellakhdar, *La pharmacopée marocaine traditionnelle*, II/1018.
29 Shem Tov ben Isaac, *Sefer ha-Shimmush*, 239–240.

(*cont.*)

Common name	Transliteration	Arabic name
Andarānī salt[30]	*milḥ andarānī*	ملح أندراني
Indian salt	*milḥ hindī*	ملح هندي
copper	*nuḥās*	نحاس
ammonia	*nūshādir*	نوشادر

3 Medico-Pharmaceutical Terms

The definitions of medico-pharmaceutical terms were taken from Chipman, *The World of Pharmacy*,[31] when it was possible. The quotations are marked with the * symbol and set in italics. General medico-pharmaceutical terms, the terms connected to the preparation of medicaments, and the terms referring to utensils are collected in their separate tables.

3.1 *Terms*

Common name (definition)	Transliteration	Arabic name
collyrium	*barūd*	برود
theriac (**a paste formerly used as an antidote to poison, esp. snake venom, made from as few as four, or as many as sixty or seventy, different drugs pulverized and mixed with honey*)	*tiryāq*	ترياق
pill (**a small pellet or tablet of medicine, taken by swallowing whole or by chewing*)	*ḥabb* (*ḥubūb*)	حَبّ (حبوب)
oil[32]	*duhn* (*adhān*)	دُهْن (أدهان)
powder	*dharūr* (*dharūrāt*)	ذِرور (ذرورات)
rob (**inspissated juice of ripe fruit, obtained by evaporation of the juice over a fire till it acquires the consistence of a syrup*)	*rubb* (*rubūb*)	رب (ربوب)

30 See Shem Tov ben Isaac, *Sefer ha-Shimmush*, 331.

31 Chipman, *The world of pharmacy*, 280–282.

32 See Ibn Sayyār al-Warrāq, *Annals*, 621; Nasrallah, *Treasure trove*, 503.

(*cont.*)

Common name (definition)	Transliteration	Arabic name
medicinal powder; catapasm (**a compound medicinal powder sprinkled externally*)	*safūf* (*safūfāt*)	سَفوف (سفوفات)
oxymel	*sikanjubīn*	سِكنجبين
dentifrice (**a substance for cleaning the teeth*)	*sanūn* (*sanūnāt*)	سَنون (سنونات)
syrup (**a concentrated sugar solution that contains medication or flavoring*)	*sharāb* (*ashriba*)	شَراب (أشربة)
dose, dosage	*sharba / shurba*	شَرْبَة / شُرْبَة
suppository; eye remedy	*shiyāf / ashyāf* (*shiyāfāt*)	شِياف / أشياف (شِيافات)
recipe	*ṣifa*	صِفة
pastille (**a small medicated or flavored tablet*)	*qurṣ* (*aqrāṣ*)	قُرص (أقراص)
qīrūṭī, cerate; from the Greek κηρωτή, a cream for wounds made of olive oil, wax and sometimes rose oil	*qayrūṭī* [as vocalised by Ibn al-Amshāṭī]	قيروطِي
collyrium (**a medical lotion applied to the eye*)	*kuḥl* (*akḥāl*)	كُحْل (أكحال)
mucilage	*luʿāb*	لِعاب
liniment (**a liquid or semifluid preparation that is applied to the skin as an anodyne or a counterirritant*)	*marham* (*marāhim*)	مَرْهم (مراهم)
electuary (**a pasty mass composed of a medicine, usually in powder form, mixed in a palatable medium, as syrup, honey, or other sweet substance*)	*maʿjūn* (*maʿājīn*)	مَعْجون (معاجين)
ratio	*nisba*	نسبة

3.2 *Preparation*

English term	Transliteration	Arabic term
to squeeze (out)	*iʿtaṣara*	إِعْتَصَرَ
to mix	*imtazaja*	إِمتزج
to file	*barada*	برد
to cook (like a jam)	*tarabbā*	تَرَبَّى

(*cont.*)

English term	Transliteration	Arabic term
to dissolve	*jāba*	جَاْبَ
embers	*jamr*	جَمْر
to mix	*jamaʿa*	جَمَعَ
to make into a pill	*ḥabbaba*	حَبَّبَ
to mix	*khalaṭa*	خَلَطَ
to ferment	*khamara*	خَمَرَ
to grind	*daqqa*	دَقَّ
to dissolve	*dhāba*	ذاب
to sprinkle	*dharra*	ذَرَّ
to boil down to	*rajaʿa ilā*	رَجَعَ إِلَى
foam	*raghwa*	رَغْوَة
to store	*rafaʿa*	رفع
to crush	*saḥaqa / tasaḥḥaqa*	سَحَقَ / تَسَحَّقَ
to pour	*ṣabba*	صَبَّ
to purify	*ṣaffā*	صَفَّى
to cook	*ṭabakha*	طَبَخَ
to knead	*ʿajana*	عَجَنَ
to wash; to clean	*ghasala*	غَسَلَ
to boil	*ghalā*	غَلَى
to make into pastilles	*qarraṣa*	قَرَّصَ
to roast	*qalā*	قَلَى
to knead	*latta*	لَتَّ
to sip	*maṣṣa*	مَصَّ
sieved	*mankhūl*	مَنْخُول
soaked (macerated)	*manqūʿ*	مَنْقُوع
to grow thin	*nakhala*	نَخَلَ
to sieve	*nakhala*	نَخَلَ
to soak	*naqaʿa*	نقع

3.3 *Utensils*

English term	Transliteration	Arabic term
kettle	*qidr*	قِدْر
soapstone pot	*qidr birām*	قِدْرِ بِرَام
rasp	*mibrad*	مِبرد

4 Medical Terms

English term	Transliteration	Arabic term
purging	*istifrāgh*	استفراغ
inhaling	*istinshāq*	استنشاق
diarrhea	*ishāl*	اسهال
cicatrization	*indimāl*	اندمال
black bile	*balgham*	بلغم
būlīmūs (bulimia)	*būlīmūs*	بوليموس
dissolution	*taḥlīl*	تحليل
fissure	*tashaqquq*	تشقّق
spasm	*tashannuj*	تشنّج
evaporisation	*taṣʿīd*	تصعيد
destillation	*taqṭīr*	تقطير
breathing	*tanaffus*	تنفّس
putrification	*tanqiya*	تنقية
scabies	*jarab*	جرب
external heat	*ḥarāra gharība*	حرارة غريبة
innate heat	*ḥarāra gharīziyya*	حرارة غريزية
bowels	*ḥashan (aḥshāʾ)*	حشا (أحشاء)
calculus, stone	*ḥaṣāt*	حصاة
itching	*ḥikka*	حكّة
fever	*ḥummā (ḥummayāt)*	حمّى (حمّيات)
hectic fever	*ḥummā al-diqq*	حمى الدقّ
putrid fever	*ḥummā ʿafīn*	حمى عفين
heated fever	*ḥummā al-musakhkhin*	حمى المسخّن
heartbeat	*khafaqān*	خفقان
humour	*khilṭ (akhlāṭ)*	خلط (أخلاط)

(*cont.*)

English term	Transliteration	Arabic term
fine humour	*khilṭ rafīq*	خلط رقيق
brain	*dimāgh*	دماغ
epiphora	*damʿa*	دمعة
worm	*dūd*	دود
fluids	*ruṭūbāt*	رطوبات
eye inflammation, ophthalmia	*ramad*	رمد
spirit	*rūḥ*	روح
burning winds	*riyāh multahiba*	رياح ملتهبة
abrasion	*saḥj*	سحج
sirsām; phrenitis, inflammation of (the meninges of) the brain caused by yellow bile[33]	*sirsām*	سرسام
cough	*suʿāl*	سعال
roughness in the eyelids (by reason of a corrosive matter which causes them to become red and occasions the falling off of the eyelashes and then the ulceration of the edges of the eyelids)	*sulāq*	سلاق
incontinence of urine	*salas*	سلس
samūm	*samūm*	سموم
black bile	*sawdāʾ*	سوداء
headache	*ṣūdāʿ*	صداع
temple	*ṣudgh*	صدغ
yellow bile	*ṣafrāwī*	صفراوي
bandage	*ḍimād*	ضماد
natural disposition	*ṭabʿ*	طبع
constitution	*ṭabīʿa*	طبيعة
limb	*ṭaraf* (*aṭrāf*)	طرف (أطراف)
symptom	*ʿaraḍ* (*aʿrāḍ*)	عرض (أعراض)
sap	*ʿuṣāra* (*ʿuṣārāt*)	عصارة (عصارات)
nerves	*ʿaṣab*	عصب
muscles	*ʿaḍal*	عضل

33 See Dols, *Majnūn*, 57–58.

(*cont.*)

English term	Transliteration	Arabic term
organ	*ʿuḍw (aʿḍāʾ)*	عضو (أعضاء)
putrid	*ʿafin*	عفن
leech	*ʿalaq*	علق
nausea	*ghathayān*	غثيان
nutritive substances	*ghidāʾiyya*	غذائية
gluing agent	*ghirawiyya*	غروية
decay	*fasād*	فساد
bloodletting	*faṣd*	فصد
cardia	*fam al-maʿida*	فم المعدة
costive	*qābiḍ*	قابض
ulcer	*qarḥ (qurūḥ)*	قرح (قروح)
heart	*qalb*	قلب
colic	*qūlanj*	قولنج
colon	*qūlūn*	قولون
strength	*quwwa*	قوة
vomiting	*qayʾ*	قيء
spasms	*kuzāz*	كزاز
cauterisation	*kayy*	كي
kernel	*lubb*	لب
complexion	*lawn*	لون
melancholia	*mālīkhūliyā*	ماليخوليا
drying agents	*mujaffifāt*	مجففات
disease	*maraḍ (amrāḍ)*	مرض (امراض)
warm (temperament)	*(al-mizāj) al-ḥārr*	(المزاج) الحار
moist (temperament)	*(al-mizāj) al-raṭb*	(المزاج) الرطب
dry (temperament)	*(al-mizāj) al-yābis*	(المزاج) اليابس
cold (temperament)	*(al-mizāj) al-bārid*	(المزاج) البارد
pores	*masāmm*	مسام
stomach	*maʿida (miʿad)*	معدة (معد)
intestines	*miʿāʾ (amʿāʾ)*	معاء (أمعاء)
rectum	*miʿāʾ mustaqīm*	معاء مستقيم
gripes	*maghṣ*	مغص
sciatica	*nasā*	نسا
digestion	*haḍm*	هضم
summer cholera	*hayḍa*	هيضة
swelling	*waram (awrām)*	ورم (أورام)

Bibliography

List of Manuscripts Consulted

MS Cairo, Dār al-Kutub, majāmīʿ 210/16

MS Dublin, Chester Beatty Library, Ar 4027

MS Istanbul, Millet Kütüphanesi, Feyzullah Efendi 848

MS Istanbul, Millet Kütüphanesi, Feyzullah Efendi 1319

MS Istanbul, Süleymaniye Kütüphanesi, Shahīd ʿAlī 2006

MS Mashhad, Āstān-e Qods-e Rażavī 6339

MS Mosul, Madrasat Yahyā Bāshā 175/9

MS Paris, Bibliothèque nationale de France, Arabe 3025

MS Princeton, Princeton University Library, Garrett 570H

MS Tarīm, Maktabat al-Aḥqāf, majmūʿat Āl Yaḥyā, 123 majāmīʿ (123/11)

Abbreviations

EI^2 *The Encyclopaedia of Islam, New Edition*, 12 vols. Ed. Hamilton A. Gibb et al. Leiden: E.J. Brill, 1960–2004.

EI^3 *The Encyclopaedia of Islam, Three*. Ed. Marc Gaborieau et al. Leiden: Brill, 2007–.

EIr *Encyclopædia Iranica*, vol. I–, London, 1982–.

GAL Brockelmann, Carl, *Geschichte der arabischen Litteratur*, 2 vols., Leiden–Boston: Brill, 2012 [originally published: Leiden: E.J. Brill, 1943].

GAL S Brockelmann, Carl, *Geschichte der arabischen Litteratur, Supplement*, 3 vols., Leiden–Boston: Brill, 2012 [originally published: Leiden: E.J. Brill, 1943].

GAS III Sezgin, Fuat, *Geschichte der arabischen Schrifttums*, vol. 3, Leiden: E.J. Brill, 1970.

LHOM *A Literary History of Medicine, The ʿUyūn al-anbāʾ fī ṭabaqāt al-aṭibbāʾ of Ibn Abī Uṣaybiʿah*, 5 vols., ed., transl. Emilie Savage-Smith—Simon Swain—Geert Jan van Gelder et al., Leiden: Brill, 2020. Open access: A Literary History of Medicine Online, https://scholarlyeditions.brill.com/lhom/ [The online version was consulted.]

Primary Sources

al-ʿAsqalānī, *al-Durar* = Ibn Ḥajar al-ʿAsqalānī, *al-Durar al-kāmina fī aʿyān al-miʾa al-thāmina*, 4 vols., Haydarabad: Dāʾirat al-Maʿārif al-ʿUthmāniyya, 1929–1931.

al-Baghdādī, *Hadiyyat* = al-Baghdādī, Ismāʿīl Bāshā, *Hadiyyat al-ʿārifīn, Asmāʾ al-muʾallifīn wa-āthār al-muṣannifīn*, 2 vols., Beirut: Dār Iḥyāʾ al-Turāth al-ʿArabī, n.d. [reprint of the 1955 Istanbul edition].

al-Baghdādī, *Īḍāḥ* = al-Baghdādī, Ismāʿīl Bāshā, *Īḍāḥ al-maknūn fī al-dhayl ʿalā Kashf al-ẓunūn ʿan asāmī al-kutub wa-al-funūn*, 2 vols., Beirut: Dār Iḥyāʾ al-Turāth al-ʿArabī, n.d.

al-Biqāʿī, *Iẓhār* = al-Biqāʿī, Ibrāhīm ibn ʿUmar, *Iẓhār al-ʿaṣr li-asrār ahl al-ʿaṣr*, 3 vols., ed., Riyadh, 1992–1993.

al-Biqāʿī, *ʿUnwān al-ʿunwān* = al-Biqāʿī, Ibrāhīm ibn ʿUmar, *ʿUnwān al-ʿunwān aw al-Muʿjam al-ṣaghīr*, 2nd ed., ed. Ḥasan Ḥabashī, Cairo: Dār al-Kutub wa-al-Wathāʾiq al-Qawmiyya, 2010.

al-Biqāʿī, *ʿUnwān al-zamān* = al-Biqāʿī, Ibrāhīm ibn ʿUmar, *ʿUnwān al-zamān bi-tarājim al-shuyūkh wa-al-aqrān*, 4 vols., ed. Ḥasan Ḥabashī, Cairo: Dār al-Kutub wa-al-Wathāʾiq al-Qawmiyya, 2001–2006.

Dietrich, *Dioscurides triumphans* = Dietrich, Albert, *Dioscurides triumphans, Ein anonymer arabischer Kommentar (Ende 12. Jahrh. n. Chr.) zur Materia medica, Arabischer Text nebst kommentierter deutscher Übersetzung*, 2 vols., Göttingen: Vandenhoeck & Ruprecht, 1988.

Gibb, *The travels of Ibn Baṭṭūṭa*, II = Gibb, Hamilton Alexander Rosskeen, *The travels of Ibn Baṭṭūṭa, A.D. 1325–1354, Translated with revisions and notes from the Arabic text edited by C. Defrémery and B.R. Sanguinetti*, vol. 2, Cambridge: Cambridge University Press, 1962.

Ḥājjī Bāshā, *Sihfāʾ al-aqsām* = Ḥājjī Bāshā, Jalāl al-Dīn al-Khiḍr al-Aydīnī, *Sihfāʾ al-aqsām wa-dawāʾ al-ālām, al-Maqāla al-ūlā: fī ʿilm al-ṭibb*, eds. Sayyida Ḥāmid ʿAbd al-ʿĀl—Mahā Maẓlūm Khiḍr, Cairo: Maṭbaʿat Dār al-Kutub wa-al-Wathāʾiq al-Qawmiyya, 2016.

Ḥājjī Khalīfa, *Kashf* = Ḥājjī Khalīfa, Muṣṭafā ibn ʿAbd Allāh, *Kashf al-ẓunūn ʿan asāmī al-kutub wa-al-funūn = Keşf-el-zunun, Birinci cilt Kâtib Çelebi*, 2 vols., eds. Şerefettin Yaltkaya—Kilisli Rifat Bilge, Istanbul: Milli Eğitim Basımevi, 1971–1972.

Ḥājjī Khalīfa, *Sullam* = Ḥājjī Khalīfa, Muṣṭafā ibn ʿAbd Allāh, *Sullam al-wuṣūl fī ṭabaqāt al-fuḥūl*, 6 vols., eds. Ṣāliḥ Saʿdāwī Ṣāliḥ—Akmal al-Dīn Iḥsān Oghlū—Muḥamad ʿAbd al-Qādir al-Arnāʾūṭ, Istanbul: Markaz al-Abḥāth li-l-Taʾrīkh wa-al-Funūn wa-al-Thaqāfa al-Islāmiyya, 2010.

Ibn al-Amshāṭī, *al-Qawl al-sadīd* = Ibn al-Amshāṭī, Maḥmūd ibn Aḥmad al-ʿAyntābī, *al-Qawl al-sadīd fī ikhtiyār al-imāʾ wa-al-ʿabīd*, ed. Muḥammad ʿĪsā Ṣāliḥiyya, Beirut: Muʾassasat al-Risāla, 1996.

Ibn al-Athīr, *al-Mathal al-sāʾir* = Ibn al-Athīr, Ḍiyāʾ al-Dīn Naṣr Allāh ibn Muḥammad, *al-Mathal al-sāʾir fī adab al-kātib wa-al-shāʿir*, 4 vols., eds. Aḥmad al-Ḥūfī—Badawī Ṭabāna, Cairo: Dār Nahḍat Miṣr, 1959–1965.

Ibn al-Jazzār, *Ibn al-Jazzār on sexual diseases* = Ibn al-Jazzār, Abū Jaʿfar Aḥmad ibn Abī

Khālid al-Qayrawānī, *Ibn al-Jazzār on sexual diseases and their treatment, A critical edition of Zād al-musāfir wa-qūt al-ḥāḍir, Provisions for the traveller and nourishment for the sedentary, Book 6*, ed., transl. Gerrit Bos, London–New York: Routledge, 2010 (first published in 1997).

Ibn al-Jazzār, *Ibn al-Jazzār's Zād al-musāfir* = Ibn al-Jazzār, Abū Jaʿfar Aḥmad ibn Abī Khālid al-Qayrawānī, *Ibn al-Jazzār's Zād al-musāfir wa-qūt al-ḥāḍir, Provisions for the traveller and nourishment for the sedentary, Book 7 (7–30)*, ed., transl. Gerrit Bos, Leiden–Boston: Brill, 2015.

Ibn al-Jazzār, *Ibn al-Jazzār's Zād al-musāfir I–II* = Ibn al-Jazzār, Abū Jaʿfar Aḥmad ibn Abī Khālid al-Qayrawānī, *Ibn al-Jazzār's Zād al-musāfir wa-qūt al-ḥāḍir, Provisions for the Traveller and Nourishment for the Sedentary, Books I and II: Diseases of the Head and the Face*, ed., transl. Gerrit Bos—Fabian Käs, Leiden–Boston: Brill, 2022.

Ibn al-Khaṭīb, *al-Wuṣūl* = Ibn al-Khaṭīb, Abū ʿAbd Allāh Lisān al-Dīn, *Libro del cuidado de la salud durante las estaciones del año o "Libro de la higiene" = Kitāb al-wuṣūl li-ḥifẓ al-ṣiḥḥa fī al-fuṣūl*, ed., transl. María de la Concepción Vázquez de Benito, Salamanca: Ediciones Universidad de Salamanca, 1984.

Ibn Mājah, *Sunan* = Ibn Mājah, Abū ʿAbd Allāh Muḥammad ibn Yazīd, *Sunan Ibn Mājah*, 4 vols., ed. Khalīl Ma'mūn Shīḥā, Beirut: Dār al-Maʿrifa, 1998.

Ibn al-Nadīm, *Fihrist* = Ibn al-Nadīm, Abū al-Faraj Muḥammad ibn Isḥāq, *Kitāb al-Fihrist*, 4 vols., ed. Ayman Fu'ād Sayyid, London: Al-Furqān Islamic Heritage Foundation, 2014.

Ibn al-Qifṭī, *Ta'rīkh al-ḥukamā'* = Ibn al-Qifṭī, Jamāl al-Dīn ʿAlī ibn Yūsuf, *Ta'rīkh al-ḥukamā'*, ed. Julius Lippert, Leipzig: Dieterich'sche Verlagsbuchhandlung, 1903.

Ibn al-Quff, *Jāmiʿ al-gharaḍ* = Ibn al-Quff, Amīn al-Dawla Abū al-Faraj ibn Muwaffaq al-Dīn Yaʿqūb ibn Isḥāq al-Malakī al-Masīḥī al-Karakī, *Jāmiʿ al-gharaḍ fī ḥifẓ al-ṣiḥḥa wa-dafʿ al-maraḍ*, ed. Sāmī Khalaf al-Ḥamārnah, ʿAmmān: Manshūrāt al-Jāmiʿa al-Urduniyya, 1989.

Ibn Sayyār al-Warrāq, *Annals* = Ibn Sayyār al-Warrāq, *Annals of the caliphs' kitchens, Ibn Sayyār al-Warrāq's tenth-century Baghdadi cookbook*, transl., introd. Nawal Nasrallah, Leiden–Boston: Brill, 2010.

Ibn Sīnā, *al-Qānūn* = Ibn Sīnā, Abū ʿAlī al-Ḥusayn ibn ʿAbd Allāh, *al-Qānūn fī al-ṭibb*, 4 vols., ed. Saʿīd Laḥḥām, Beirut: Dār al-Fikr, 1994.

Ibn Taghribirdī, *al-Manhal* = Ibn Taghribirdī, Jamāl al-Dīn Abū al-Maḥāsin Yūsuf, *al-Manhal al-ṣāfī wa-al-mustawfī baʿd al-wāfī*, 13 vols., eds. Muḥammad Muḥammad Amīn—Nabīl Muḥammad ʿAbd al-ʿAzīz, Cairo: Dār al-Kutub wa-al-Wathā'iq al-Qawmiyya, 1984–2009.

Ibn Taghribirdī, *al-Nujūm* = Ibn Taghribirdī, Jamāl al-Dīn Abū al-Maḥāsin Yūsuf, *al-Nujūm al-zāhira fī mulūk Miṣr wa-al-Qāhira*, 16 vols., eds. Fahīm Muḥammad Shaltūt et al., Cairo: al-Hay'a al-Miṣriyya al-ʿĀmma, 1963–1972.

Ibn al-Tilmīdh, *Dispensatory* = Ibn al-Tilmīdh, Hibat Allāh ibn Ṣaʿīd, *The dispensatory of Ibn at-Tilmīḏ, Arabic text, English translation, study and glossaries*, ed., transl. Oliver Kahl, Leiden–Boston: Brill, 2007.

al-Tirmidhī, *Sunan* = al-Tirmidhī, Muḥammad ibn ʿĪsā, *Sunan al-Tirmidhī, al-Musammā bi-Jāmiʿ al-Tirmidhī*, 3 vols., Cairo: Sharikat al-Quds, 2009.

Jones, *Hippocrates*, I = Jones, W.H.S. (transl.), *Hippocrates*, vol. I, Cambridge, MA–London: Harvard University Press, 1923.

Kaḥḥāla, *Muʿjam* (1957) = Kaḥḥāla, ʿUmar Riḍā, *Muʿjam al-muʾallifīn, Tarājim muṣannifī al-kutub al-ʿarabiyya*, 15 vols. in 7, Beirut: Dār Iḥyāʾ al-Turāth al-ʿArabī, 1957–1961.

Kaḥḥāla, *Muʿjam* (1993) = Kaḥḥāla, ʿUmar Riḍā, *Muʿjam al-muʾallifīn, Tarājim muṣannifī al-kutub al-ʿarabiyya*, 4 vols., Beirut: Muʾassasat al-Risāla, 1993.

al-Kūhīn al-ʿAṭṭār, *Minhāj al-dukkān* = al-Kūhīn al-ʿAṭṭār, Abū al-Munā Dāwud ibn Abī Naṣr al-Hārūnī al-Isrāʾīlī, *Minhāj al-dukkān wa-dustūr al-aʿyān fī aʿmāl wa-tarākīb al-adwiya al-nādiʿa li-l-insān*, Cairo: Dār al-Kitāb al-ʿArabiyya al-Kabirī, 1911.

al-Majūsī, *Kāmil al-ṣināʿa* = al-Majūsī, ʿAlī ibn al-ʿAbbās, *Kāmil al-ṣināʿa al-ṭibbiyya*, 2 vols., Būlāq, 1294/1877 (repr. Frankfurt am Main: Institute for the History of Arabic-Islamic Sciences at the Johann Wolfgang Goethe University, 1996).

Maimonides, *On the elucidation of some symptoms* = Maimonides, Moses, *On the elucidation of some symptoms and the response to them, (formerly known as On the causes of symptoms)*, ed., transl. Gerrit Bos, Leiden–Boston: Brill, 2019.

al-Malaṭī, *Nayl al-amal* = al-Malaṭī, ʿAbd al-Bāsiṭ ibn Khalīl, *Nayl al-amal fī dhayl al-duwal*, 9 vols., ed. ʿUmar Tadmurī, Sidon–Beirut: al-Maktaba al-ʿAṣriyya, 2002.

al-Maqrīzī, *Durar* = al-Maqrīzī, Taqī al-Dīn Aḥmad ibn ʿAlī, *Durar al-ʿuqūd al-farīda fī tarājim al-aʿyān al-mufīda*, 4 vols., ed. Maḥmūd al-Jalīlī, Beirut: Dār al-Gharb al-Islāmī, 2002.

al-Maqrīzī, *al-Khiṭaṭ* = al-Maqrīzī, Taqī al-Dīn Aḥmad ibn ʿAlī, *al-Mawāʿiẓ wa-al-iʿtibār fī dhikr al-khiṭaṭ wa-al-āthār*, 5 vols., ed. Ayman Fuʾād Sayyid, London: Al-Furqān Islamic Heritage Foundation Centre for the Study of Islamic Manuscripts, 2013.

Nasrallah, *Treasure trove* = Nasrallah, Nawal (transl., introd.), *Treasure trove of benefits and variety at the table, A fourteenth-century Egyptian cookbook*, Leiden–Boston: Brill, 2018.

al-Qalqashandī, *Ṣubḥ al-aʿshā* = al-Qalqashandī, Abū al-ʿAbbās Aḥmad, *Kitāb ṣubḥ al-aʿshā*, 14 vols., Cairo: Dār al-Kutub al-Khidīwiyya, 1913–1922.

Qusṭā ibn Lūqā, *Qusṭā ibn Lūqā's medical regime* = Qusṭā ibn Lūqā, al-Baʿlabakkī, *Qusṭā ibn Lūqā's medical regime for the pilgrims to Mecca, The Risāla fī tadbīr safar al-ḥajj*, ed., transl. Gerrit Bos, Leiden–New York–Köln: E.J. Brill, 1992.

Qusṭā ibn Lūqā, *Qusṭā ibn Lūqā on purgative drugs and purgation* = Qusṭā ibn Lūqā, al-Baʿlabakkī, *Qusṭā ibn Lūqā on purgative drugs and purgation, Kitāb Qusṭā ibn Lūqā fī l-Adwiya al-mushila wa-l-ʿilāǧ bi-l-ishāl*, ed., transl. Lena Ambjörn, Frankfurt am Main: Institute for the History of Arabic-Islamic Science at the Johann Wolfgang Goethe University, 2004.

Qusṭā ibn Lūqā, *Qusṭā ibn Lūqā on the preparation of purgative drugs* = Qusṭā ibn Lūqā, al-Baʿlabakkī, "Qusṭā ibn Lūqā on the preparation of purgative drugs, Edition, translation and commentary", ed., transl. Lena Ambjörn, *Zeitschrift für Geschichte der arabisch-islamischen Wissenschaften* 17 (2006/2007), 125–197.

al-Rāzī, *al-Manṣūrī* = al-Rāzī, Abū Bakr Muḥammad ibn Zakariyyāʾ, *al-Manṣūrī fī al-ṭibb*, ed. Ḥāzim al-Bakrī Ṣiddīqī, al-Kuwayt: Maʿhad al-Makhṭūṭāt al-ʿArabiyya, 1987.

al-Rāzī, *al-Ḥāwī* = al-Rāzī, Abū Bakr Muḥammad ibn Zakariyyāʾ, *al-Ḥāwī fī al-ṭibb*, ṭabʿa jadīda muṣaḥḥaḥa, 23 vols. in 7, ed. Haytham Khalīfa Ṭuʿaymī, Beirut: Dār Iḥyāʾ al-Turāth al-ʿArabī, 2002.

Sābūr ibn Sahl, *Sābūr ibn Sahl's dispensatory* = Sābūr ibn Sahl, *Sābūr ibn Sahl's dispensatory in the recension of the ʿAḍudī Hospital*, ed., transl. Oliver Kahl, Ledien–Boston: Brill, 2009.

al-Sakhāwī, *al-Ḍaw'* = al-Sakhāwī, Shams al-Dīn Muḥammad ibn ʿAbd al-Raḥmān, *al-Ḍawʾ al-lāmiʿ li-ahl al-qarn al-tāsiʿ*, 12 vols., Beirut: Dār al-Jīl, 1992.

al-Sakhāwī, *al-Dhayl* = al-Sakhāwī, Shams al-Dīn Muḥammad ibn ʿAbd al-Raḥmān, *al-Dhayl ʿalā Rafʿ al-iṣr aw Bughyat al-ʿulamāʾ wa-al-ruwāt*, eds. Jawdah Hilāl—Muḥammad Maḥmūd Ṣubḥ, Cairo: al-Dār al-Miṣriyya li-l-Taʾlīf wa-al-Tarjama, 1966.

al-Sakhāwī, *Wajīz al-kalām* = al-Sakhāwī, Shams al-Dīn Muḥammad ibn ʿAbd al-Raḥmān, *Wajīz al-kalām fī al-dhayl ʿalā Duwal al-islām*, 4 vols., eds. Bashshār ʿAwwād Maʿrūf—ʿIṣām Fāris al-Ḥarastānī—Aḥmad al-Khuṭaymī, Beirut: Muʾassasat al-Risāla, 1995.

al-Ṣayrafī, *Inbāʾ al-haṣr* = al-Ṣayrafī, ʿAlī ibn Dāwūd al-Jawharī, *Inbāʾ al-haṣr bi-abnāʾ al-ʿaṣr*, ed. Ḥasan Ḥabashī, Cairo: al-Hayʾa al-Miṣriyya al-Āmma li-l-Kitāb, 2002.

Shams al-Dīn, *al-Madhhab al-tarbawī* = Shams al-Dīn, ʿAbd al-Amīr, *al-Madhhab al-tarbawī ʿinda Ibn Sīnā, Min khilāl falsafatihi al-ʿamaliyya*, Beirut: al-Sharika al-ʿĀlamiyya li-l-Kitāb, 1988.

al-Shawkānī, *Badr* = al-Shawkānī, Muḥammad ibn ʿAlī, *al-Badr al-ṭāliʿ bi-mahāsin man baʿda al-qarn al-sābiʿ*, 2 vols., Cairo: Dār al-Kitāb al-Islāmī, n.d.

Shem Tov ben Isaac, *Sefer ha-Shimmush* = Shem Tov ben Isaac, of Tortosa, *Medical synonym lists from medieval Provence, Shem Tow ben Isaac of Tortosa, Sefer ha-Shimmush, Book 29, Part 1: Edition and commentary of List 1* (*Hebrew–Arabic–Romance/Latin*), ed., transl. Gerrit Bos—Martina Hussein—Guido Mensching—Frank Savelsberg, Leiden–Boston: Brill, 2011.

al-Suyūṭī, *Naẓm* = al-Suyūṭī, Jalāl al-Dīn ʿAbd al-Raḥmān ibn Abī Bakr, *Naẓm al-ʿiqyān fī aʿyān al-aʿyān*, ed. Philip Hitti, New York, NY: al-Maṭbaʿa al-Sūiryya al-Amrīkiyya, 1927.

al-Ṭabarī, *Firdaws al-ḥikma* = al-Ṭabarī, Abū al-Ḥasan ʿAlī ibn Sahl Rabban, *Firdaws al-ḥikma = Firdausu'l-Ḥikmat or Paradise of Wisdom of ʿAlī b. Rabban-al-Ṭabarī*, ed. Muḥammad Zubayr Ṣiddiqī, Berlin-Charlottenburg: Buch- u. Kunstdruckerei "Sonne" G.m.b.H., 1928.

al-Ṭabarī, *The polemical works* = al-Ṭabarī, Abū al-Ḥasan ʿAlī ibn Sahl Rabban, *The polemical works of ʿAlī al-Ṭabarī*, eds. Rifaat Ebied—David Thomas, Leiden–Boston: Brill, 2016.

al-Ṭabarī, *Health regimen* = al-Ṭabarī, Abū al-Ḥasan ʿAlī ibn Sahl Rabban, *ʿAlī ibn Sahl Rabban aṭ-Ṭabarī's Health regimen or "Book of the pearl", Arabic text, English translation, introduction and indices*, ed., transl. Oliver Kahl, Leiden–Boston: Brill, 2021.

al-Ziriklī, *al-Aʿlām* = al-Ziriklī al-Dimashqī, Khayr al-Dīn ibn Maḥmūd ibn Muḥammad ibn ʿAlī ibn Fāris, *al-Aʿlām, Qāmūs tarājim li-ashhur al-rijāl wa-al-nisāʾ min al-ʿarab wa-al-mustaʿribīn wa-al-mustashriqīn*, 16 vols., Beirut: Dār al-ʿIlm li-l-Malāyīn, 2002.

Catalogues

ʿAbd al-Bāsiṭ, *Fihris* = ʿAbd al-Bassāṭ, Aḥmad, *Fihris majāmīʿ al-maktabāt al-khāṣṣa bi-Dār al-Kutub al-Miṣriyya*, 8 vols., London: al-Furqān Islamic Heritage Foundation, 2015.

Arberry, *Cambridge* = Arberry, Arthur John, *A second supplementary hand-list of the Muhammadan manuscripts in the University & Colleges of Cambridge*, Cambridge: Cambridge University Press, 1952.

Arberry, *Chester Beatty* = Arberry, Arthur John, The Chester Beatty Library, A handlist of the Arabic manuscripts, 8 vols, Dublin: Emery Walker (vols. 1–2)—Hodges Figgis & Co (vols. 3–8), 1955–1966.

ʿArshī, *Catalogue* = ʿArshī, Imtiyāz ʿAlī, *Catalogue of the Arabic manuscripts in Raza Library, Rampur*, 6 vols., Rampur, UP: Raza Library Trust, 1963–1977.

al-ʿAydarūs, *Fihris* = al-ʿAydarūs, ʿAbd Allāh ibn Ḥusayn ibn Muḥammad—Ibn Shihāb, ʿAbd al-Qādir ibn Ṣāliḥ—al-Saqqāf, ʿAbd al-Raḥmān (eds.), *Fihris al-makhṭūṭāt al-Yamaniyya li-Maktabat al-Aḥqāf bi-muḥāfaẓat Ḥaḍramawt—al-Jumhūriyya al-Yamaniyya*, 3 vols., Qum–Tehran: Maktabat Samāḥat Āyat Allāh al-Marʿashī al-Najafī al-Kubrā, al-Khizāna al-ʿĀlamiyya li-l-Makhṭūṭāt al-Islāmiyya–Markaz al-Wathāʾiq wa-al-Taʾrīkh al-Diblūmāsī, Wizārat al-Khārijiyya bi-al-Jumhūriyya al-Islāmiyya al-Īrāniyya, 2009.

Biesterfeldt—Haddad, *Fihris* = Biesterfeldt, Hans Hinrich—Haddad, Farid Sami, *Fihris al-makhṭūṭāt al-ṭibbiyya al-ʿarabiyya fī maktabat al-duktūr Sāmī Ibnrāhīm Ḥaddād*, Aleppo: Aleppo University Press, 1984.

Dirāyatī, *Fihristagān* = Dirāyatī, Muṣṭafā (ed.), *Fihristagān-i nuskhahā-yi khaṭṭī-yi Īrān*, 34 vols, Tehran: Sāzmān-i Asnād wa Kitābkhāna-yi Millī-yi Jumhurī-yi Islāmī-yi Īrān, 2012.

Fihris Dār al-Kutub 1921 = *Fihris al-kutub al-ʿarabiyya al-mawjūda bi-al-Dār li-ghāyat sanat 1921, Wa-mulḥaq bi-al-kutub al-ʿarabiyya al-wārida li-l-Dār fī sanatay 1922 wa-1923 wa-al-sittat al-shuhūr al-ūlā min sanat 1924*, 9 vols, Cairo: Maṭbaʿat Dār al-Kutub al-Miṣriyya, 1342/1924.

Fihrist al-kutub al-ʿarabiyya = al-Qism al-ʿArabī bi-al-Kutubkhāna al-Khidīwiyya, *Fihrist al-kutub al-ʿarabiyya al-maḥfūẓa bi-al-Kutubkhāna al-Khidīwiyya al-Miṣriyya*, 7 vols., Egypt: s.n., 1888–1893.

al-Fihris al-tamhīdī = Maʿhad al-Makhṭūṭāt al-Muṣawwara, *al-Fihris al-tamhīdī li-l-makhṭūṭāt al-muṣawwara ḥattā awākhir shahr Uktūbar (Tishrīn al-Awwal) 1948*, Cairo: Jāmiʿat al-Duwal al-ʿArabiyya, 1948.

al-Halwaji, *Catalogue* = al-Halwaji, Abd al-Sattar (ed.), *Catalogue of Arabic Manuscripts in the Egyptian National Library (Dār al-Kutub al-Miṣriyyah), Collections (Majāmīʿ)*, 4 vols., Cairo–London: Egyptian National Library & Archives–Al-Furqān Islamic Heritage Foundation, 2011.

Hitti, *Garrett* = Hitti, Philip K.—Faris, Nabih Amin—ʿAbd al-Malik, Buṭrus, *Descriptive catalog of the Garrett Collection of Arabic manuscripts in the Princeton University Library*, Princeton, NJ: Princeton University Press, 1938.

İhsanoğlu, *Fihris* = İhsanoğlu, Ekmeleddin, *Fihris makhṭūṭāt al-ṭibb al-islāmī bi-al-lughāt al-ʿarabiyya wa-al-turkiyya wa-al-fārisiyya fī maktabāt Turkiyā = Catalogue of Islamic medical manuscripts (in Arabic, Turkish & Persian) in the libraries of Turkey*, Istanbul: IRCICA, 1984.

al-Jalabī, *Makhṭūṭāt* = al-Jalabī al-Mawṣilī, Dāwud, *Kitāb makhṭūṭāt al-Mawṣil, Wa-fīhi baḥth ʿan madārisihā al-dīniyya wa-madāris mulḥaqātihā*, Baghdad: Maṭbaʿat al-Furāt, 1927.

al-Khaṭṭābī, *Fahāris* = al-Khaṭṭābī, Muḥammad al-ʿArabī, *Fahāris al-Khizāna al-Malakiyya, al-Mujallad al-thānī, al-Ṭibb wa-al-ṣaydala wa-al-bayṭara wa-al-ḥayawān wa-al-nabāt*, Rabat, 1982.

al-Munajjid, *Maṣādir jadīda* = al-Munajjid, Ṣalāḥ al-Dīn, "Maṣādir jadīda ʿan taʾrīkh al-ṭibb ʿinda al-ʿarab", *Majallat Maʿhad al-Makhṭūṭāt al-ʿArabiyya* 5/2 (1959), 229–348.

Pertsch, *Die arabischen Handschriften* = Pertsch, Ludwig Karl Wilhelm, *Die arabischen Handschriften der herzoglichen Bibliothek zu Gotha*, 4 vols, Gotha: Friedr. Andr. Perthes, 1878–1883.

Qaṭāya, *Makhṭūṭāt al-ṭibb* = Qaṭāya, Salmān, *Makhṭūṭāt al-ṭibb wa-al-ṣaydala fī al-maktabāt al-ʿāmma bi-Ḥalab*, Aleppo: Jāmiʿat Ḥalab, aʿhad al-Turāth al-ʿIlmī al-ʿArabī, 1976.

Savage-Smith, *A new catalogue* = Savage-Smith, Emilie, *A new catalogue of Arabic manuscripts in the Bodleian Library, University of Oxford*, Volume 1: Medicine, Oxford: Oxford University Press, 2011.

Slane, *Catalogue* = Slane, William MacGuckin, baron de, *Catalogue des manuscrits arabes*, Paris: Imprimerie nationale, 1883–1895.

The contributions = *The contributions of the Arab and Islamic civilizations to medical sciences*, Cairo: Dār al-Kutub–UNESCO–CultNat, 2002.

Secondary Literature

ʿAbd al-Wahhāb, *Kitāb al-ʿumr* = ʿAbd al-Wahhāb, Ḥasan Ḥusnī, *Kitāb al-ʿumr fī al-muṣannafāt wa-al-muʾallifīn al-tūnīsiyyīn*, 2 vols., Beirut: Dār al-Gharb al-Islāmī, 1990.

Adamson, *Al-Rāzī* = Adamson, Peter, *Al-Rāzī*, New York, NY: Oxford University Press, 2021.

Aerts, *Imām (technical term)* = Aerts, Stijn, "Imām (technical term)", in EI^{3} 2020–4/pp.

Afsaruddin, *Garden* = Afsaruddin, Asma, "Garden", in Jane Dammen McAuliffe (ed.), *Encyclopaedia of the Qurʾān*, II, Leiden–Boston–Köln: Brill, 2002, 282–287.

Álvarez Millán, *Zuhr, Banū* = Álvarez Millán, Christina, "Zuhr, Banū", in EI^{3} 2019–2/145–153.

Arnaldez, *Ibn Rus̲h̲d* = Arnaldez, R., "Ibn Rus̲h̲d", in EI^{2} III/909–920.

Azar, *The sage of Seville* = Azar, Henry, *The sage of Seville, Ibn Zuhr, his time, and his medical legacy*, Cairo—New York, NY: The American University in Cairo Press, 2008.

Badawi—Abdel Haleem, هـ/م/ر *h–m–r* = Badawi, Elsaid M.—Abdel Haleem, Muhammad, "هـ/م/ر h–m–r", in Elsaid M. Badawi—Muhammad Abdel Haleem (eds.), *Dictionary of Qurʾanic Usage*; http://dx.doi.org/10.1163/1875-3922_dqu_SIM_001811 (last accessed 18 March 2021).

Badawi—Abdel Haleem, م/ح/و *m–ḥ–w* = Badawi, Elsaid M.—Abdel Haleem, Muhammad, "م/ح/و m–ḥ–w", in Elsaid M. Badawi—Muhammad Abdel Haleem (eds.), *Dictionary of Qurʾanic Usage*; http://dx.doi.org/10.1163/1875-3922_dqu_SIM_001583 (last accessed 18 March 2021).

Badawi—Abdel Haleem, ن/ج/و *n–j–w* = Badawi, Elsaid M.—Abdel Haleem, Muhammad, "ن/ج/و n–j–w", in Elsaid M. Badawi—Muhammad Abdel Haleem (eds.), *Dictionary of Qurʾanic Usage*; http://dx.doi.org/10.1163/1875-3922_dqu_SIM_001669 (last accessed 18 March 2021).

Badawi—Abdel Haleem, س/ف/ر *s–f–r* = Badawi, Elsaid M.—Abdel Haleem, Muhammad, "س/ف/ر s–f–r", in Elsaid M. Badawi—Muhammad Abdel Haleem (eds.), *Dictionary of Qurʾanic Usage*; http://dx.doi.org/10.1163/1875-3922_dqu_SIM_000821 (last accessed 18 March 2021).

Bauer, *Mamluk literature* = Bauer, Thomas, "Mamluk literature, Misunderstandings and new approaches", *Mamlūk Studies Review* 9/2 (2005), 105–132.

Behrens-Abouseif, *The book* = Behrens-Abouseif, Doris, *The book in Mamluk Egypt and Syria (1250–1517), Scribes, libraries and market*, Leiden–Boston: Brill, 2018.

Bellakhdar, *La pharmacopée marocaine traditionnelle* = Bellakhdar, Jamal, *La pharmacopée marocaine traditionelle, Médecine arabe ancienne et savoirs populaires*, 2 vols., Casablanca: Éditions Le Fennec, 2020.

Ben Abdesselem, *Sad̲j̲ʿ* = Ben Abdesselem, Afif, "Sadjʿ, 3. In Arabic literature of the Islamic period", in EI^{2} VIII/734–738.

Berkey, *The transmission* = Berkey, Jonathan Porter, *The transmission of knowledge in medieval Cairo, A social history of Islamic education*, Princeton, NJ: Princeton University Press, 1992.

Bonebakker, *Ibtidāʾ* = Bonebakker, S.A., "Ibtidāʾ", in EI² III/1006.

Borg, *Sajʿ* = Borg, Gert, "Sajʿ", in Kees Versteegh (ed.), *Encyclopedia of Arabic language and linguistics*, IV, Leiden–Boston: Brill, 2009, 103–106.

Borrmans, *Salvation* = Borrmans, Maurice, "Salvation", in Jane Dammen McAuliffe (ed.), *Encyclopaedia of the Qurʾān*, III, Leiden–Boston–Köln: Brill, 2004, 522–524.

Bosch-Vilá, *Ibn al-Khaṭīb* = Bosch-Vilá, Jacinto, "Ibn al-Khaṭīb", in EI² III/835–837.

Bosworth, *al-Ḳalḳashandī* = Bosworth, C.E., "al-Ḳalḳashandī", in EI² IV/509–511.

Bosworth—Latham, *al-Thughūr* = Bosworth, C.E.—Latham, J.D., "al-Thughūr", in EI² X/446–449.

Böwering, *God and his attributes* = Böwering, Gerhard, "God and his attributes", in Jane Dammen McAuliffe (ed.), *Encyclopaedia of the Qurʾān*, II, Leiden–Boston–Köln: Brill, 2002, 316–331.

Brain, Peter, *Galen on bloodletting, A study of the origins, development and validity of his opinions, with a translation of the three works*, Cambridge: Cambridge University Press, 1986.

Bray, *Literary approaches* = Bray, Julia, "Literary approaches to medieval and early modern Arabic biography", *Journal of the Royal Asiatic Society, Third Series*, 20/3 (2010), 237–253.

Brentjes, *Research foci* = Brentjes, Sonja, "Research foci in the history of ccience in past Islamicate societies", Histories 2/3 (2022), 270–287.

Brentjes, *The prison of categories* = Brentjes, Sonja, "The prison of categories—'Decline' and its company", in Felicitas Opwis—David Reisman (eds.), *Islamic Philosophy, Science, Culture, and Religion, Studies in Honor of Dimitri Gutas*, Leiden–Boston: Brill, 2012, 131–156.

Brinner, *Ibn Iyās* = Brinner, W.M., "Ibn Iyās", in EI² III/812–813.

Broadbridge, *Academic* rivalry = Broadbridge, Anne F., "Academic rivalry and the patronage system in fifteenth-century Egypt, Al-ʿAynī, al-Maqrīzī, and Ibn Ḥajar al-ʿAsqalānī", *Mamlūk Studies Review* 3 (1999), 85–107.

Browne, *Arabian medicine* = Browne, Edward Granville, *Arabian medicine*, Cambridge: Cambridge University Press, 1962.

Buck—Steffen, *History of the development of travel medicine* = Buck, Gabriela—Steffen, Robert, 'History of the development of travel medicine as a new discipline', in Annelies Wilder-Smith—Eli Schwartz—Marc Shaw (eds.), *Travel medicine, Tales behind the science*, Amsterdam: Elsevier, 2007, 7–12.

Chaumont, *ʿUmra* = Chaumont, "ʿUmra", in EI² X/864–866.

Chipman, *The world of pharmacy* = Chipman, Leigh, *The world of pharmacy and pharmacists in Mamlūk Cairo*, Leiden–Boston: Brill, 2010.

Csorba, *The genre of travel regimens* = Csorba, Zsuzsanna, *The genre of travel regimens in medieval Arabic medicine, With a critical edition and translation of Ibn al-Amshāṭī's al-Isfār ʿan ḥikam al-asfār*, PhD dissertation, Budapest: Eötvös Loránd University, 2021.

Dekkiche, *Crossing the line* = Dekkiche, Malika, "Crossing the line, Mamluk response to Qaramanid threat in the fifteenth century according to MS ar. 4440 (Paris, BnF)", *Bulletin of the School of Oriental and African Studies* 80/2 (2017), 253–281.

Dietrich, *Halīladj* = Dietrich, Albert, "Halīladj", in EI² XII/349–350.

Dietrich, *Ṣamgh* = Dietrich, Albert, "Ṣamgh", in EI² VIII/1042–1043.

Dols, *Majnūn* = Dols, Michael W., *Majnūn: the madman in medieval Islamic society*, Oxford: Clarendon Press, 1992.

Drory, *Models and contacts* = Drory, Rina, *Models and contacts, Arabic literature and its impact on medieval Jewish culture*, Leiden–Boston–Köln: Brill, 2000.

Ende, *Mudjāwir* = Ende, W., "Mudjāwir", in EI² VII/293–294.

Fancy, *Science and religion* = Fancy, Nahyan, *Science and religion in Mamluk Egypt, Ibn al-Nafīs, pulmonary transit and bodily resurrection*, London–New York, NY: Routledge, 2013.

Freimark, *Das Vorwort* = Freimark, Peter, *Das Vorwort als literarische Form in der arabischen Literatur*, PhD dissertation, Münster: Westfälische Wilhelms-Universität Münster, 1967.

Freimark, *Muḳaddima* = Freimark, Peter, "Muḳaddima", in EI² VII/495–496.

Frolov, *Classical Arabic verse* = Frolov, Dmitry, *Classical Arabic verse, History and theory of ʿarūḍ*, Leiden–Boston–Köln: Brill, 2000.

Fuess, *Rotting ships* = Fuess, Albrecht, "Rotting ships and razed harbors, The naval policy of the Mamluks", *Mamlūk Studies Review* 5 (2001) 45–71.

Gacek, *The Arabic manuscript tradition* = Gacek, Adam, *The Arabic manuscript tradition, A glossary of technical terms and bibliography*, Leiden–Boston–Köln: Brill, 2001.

Gaffney, *Load or burden* = Gaffney, Patrick D., "Load or burden", in Jane Dammen McAuliffe (ed.), *Encyclopaedia of the Qurʾān*, III, Leiden–Boston–Köln: Brill, 2004, 227–228.

Garrison, *Notes on the history of military medicine* = Garrison, Fielding H., *Notes on the history of military medicine*, Hildesheim–New York: Georg Olms Verlag, 1970.

Goudie, *Al-Biqāʿī's self-reflection* = Goudie, Kenneth, "Al-Biqāʿī's self-reflection, A preliminary study of the autobiographical in his *ʿUnwān al-zamān*", in Hugh Kennedy (ed.), *The historiography of Islamic Egypt (c. 950–1800)*, Leiden–Boston–Köln: Brill, 2001, 377–400.

Goudie, *How to make it in Cairo* = Goudie, Kenneth, "How to make it in Cairo, The early career of Burhān al-Dīn al-Biqāʿī", *Mamlūk Studies Review* 23 (2020), 203–230.

Gully, *The culture of letter-writing* = Gully, Adrian, *The culture of letter-writing in premodern Islamic society*, Edinburgh: Edinburgh University Press, 2008.

Guo, *Al-Biqāʿī's chronicle* = Guo, Li, "Al-Biqāʿī's chronicle, A fifteenth century learned man's reflection on his time and world", in Hugh Kennedy (ed.), *The historiography of Islamic Egypt* (*c. 950–1800*), Leiden–Boston–Köln: Brill, 2001, 121–148.

Guo, *Tales of a medieval Cairene harem* = Guo, Li, "Tales of a medieval Cairene harem, Domestic life in al-Biqāʿī's autobiographical chronicle", *Mamlūk Studies Review* 9 (2005), 101–121.

Gupta et al., *Dragon's blood* = Gupta, Deepika—Bleakley, Bruce—Gupta, Rajinder K., "Dragon's blood, Botany, chemistry and therapeutic uses", *Journal of Ethnopharmacology* 115 (2008), 361–380.

Gutas, *Avicenna* = Gutas, Dimitri, *Avicenna and the Aristotelian tradition, Introduction to reading Avicenna's philosophical works, Second, revised and enlarged edition, Including an inventory of Avicenna's authentic works*, Leiden–Boston: Brill, 2014.

Haddad, *An illustrated Arabic medical manuscript* = Haddad, Farid Sami, "An illustrated Arabic medical manuscript of the fifteenth century (Amshati's Mundjiz)", *Clio Medica: Acta Academiae Internationalis Historiae Medicinae* 18 (1983), 243–252.

Hamarneh, *Ibn al-Ḳuff* = Hamarneh, Sami Khalaf, "Ibn al-Ḳuff", in EI² XII/391.

Hamarneh, *Ibn Al-Quff's writings* = Hamarneh, Sami Khalaf, "Ibn Al-Quff's writings on hygienic regulations and the preservation of health", in Adnan Hadidi (ed.), *Studies in the history and archaeology of Jordan, I*, Amman: Department of Antiquities, 1982, 373–383.

Hawting, *Pilgrimage* = Hawting, Gerald, "Pilgrimage", in Jane Dammen McAuliffe (ed.), *Encyclopaedia of the Qurʾān*, IV, Leiden–Boston–Köln: Brill, 2004, 91–100.

Hermansen, *Talent* = Hermansen, Marcia, "Talent", in Jane Dammen McAuliffe (ed.), *Encyclopaedia of the Qurʾān*, V, Leiden–Boston–Köln: Brill, 2006, 191–192.

Hinz, *Islamische Masse* = Hinz, Walther, *Islamische Masse und Gewichte, Umgerechnet ins metrische System*, Leiden: E.J. Brill, 1955.

Hirschler, *The formation* = Hirschler, Konrad, "The formation of the civilian elite in the Syrian province, The case of Ayyubid and early Mamluk Ḥamāh", *Mamlūk Studies Review* 12/2 (2008), 95–132.

Hodgson, *The venture* = Hodgson, Marshall G.S., *The venture of Islam, Conscience and history in a world civilization*, 3 vols., Chicago, IL–London: The University of Chicago Press, 1974.

Holt, *al-Muʾayyad S͟hayk͟h* = Holt, P.M., "al-Muʾayyad S͟hayk͟h", in EI² VII/271–272.

Holt, *The age of the Crusades* = Holt, P.M., *The age of the Crusades, The Near East from the eleventh century to 1517*, London–New York, NY: Routledge, 2013.

Horden, *Regimen and travel* = Horden, Peregrine, 'Regimen and travel in the Mediterranean', in Renate Schkeiser—Ulrike Zellmann (eds.), *Mobility and travel in the Mediterranean from Antiquity to the Middle Ages*, Münster: Lit Verlag, 2004, 117–132.

Horden, *Travel sickness* = Horden, Peregrine, 'Travel sickness, Medicine and mobility in the Mediterranean from Antiquity to the Renaissance', in W.V. Harris (ed.), *Rethinking the Mediterranean*, Oxford: Oxford University Press, 2005, 179–199.

Humbert, *Papiers* = Humbert, G., "Papiers non filigranés utilisés au Proche-Orient jusqu'en 1450, Essai de typologie", *Journal Asiatique* 286/1 (1998), 1–54.

al-Jalabī, *Man huwa al-Qūṣūnī* = al-Jalabī al-Mawṣilī, Dāwud, "Man huwa al-Qūṣūnī, Le Qûsûny", *Lughat al-ʿArab* 8/3 (1930), 164–167.

al-Jalabī, *Maḥmūd al-ʿAntābī al-Amshāṭī* = al-Jalabī al-Mawṣilī, Dāwud, "Maḥmūd al-ʿAntābī al-Amshāṭī wa-Sarī al-Dīn bin al-Ṣāniʿ", *Lughat al-ʿArab* 8/4 (1930), 259–260.

Jouanna, *Water, health and disease* = Jouanna, Jacques, "Water, health and disease in the Hippocratic treatise *Aris, waters, places*", in Jacques Jouanna, *Greek medicine from Hippocrates to Galen, Selected papers*, Leiden–Boston: Brill, 2012, 155–172.

Kinberg, *Piety* = Kinberg, Leah, "Piety", in Jane Dammen McAuliffe (ed.), *Encyclopaedia of the Qurʾān*, III, Leiden–Boston–Köln: Brill, 2004, 90–91.

Kozarsky—Keystone, *Introduction* = Kozarsky, Phyllis E.—Keystone, Jay S., 'Introduction to travel medicine', in Jay S. Keystone et al. (eds.), *Travel medicine*, 4th ed., Edinburgh: Elsevier, 2019, 1–2.

Lambourn, *Abraham's luggage* = Lambourn, Elizabeth A., *Abraham's luggage, A social life of things in the medieval Indian Ocean world*, Cambridge: Cambridge University Press, 2018.

Löw, *Aramaeische Pflanzennamen* = Löw, Immanuel, *Aramaeische Pflanzennamen*, Leipzig: Wilhelm Engelmann, 1881.

Marmon, *al-ʿAynī, Badr al-Dīn* = Marmon, Shaun E., "al-ʿAynī, Badr al-Dīn", in EI³ 2014–3/45–47.

Martel-Thoumian, *Les civils* = Martel-Thoumian, Bernadette, *Les civils et l'administration dans l'état militaire mamlūk (IXe/XVe siècle)*, Damascus: Institut français de Damas, 1991.

Massoud, *The chronicles* = Massoud, Sami G., *The chronicles and annalistic sources of the early Mamluk Circassian period*, Leiden–Boston: Brill, 2007.

Meloy, *Ibn Fahd* = Meloy, John Lash, "Ibn Fahd", in EI³ 2017–2/127–130.

Meyerhof, *ʿAlî aṭ-Ṭabarî's "Paradise of Wisdom"* = Meyerhof, Max, "ʿAlî aṭ-Ṭabarî's "Paradise of Wisdom", one of the oldest Arabic compendiums of medicine", in Fuat Sezgin (ed.), *ʿAli ibn Rabban al-Ṭabarī (d.c.250/864), Texts and studies*, Frankfurt am Main: Institute for the History of Arabic-Islamic Science at the Johann Wolfgang Goethe University, 1996, 90–138.

Meyerhof, *Thirty-three clinical observations* = Meyerhof, Max, "Thirty-three clinical observations by Rhazes (circa 900 A.D.)", in Fuat Sezgin (ed.), *Muḥammad ibn Zakarīyāʾ al-Rāzī (d. 313/925), Texts and studies, vol. III*, Frankfurt am Main: Institute for the History of Arabic-Islamic Science at the Johann Wolfgang Goethe University, 1996, 1–52.

Micheau, *ʿAlī b. al-ʿAbbās al-Majūsī* = Micheau, Françoise, "ʿAlī b. al-ʿAbbās al-Majūsī", in EI[3] 2009–2/76–77.

Netton, *Riḥla* = Netton, I.R., *'Riḥla'*, in EI[2] VIII/528.

Northrup, *From slave to sultan* = Northrup, Linda, *From slave to sultan, The career of al-Manṣūr Qalāwūn and the consolidation of Mamluk rule in Egypt and Syria, 678–689 A.H./1279–1290 A.D.*, Stuttgart: Franz Steiner Verlag, 1998.

Olsson, *Design, determinism and salvation* = Olsson, Joshua Thomas, *Design, determinism and salvation in the Firdaws al-Ḥikma of ʿAlī Ibn Rabban al-Ṭabarī*, PhD dissertation, Cambridge: University of Cambridge, 2015.

Orfali, *The art of the muqaddima* = Orfali, Bilal, "The art of the muqaddima in the works of Abū Manṣūr al-Thaʿālibī (d. 429/1039)", in Lale Behzadi—Waḥīd Bihmardī (eds.), *The weaving of word, Approaches to classical Arabic prose*, Beirut–Würzburg: Orient-Institut Beirut–Ergon in Kommission, 2009, 181–202.

Peterson, *Forgiveness* = Peterson, Daniel C., "Forgiveness", in Jane Dammen McAuliffe (ed.), *Encyclopaedia of the Qurʾān*, II, Leiden–Boston–Köln: Brill, 2002, 224–225.

Petry, *The civilian elite* = Petry, Carl F., *The civilian elite of Cairo in the later middle ages*, Princeton, NJ: Princeton University Press, 1981.

Popper, *Abu 'l-Maḥāsin* = Popper, "Abu 'l-Maḥāsin Djamāl al-Dīn Yūsuf b. Taghrībirdī", in EI[2] I/138.

Pormann, *Review of Ibn al-Jazzār on fevers* = Pormann, Peter E., [Review of] "Ibn al-Jazzār on Fevers. A critical edition of the *Zād al-musāfir wa-qūt al-ḥāḍir*—Provisions for the Traveller and Nourishment for the sedentary, Book 7. By Gerrit Bos, Chapters 1–6. The original Arabic text with an English translation, introduction and commentary pp. 413 (Sir Henry Wellcome Asian Series), London and New York, Kegan Paul International, 2000", *Journal of the Royal Asiatic Society* 11/1 (2001), 65–69.

Pormann—Savage-Smith, *Medieval Islamic medicine* = Pormann, Peter E.—Savage-Smith, Emilie, *Medieval Islamic medicine*, Cairo: The American University in Cairo Press, 2007.

Ranking, *The life and works of Rhazes* = Ranking, George Spiers A., "The life and works of Rhazes (Abū Bakr Muḥammad bin Zakarīya ar-Rāzī)", in Fuat Sezgin (ed.), *Muḥammad ibn Zakarīyāʾ al-Rāzī (d. 313/925), Texts and studies, vol. II*, Frankfurt am Main: Institute for the History of Arabic-Islamic Science at the Johann Wolfgang Goethe University, 1996, 73–104.

Reisman, *A holograph MS* = Reisman, David C., "A holograph MS of Ibn Qāḍī Shuhbah's *"Dhayl"* ", *Mamlūk Studies Review* 2 (1998), 19–49.

Renard, *Deliverance* = Renard, John, "Deliverance", in Jane Dammen McAuliffe (ed.), *Encyclopaedia of the Qurʾān*, I, Leiden–Boston–Köln: Brill, 2001, 518–519.

Rosenthal, *Ibn Hadjar al-ʿAskalānī* = Rosenthal, Franz, "Ibn Hadjar al-ʿAsḳalānī", in EI[2] III/776–778.

Rosenthal, *On the Semitic root s/š-p-r* = Rosenthal, Franz, "On the Semitic root s/š-p-r and Arabic safar, "travel" ", *Jerusalem Studies in Arabic and Islam* 24 (2000), 4–21.

Rubin, *Sacred precincts* = Rubin, Uri, "Sacred precincts", in Jane Dammen McAuliffe (ed.), *Encyclopaedia of the Qur'ān*, III, Leiden–Boston–Köln: Brill, 2004, 513–516.
Saleh, *al-Biqāʿī* = Saleh, Walid, "al-Biqāʿī", in EI³ 2010–2/119–115.
Saleh, *In defense of the Bible* = Saleh, Walid, *In defense of the Bible, A critical edition and introduction to al-Biqāʿī's Bible treatise*, Leiden–Boston: Brill, 2008.
Sato, *Sugar* = Sato, Tsugitaka, *Sugar in the social life of medieval Islam*, Leiden–Boston: Brill, 2015.
Schacht, *Ibn Buṭlān* = Schacht, Paul, "Ibn Buṭlān", in EI² III/740–742.
Schadewaldt, *Ärztliche Regimina* = Schadewaldt, Hans, "Ärztliche Regimina für Pilgerreisen", in Barbara Haupt—Wilhelm G. Busse (eds.), *Pilgerreisen im Mittelalter und Renaissance*, Düsseldorf: Droste Verlag, 2006, 213–220.
Sellheim, *al-Samʿānī* = Sellheim, Rudolf, "al-Samʿānī", in EI² VIII/1024–1025.
Shefer-Mossensohn, *Ḥājjī Pasha* = Shefer-Mossensohn, Miri, "Ḥājjī Pasha", in EI³ 2017–3/22–24.
Sobernheim, *Čaḳmaḳ* = Sobernheim, M., "*Čaḳmaḳ*", in EI² II/6.
Sourdel, *Ibn Makhlad* = Sourdel, Dominique, "Ibn Makhlad", in EI² III/859.
Steffen—DuPont, *Manual of travel medicine* = Steffen, Robert—DuPont, Herbert L. (eds.), *Manual of travel medicine and health*, 2nd ed., Hamilton–London: BC Decker Inc, 2003.
Stewart, *Sajʿ in the Qur'ān* = Stewart, Devin J., "Sajʿ in the Qur'ān, Prosody and structure", *Journal of Arabic Literature* 21/2 (1990), 101–139.
Strohmaier, *Galen the pagan* = Strohmaier, Gotthard, "Galen the pagan and Ḥunayn the Christian, Specific transformations in the commentaries on Airs, Waters, Places and the Epidemics", in: Peter Pormann (ed.), *Epidemics in context, Greek Commentaries on Hippocrates in the Arabic Tradition*, Berlin–Boston: De Gruyter, 2012, 171–184.
Strohmaier, Galen's not uncritical commentary = Strohmaier, Gotthard, "Galen's not uncritical commentary on Hippocrates' *Airs, waters, places*", *Bulletin of the Institute of Classical Studies, Supplement*, 84 (2004), 1–9.
Sudhoff, *Ärztliche Regimina* = Sudhoff, Karl, "Ärztliche Regimina für Land- und Seereisen aus dem 15. Jahrhundert", *Archiv für Geschichte der Medizin*, 4/4 (1910), 263–281.
Thomas, *al-Ṭabarī* = Thomas, D., "al-Ṭabarī", in EI² X/17–18.
Toorawa, *Travel in the medieval Islamic world* = Toorawa, Shawkat M., 'Travel in the medieval Islamic world, The importance of patronage, as illustrated by ʿAbd al-Latif al-Baghdadi (d. 629/1231) (and other littérateurs)', in Rosamund Allen (ed.), *Eastward bound, Travel and travellers*, Manchester: Manchester University Press, 2004, 53–70.
Troupeau, *Manuscripts* = Troupeau, Gérard, "Manuscripts of the Kāmil aṣ-ṣināʿa", in Charles Burnett—Danielle Jacquart (eds.), *Constantine the African and ʿAlī ibn al-ʿAbbās al-Mağūsī, The Pantegni and related texts*, Leiden–New York, NY–Köln: E.J. Brill, 1994, 303–315.

Ullmann, *Die Medizin* = Ullmann, Manfred, *Die Medizin im Islam*, Leiden–Köln: E.J. Brill, 1970.

Ullmann, *Islamic medicine* = Ullmann, Manfred, *Islamic medicine*, Edinburgh: Edinburgh University Press, 1978.

Van den Boogert, *The manuscript library of Tarīm* = Van den Boogert, Nico, "The manuscript library of Tarīm in Wāḍī Ḥaḍramawt", *Manuscripts of the Middle East* 6 (1992), 155–157.

Vidal-Castro, *Ibn al-Khaṭīb* = Vidal-Castro, Francisco, "Ibn al-Khaṭīb, Lisān al-Dīn", in EI³ 2017–5/116–123.

Wakelnig, *Al-Ṭabarī and al-Ṭabarī* = Wakelnig, Elvira, "Al-Ṭabarī and al-Ṭabarī. Compendia between medicine and philosophy", in Peter Adamson—Peter E. Pormann (eds.), *Philosophy and medicine in the formative period of Islam*, London: The Warburg Institute, 2017, 218–254.

"Manuscripts of the Kāmil aṣ-ṣināʿa", in Charles Burnett—Danielle Jacquart (eds.), *Constantine the African and ʿAlī ibn al-ʿAbbās al-Maǧūsī, The Pantegni and related texts*, Leiden–New York, NY–Köln: E.J. Brill, 1994, 303–315.

Walsh, *Ḥādjdjī Pasha* = Walsh, James, "Ḥādjdjī Pasha", in EI² III/45.

Wensinck, *Samūm* = Wensinck, "Samūm", in EI² VIII/1056.

Wiet, *Barsbāy* = Wiet, G., "Barsbāy", in EI² I/1053–1054.

Witkam, *Establishing* = Witkam, Jan Just, "Establishing the stemma, Fact or fiction?", *Manuscripts of the Middle East* 3 (1988), 88–101.

Witkam, *Ibn al-Akfānī* = Witkam, Jan Just, "Ibn al-Akfānī", in EI² XII/381.

Witkam, *The philologist's stone* = Witkam, Jan Just, "The philologist's stone, The continuing search for the stemma", *Comparative Oriental Manuscript Studies Newsletter* 6 (2013), 34–38.

Witt, *Al-Rāzīs Kitāb al-Hāwī* = Witt, Mathias, "Al-Rāzī's *Kitāb al-Hāwī* (Rhazes, *Liber Continens*), Eine Konkordanz der arabischen und lateinischen Fassung samt Bemerkungen zu 13 arabisch unedierten Kapiteln", *Zeitschrift der Deutschen Morgenländischen Gesellschaft* 171/2 (2021), 323–342.

Index of *Materia medica*

The indices cover only those *materia medica* and medical terms which appear in Ibn al-Amshāṭī's *al-Isfār ʿan ḥikam al-asfār*. Page numbers are listed for the English terms but their Arabic equivalents are given in parentheses. The page numbers of the English translation of Ibn al-Amshāṭī's *Isfār* are set in bold. In case of *materia medica* appearing as an ingredient of a recipe or a medical term being included in the indication of the recipe, the ID of the recipe is also provided in parentheses. There is also an alphabetic list of the Arabic terms so that the reader can easily find the English terms to look for.

1 English–Arabic

2 Arabic–English

Index of Medical Terms

1 English–Arabic

2 Arabic–English

Printed in the United States
by Baker & Taylor Publisher Services